Other books by Thomas Merton

PROSE

My Argument with the Gestapo
Conjectures of a Guilty Bystander
Faith and Violence
Seeds of Destruction
New Seeds of Contemplation
The Sign of Jonas
The Seven Storey Mountain

POETRY

Cables to the Ace
Emblems of a Season of Fury
The Geography of Lograire
Original Child Bomb
Raids on the Unspeakable
Selected Poems

THOMAS MERTON ON PEACE

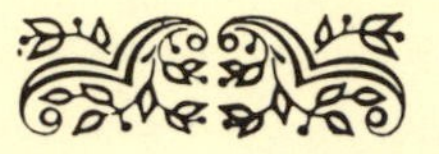

THOMAS MERTON ON PEACE

With an Introduction by Gordon C. Zahn

The McCall Publishing Company

NEW YORK

Many of these pieces were first published in such periodicals as *Blackfriars, Peace News, Ramparts, Commonweal,* the *Catholic Worker, Jubilee, Fellowship, Saturday Review, Peace,* and later, in some instances, substantially rewritten for inclusion in collections of the author's work.

Published simultaneously in Canada by Doubleday Canada Ltd., Toronto.

Library of Congress Catalog Card Number: 75–122148

SBN 8415–0060–6

The McCall Publishing Company
230 Park Avenue
New York, N.Y. 10017

PRINTED IN THE UNITED STATES OF AMERICA

Design by Tere LoPrete

Contents

Original Child Monk: An Appreciation, by Gordon C. Zahn IX

I PRINCIPLES OF PEACE

Original Child Bomb 3
Peace: Christian Duties and Perspectives 12
The Christian in World Crisis: Reflections on the Moral Climate of the 1960s 20
Preface to Vietnamese Translation of No Man Is An Island 63
Peace and Protest: A Statement 67
Peace and Revolution: A Footnote from Ulysses 70
Breakthrough to Peace 76
Christian Ethics and Nuclear War 82
Christianity and Defense in the Nuclear Age 88
Target Equals City 94
The Machine Gun in the Fallout Shelter 103
Peace: A Religious Responsibility 107
Passivity and Abuse of Authority 129
An Enemy of the State 134
A Martyr for Peace and Unity 139
The Answer of Minerva 144
Auschwitz: A Family Camp 150
A Devout Meditation in Memory of Adolf Eichmann 160

II THE NONVIOLENT ALTERNATIVE

Danish Nonviolent Resistance to Hitler 165
Man Is a Gorilla with a Gun 168
Saint Maximus the Confessor on Nonviolence 172
A Tribute to Gandhi 178
Faith and Violence 185
One: Toward a Theology of Resistance 186
Two: Vietnam: An Overwhelming Atrocity 192
Three: From Nonviolence to Black Power 198
Four: Violence and the Death of God: Or God as Unknown Soldier 202
Blessed Are the Meek: The Christian Roots of Nonviolence 208
Christian Action in World Crisis 219
Note on Civil Disobedience and Nonviolent Revolution 227
Note for Ave Maria 231
War and the Crisis of Language 234
Ishi: A Meditation 248

III INCIDENTAL WRITINGS

In Acceptance of the Pax Medal, 1963 257
Retreat, November, 1964: Spiritual Roots of Protest 259
Message aux Amis de Gandhi, January 31, 1965 261
Nhat Hanh Is My Brother 262
Notes for a Statement on Aid to Civilian War Victims in Vietnam 264
Prayer for Peace 267

THOMAS MERTON ON PEACE

Original Child Monk: An Appreciation

It would amuse Tom Merton that this introductory essay to a volume of his writings on war and peace is being written by a pacifist and a sociologist since he was always so careful to point out that he was neither—on one occasion even going so far as to thank God that he was not burdened with the latter designation. The remarkable thing, of course, is that in a very special sense he was both. His careful elaboration of what he considered to be the Christian's mission with respect to war and peace was, to this observer's way of thinking, profoundly pacifist. Similarly, however much he may have lacked and shunned the formal credentials for admission to the august fraternity of sociologists, his perceptive grasp of events and their consequences, his extensive familiarity and critical interest in other cultures and societies together with his cogent comparisons between them and the strengths and weaknesses of our own made him more than eligible for honorary membership as an exceptionally gifted, though amateur, practitioner of that much scorned discipline.

If I can claim any particular qualification for taking on this task it would be that Merton and I shared a commitment to a surprisingly similar interpretation of Christian social teachings and obligations and did so at a time when that interpretation, now much more widely held, was highly suspect and, to some of our fellow Catholics, probably on the fringes of heresy. Reviewing his writings in this area—including some, I must add, that are not included in this volume—proved to be a singularly moving experience and a gratifying one as I encountered new or forgotten evidence of how close our agreement really was.

If memory serves me right, our correspondence began in 1961 or so with a favorable comment by him on something I had published, possibly my first book, and an invitation to contribute an essay to a book he was planning to edit under the tentative title "The Human Way Out." This was the book which finally appeared after some delay and no little difficulty as *Breakthrough to Peace* (New Directions, 1962). From time to time the mail would bring a copy of a poem or essay he had written or some more substantial item like the collection of his "cold war letters" [1] or "The Christian in World Crisis."

From the confines of his monastic cell Merton had somehow managed to fashion a circle of correspondents that linked hundreds of us together in a community of concern without our knowing it. It was a broadly inclusive community, one which spread across all the usual divisions of race, religion, state of life, etc. Scholars, religious writers, poets and politicians—all these and many more found their place in that network, sharing with him their thoughts and worries and receiving, in turn, his not always cheering assessment of the perilous situation facing the church, the nation, and the entire world in the aftermath of the Second World War.[2]

The universality reflected in his list of correspondents is matched by, and undoubtedly related to, the universality of his social interests. Anyone operating (as I confess I did) under the fixed stereotype of the Trappist monk as a man who had "foresworn" the world and its transient concerns and by so doing separated himself from all interest, and certainly involvement, in contemporary events and the social problems existing outside of the monastery walls found it difficult to understand how *this* Trappist monk managed to keep abreast of them and to help others to recognize and deal with those events and problems in the context of their Christian beliefs and obligations. This interest and influence, it should not be necessary to add, were not limited to the issues of war and peace with which we shall be dealing here. His writings on the American race problem, his profoundly prophetic "Letters to a White Liberal" to mention only one,[3] reveal a depth and accuracy of analysis that often enough were to find verification in blood and fire years later, as the ghettoes of our major cities exploded.

The important point, of course, is not that he was, as we so often like to put it, "ahead of his time." Rather it is that he, so much more than others, was so truly in tune with his time, so alert to what was wrong at that precise moment, and what had to be done then to correct that wrong if we were to escape the price for failing to do so. Nowhere is this perception of the hour and its urgent needs more impressive than in his writings on war and peace. If we concentrate upon them in this volume it is not to ignore his writings on race or on feminism or his more general analyses of the fatal flaws in our

1. Published in *Seeds of Destruction* (New York: Farrar, Straus & Giroux, Inc., 1964).
2. It would be impossible to include the names of all of his correspondents in this paper, especially since some of the letters were not in the group he later released for publication. Among them were such luminaries as Erich Fromm, Dorothy Day, John Tracy Ellis, W. H. Ferry, Leo Szilard, Leslie Dewart, Walter Stein, Karl Stern, Mrs. Robert Kennedy, James Forest.
3. This essay (and a selection from the "cold war letters" as well) appeared in *Seeds of Destruction* (New York: Farrar, Straus & Giroux, 1964).

materialistic culture and the parallels he drew with past cultures in their period of decline. Hopefully these will be given treatment in their deserved fullness in other collections of Merton's work. Even were this not done, however, the special focus of this essay and the volume it introduces would still be justified, if only by the extra note of urgency he put into his efforts to awaken Christians to their "grave responsibility to protest clearly and forcibly against trends that lead inevitably to crimes which the Church deplores and condemns." The crimes to which he was referring were the crimes of wars past and wars future, especially the latter, which, he felt, would rank "second only to the Crucifixion" itself.

So prolific and wide-ranging were these writings on peace that it is all but impossible to bring them within the confines of a single commentary. A chronological survey will not do, if only because of the regrettable fact that so many are undated. But even if it were possible to put them in proper time sequence, it is unlikely that this would reveal anything of particular significance. The consistency of his concerns outweighs the slight differences in emphasis or attitude one might uncover over the course of time. Where some item does take on special interest because of its contemporary setting this becomes clear enough from internal evidence. One finds this, for example, in his critical rejoinder to an article justifying a violent defense of a family fallout shelter against neighbors in distress or, again, in his references to the rise of Castro and the implications of the Cuban missile crisis which entered into several of his cold war letters. It might be possible, too, by means of a chronological analysis to establish a shift toward a more frankly pacifist ("nuclear" or, in John Courtney Murray's term, "relative" pacifist) stance as he became more familiar with, and more obviously disenchanted by, the specialized jargon and overblown rhetoric of the kind of "nuclear realism" expounded by Herman Kahn and some of his more devoted Catholic imitators. Here too, however, the shift was not so pronounced as to be of major import to an understanding of his overall position.

A more promising approach, and the one to be taken here, seeks to identify and trace the principal themes recurring in the Merton peace literature. There are difficulties here as well. All of Merton's writings, whether specifically focused on spirituality and mysticism, on the liturgy and the monastic life, or on pressing social issues and problems, are of a piece. To impose one's own framework upon them, as one necessarily does when one sets out to identify and discuss separate themes, is to risk destroying the total unity which gives these writings their value and impact. Nevertheless, the risk is worth taking especially when, as here, the reader has the opportunity to check the analysis against his own reading of the material upon which it is based.

The themes, as I shall develop them in this essay, number five and shall be treated in the following order. First and most basic is his conception of the nature of the Christian mission and witness. From this we shall move to his discussion of traditional "just war" teachings and the pacifist rejection of those teachings. Two special cases are then considered: nuclear war and deterrence and, and even more restricted focus, the war in Vietnam. Finally we reach what may prove to be his most lasting contribution to Catholic thinking on war and peace, the promise and prospects of nonviolence as a Christian alternative to war. Every effort will be made to keep the discussion as true to Merton's position as possible, with frequent recourse to the writings themselves, often enough in the form of direct quotation from those writings.[4]

I: Christian Mission and Witness

In one sense, the complete Merton corpus is an extended, in-depth exploration of the meaning of Christianity for each individual believer and how it is to be translated into life-style and behavior. In the specific frame of reference of this volume, the issue is set in the most simple and direct manner conceivable: "the supreme obligation of every Christian taking precedence over absolutely everything else" is to work for the abolition of war and thereby do his bit to preserve humanity from the threat of total annihilation. Moving beyond this flat statement of responsibility, we find that two notes in particular account for the tone of urgency it reveals. First is his identification of the times in which we live as a "post-Christian era." Second and quite directly related to this is his insistence upon the eschatological perspective in any attempt to define the role the Christian is to play in the world that is no longer Christian.

He speaks, for instance, of "the dwindling and confused Christian minority in the West" and, in another place, of "a non-Christian world [which] still retains a few vestiges of Christian morality, a few formulas and clichés, which serve on appropriate occasions to adorn indignant editorials and speeches. . . ." The implications of such an awareness of exile and alienation for a Christian evaluation of war and participation in war should be evident enough. One would assume

4. It might be well at this point to clarify the manner in which I shall be using the Merton writings. Since most of the items used as sources for this essay are included in this volume, brief and fragmentary quotations from them will not be explicitly footnoted. The reason for this should be self-evident; to do otherwise would burden this essay with an extravagant number of essentially unnecessary citations. Less direct references, including Merton's quotations from other writers, will be given more explicit identification. Some of the sources that have been used, most notably "cold war letters" circulated only in mimeographed form, are not available for direct and identified quotation because of legal restrictions included by Merton himself in the documents establishing the Merton Legacy. Where such items are used, their contents will usually be given in paraphrase and, of course, without citation.

that in a "post-Christian" world the appropriate relationship between the secular and religious communities would be one which would define for the citizen-believer a position closer to his counterpart in pre-Constantinian Rome than to the Christians of the intervening centuries who might have had some excuse, if not justification, for blindly acquiescing in whatever calls to service might be issued by their temporal lords and masters. Theological fiction though he may have been, the so-called Christian prince would have been expected to govern his policies and his actions according to moral precepts and restrictions, an expectation that would have no reasonable basis at all in the aggressively anti-Christian pre-Constantinian days or in the morally indifferent setting of the present. Indeed, one can argue—and at times Merton does so quite explicitly—that the individual Christian ought to look upon the acts and demands of his nation's leaders with intense suspicion, recognizing in them a highly probable challenge to his personal spiritual responsibilities and well-being. In a world poised for the final clash between Gog, the Giant of the East, and Magog, the Giant of the West, Merton, writing "from Magog's country," warns us not to be deceived by the giants or by their thunderous denunciations of one another and their preparations for mutual destruction. "The fact that they are powerful does not mean that they are sane, and the fact that they speak with intense conviction does not mean that they speak the truth."

This poetic expression of a titanic struggle already in progress is but one statement of Merton's conviction that the Christian attitude toward war, as indeed toward everything else, must be "fundamentally eschatological." Viewed in this context, the Christian does not need to fight and should not fight. From the Book of the Apocalypse he draws the picture of the Kingdom as one "of saints and martyrs, priests and witnesses, whose main function is to bide their time in faith, loving one another and the truth, suffering persecution in the furious cataclysm which marks the final testing of earthly society. They will take no direct part in the struggles of earthly kingdoms. Their life is one of faith, gentleness, meekness, patience, purity. They depend on no power other than the power of God, and it is God they obey rather than the state, which tends to usurp the powers of God and to blaspheme Him, setting itself up in His stead as an idol and drawing to itself the adoration and worship that are due to Him alone." To many the continual harping on "the approaching end," the characterization of these as days of "bad dreams," and other equally dismal figures of speech may seem to carry overtones of a black pessimism bordering on despair; but, of course, this would be a complete misreading of the essential point. Nowhere are we to lose sight of the certain, and favorable, outcome. As he put it in his "Letter to a White Liberal," "Christianity is the victory of Christ in the World, that is to say in history." Given this fact that the victory is assured and, in a sense, has already been won for us, the "last day" in anticipation of which all our acts should be performed will be one of confirmation. It thus becomes the special privilege and responsibility of the Christian "to manifest the mercy and truth of God in history."

No small order that, and one which, we are increasingly being made aware, is likely to carry overtones of resistance, possibly even revolution. It is not at all surprising, then, to find so much of Merton's writings in this area celebrating the words and sacrifices of those authentic Christian witnesses of our day who dared defy the totalitarian power of the rulers of Nazi Germany: Alfred Delp, Max Josef Metzger, Franz Jägerstätter—martyrs all. "They refused to submit to a force which they recognized as antihuman and utterly destructive. They refused to accept this evil and to palliate it under the guise of 'legitimate authority.' In doing so they proved themselves better theologians than the professionals and the pontiffs who supported that power and made others obey it, thus cooperating in the evil."

This recognition of the protest dimension of Christianity dominates many of his letters and incidental essays. In November, 1964, he directed what must have been a memorable retreat on the "Spiritual Roots of Protest"—memorable if only for the fact that at least five of the participants would later be in prison for "crimes" of resistance.[5] Again and again in his writings one encounters some version of the anguished lament over "the almost total lack of protest on the part of religious people and clergy, in the face of enormous social evils," a lack he ascribed not to inherent wickedness or perversity but simply to the fact that "they are no longer capable of *seeing and evaluating* certain evils as they truly are, as crimes against God and as betrayals of the Christian ethic of love."

Strong and consistent though his stress on protest may have been, he did not encourage free improvisation or open-ended resistance. Several of his letters criticize such actions as the burning of draft cards or, in a more facetious vein, swimming out to Polaris submarines with a banner between one's teeth. As we shall see in another context, he held rather firm convictions as to the crucial importance of the communication aspect of dissent and civil disobedience and counseled against protests that were too ambiguous or too threatening. Something like the "Peace Hostage Exchange" project, on the other hand, impressed him so deeply that he gave consideration to finding some way in which he could become personally involved, finally deciding with some regret that it was out of the question for him. His criticisms of the more extreme actions were balanced by his awareness of the difficulties of getting the peace message across to a mass audience. "When protest becomes desperate and seemingly extreme," he observed, "then

5. The participants included—along with distinguished Protestant peace leaders A. J. Muste and John Howard Yoder—Revs. Daniel Berrigan, S.J., and Philip Berrigan, S.S.J., of the "Baltimore Four" and "Catonsville Nine"; Rev. Robert Cunnane and James Forest of the "Milwaukee Fourteen"; and Thomas Cornell, draft-card burner.

perhaps one reason for this is that the ones protesting have given up hope of a fair hearing, and therefore seek only to shock or to horrify." He was not ready to approve, but neither was he going to condemn such actions.

As time went on some of the more "desperate and extreme" actions would involve and even be led by Catholics, including, surprisingly enough, Catholic priests and nuns. Catholics played a leading part, for example, in the demonstrations of civil disobedience protesting New York air raid tests and in the first flurry of draft-card burnings. Though he had some reservations about the latter, he had nothing but praise for the courage and determination of Dorothy Day and several of her young followers at the *Catholic Worker* who defied the orders to take shelter when the sirens sounded and joined with representatives of other peace groups in a public protest meeting instead.

The problem as he saw it, however, was not to be found in the Catholics who carried their protest to extremes but, rather, was represented by the great majority of American Catholics who "went along," as Catholics of all nations have always gone along, supporting war and preparations for war without question. Some of Merton's bitterest comments were reserved for this lamentable failure of his Church to inspire its members to oppose the militaristic ethos and the arms race. The Catholic, he felt, had to develop ways to translate his inescapable moral obligation to work for peace into effective and practical steps. Among the steps he recommended were such things as refusing to vote for "belligerent politicians," working to promote and support the Peace Corps, and, most important, freeing themselves from the "crusading spirit that thinks our problems can be solved by nuclear war."

A particularly grim example of this spirit was a letter he received from a woman he categorized as a "devout she-wolf." Writing from France—and a total stranger to Merton—she asked him to solicit the prayers of the Gethsemani community that America might finally launch a full-scale nuclear war against Russia! Shocked as he was by such excesses, he saw the real problem as something much more subtle. Drawing upon classical imagery, he traced the true origins of such thinking to a time when Christians began to look upon Christ as a Prometheus figure; this opened the way, first, to the justification of war, then the crusades, and finally to the epitome of violence in the double atrocities of Auschwitz and Hiroshima. Michelangelo's *Christ of the Sistine Chapel* fit into this Promethean image, "whipping sinners with his great Greek muscles." Through the idealization of force and power Catholics found it possible to contemplate even the (nuclear) destruction of the entire world as a kind of Last Judgment. And he was willing to grant that they might be right, though not exactly in the way they had in mind. "Well, that's the way it is the Judgment and that's the way men judge themselves, and that's the way the poor and the helpless and the maimed enter into the Kingdom: when the Prometheus types blow the door wide open for them."

The intensity of feeling that such a caustic conclusion reveals was in large part a reflection of the difficulties Merton was experiencing in his efforts to give voice to what he felt had to be said. It was not an easy time for him; in fact, there are occasional hints in some of his correspondence that his sense of vocation was being put to an excruciating test. There were frequent references to the obstacles he was encountering: official disapproval, both from his own superiors and from bishops and others on the outside; long delays in getting clearance from his censors; even the quite nonsensical charge (taken all too seriously by his religious superiors) that he was contributing articles to a Communist-controlled publication—the *Catholic Worker!* He was most concerned at this time with the fate of his *Breakthrough* volume, but even his shorter pieces were being held up or blocked altogether. In April, 1962, and as no surprise to him, the ax fell and he was forbidden to publish material dealing with the issues of war and peace. It was still possible to circulate mimeographed articles and the like privately, but this too had to be done with care and circumspection lest the order be extended to cover that as well. His acceptance in obedience while appealing to higher spiritual authorities became a matter of some concern to his correspondents, and the thought that he might be giving in too easily on a matter of conscience troubled him to some extent. Be that as it may, he was determined to continue his efforts within the newly imposed limitations: printing forbidden, then he would mimeograph; mimeographing forbidden, then he would write on the backs of envelopes. Later more permissive superiors and, of course, the impact of John XXIII would free him from these restraints; but while they remained in effect, one of the Church's most influential voices for peace would be muted though not stilled.

How, one must ask, could it have been considered "unseemly" by Catholics, including bishops and his Trappist superiors, for a monk to address himself to so crucial a moral issue? Several answers suggest themselves, but two in particular deserve consideration here. One was his apparent departure from the "just war" morality and what was generally considered to be the "orthodox" position rejecting pacifism; this will be discussed below as the second major theme with which we are concerned. The other had more to do with the Communist "menace" and Merton's consistent criticism of Catholic willingness to accept the cold-war rhetoric as the only acceptable response to that menace. Merton, it must be noted at once, was not at all favorable toward Communism either as political system or as ideology. As much as anyone, he recognized the dangers to the security of the United States and other nations posed by the Soviet "Gog," and he frequently voiced his appreciation of the opportunities and advantages provided by a democratic system. The antireligious commitment of the Soviet Union and, in particular, its proclaimed enmity toward Christianity was a known evil as far as he was concerned, though he was prepared to recognize the *possibility* of a Christian-Marxist dialogue at a time when even the more liberal segments of American Catholicism continued to bind themselves and their thought to narrow and rigid interpretations of the "condemnations" included in the social encyclicals. To Merton the Communists were not only a menace but a terrible menace and a permanent one.

At the same time, however, he refused to go along with what he regarded as "the great illusion" that the United States was a paragon of virtue, the lover of peace, and always right while the Communists were the embodiment of everything evil and base. The national fixation on this kind of oversimple, saint-vs-demon dichotomy could only lead, he insisted, to an anticommunism that was unwise, undisciplined, and rooted in emotion rather than reason. What was needed in its place was "moderation, rationality, objective thought, and above all a firm continued reliance on the very things which are our strength: constitutional processes of government, respect for the rights we want to defend, rational discussion, freedom of opinion, and a deep loyalty to our inherited ideals." A respectable enough formula, one would think, yet it was precisely this stance that far too many of his fellow Catholics—including some in positions of ecclesiastical and political power—were ready to denounce as being "soft on Communism" if not, indeed, something even more sinister. These hard-liners are still with us today, of course, less numerous perhaps and certainly no longer representative of the "official" attitude of the Catholic Church; but at the time Merton set out to correct what he recognized to be a shortsighted and essentially unchristian attitude that threatened to bring about a total disaster for Church, nation, and world, their voice and their influence was decisive, decisive enough at least to have him silenced.

II: The "Just War" and Pacifism

The second major source of the disapproval which greeted Merton's peace writings, as noted above, was their apparent departure from the traditional teachings on the morality of war as set forth originally by Saint Augustine, confirmed by Saint Thomas Aquinas, and then expanded and elaborated upon by the neo-Scholastics. In the strictest sense this was a grossly unjust misunderstanding of his position. Repeatedly he took special pains to emphasize the fact that he was not a pacifist, that he did not hold that the Christian was forbidden ever to fight or that no war could ever be just. At the same time, it is true that these disclaimers were fixed at the level of *theory;* when it came to questions of actual or potential *practice,* that is to the kinds of wars actually being fought or likely to be fought in the future, he considered them "shot through and through" with evil, falsity, and sin.

There was no doubt that his active sympathy and open support were given to people like Dorothy Day and the others who did go much further than Merton himself in proclaiming an outright pacifist commitment. Finally, even at the level of theory one can find hints of inconsistency in his discussions of pacifism and the just war which suggest that his heart really did belong to the former and his fervent protestations to the contrary were largely a matter of semantics.

At one point, for example, he warns that pacifists are likely to face more difficulties in the "cold war" situation than they had encountered in World War II, an observation which led him to confess that he had been a "modified" pacifist in that conflict. In another letter he took the position that there was a place for Christians who were totally committed to the rejection of war and violence, that they would serve as an example to others, a thought which led him to the frank admission that, for himself, he would not consider it licit for him as a monk ever to kill another human being even in self-defense. He was much concerned about the failure of the Catholic community to recognize the conscientious objector option as legitimate for its young men who were subject to the draft. This was just another evidence of the hard and tough "realism" exhibited by the Catholic Church in America which he took to be a scandalous disregard of the many urgent statements issued by the popes calling for peace and disarmament throughout the world. All of these were taken to reflect a degeneration of moral teaching which had brought us to the point where "the Christian gave heroic witness to his God and his faith by a meek, unquestioning obedience even unto death in submission to a Church authority that ordered him to submit to a civil authority that was not necessarily Christian—perhaps even anti-Christian." The net result was that "in fact God was drafted into all the armies and invited to get out there and kill himself."

Merton's rejection of pacifism was directed principally against what he identified as total, or absolute, pacifism and at a peace movement which he considered so superficial as to bring its own basic principles into disrepute. He dismissed unilateralism as a hopeless cause, ruefully admitting as he did so that the ideals of its proponents "cannot but win my heartfelt sympathy." In much the same vein he found "something attractive and comforting" about the young people who were moving into nonviolent resistance, seeing in them the same kind of enthusiasm with which he had joined in the "left wing action" of the 1930s. The special measure of admiration and affection he felt for Dorothy Day was inspired in great part by her willingness to go to jail for her convictions; as far as he was concerned, her brand of peace activity (clearly pacifist) was "more significantly Christian than the rather subtle and comfy positions of certain casuists."

In 1962 when PAX, a Catholic peace association affiliated with the English society founded by Donald Attwater and others, was organized in New York, Merton was one of its sponsors, and he remained in active contact with the group until the time of his death. Similarly, when the Catholic Peace Fellowship was organized a short time later with ties to the nondenominational and explicitly pacifist Fellowship of Reconciliation, he joined the Berrigan brothers and others as sponsor of it as well. Merton, it would seem from this, was really more of a pacifist than his frequent and earnest disclaimers would lead one to believe. But his was a relative pacifism, a position which always left room, in theory at least, for even a defensive nuclear war. Absolute pacifism, that is pacifism "in a completely unqualified form," had, he felt, been officially reproved. "A Catholic may not hold," he wrote, "that all war under no matter what conditions is by its very nature unjust and evil. A Catholic may not formally deny that a community has the right to defend itself by force if other means do not avail. . . ."

Viewed in retrospect (and from my own pacifist perspective), it would appear that Merton's attachment to the "just war" formulations was formal and academic, almost, one might say, a "hang-up" on traditional theology with little or no foundation in intellectual conviction. Only at one point did he seem ready to grant them any true relevance to the real order, and that was in a passing allusion to the abortive 1956 uprising in Hungary as one possible example of a situation in which "some persons" might licitly wage war to defend themselves. In most of his writings the emphasis lay in the other direction altogether; he seemed to reject any possibility of an actual war ever meeting the conditions of the just war. It was with obvious approval (and probably some relief) that he quoted Cardinal Ottaviani's judgment that because of changes in the nature of war "modern wars can never fulfill the conditions which govern, theoretically, a just and lawful war. Moreover no conceivable cause could ever be sufficient justification for the evils, the slaughter, the moral and religious upheavals which war today entails." [6]

So strong a declaration by a man who was known not only as a distinguished moral theologian but as perhaps the foremost spokesman for the more conservative, if not reactionary, forces within the Catholic Church was encouragement indeed. However Merton could find little comparable comfort in the statements and actions of the influential leaders and theologians of the Church in America. They were much too ready to go along with the policies and judgments of the nation's political and military leaders, converting themselves and most of their following into models of conformity and complicity. By so doing they failed to provide the spiritual strength and leadership that was needed. "Although many churchmen, moved apparently by force of habit, continue to issue mechanical blessings upon these draftees and upon the versatile applications of science to the art of killing, it is evident that this use of force does not become moral just because the government and the mass media have declared the cause to be patriotic. The cliché

6. Merton cites Ottaviani, *Public Laws of the Church* (Rome, 1947) as his source for this quotation.

'My country right or wrong' does not provide a satisfactory theological answer to the moral problems raised by the intervention of American power in all parts of the Third World."

Stated more bluntly, "The current war ethic is pagan and less than pagan. There is little of Christianity left in it anywhere. The truth and justice have been drained out of it. It is a lie and a blasphemy, and this has to be said." Merton was determined to say it. He knew it would make him unpopular; and it did. He knew his ecclesiastical superiors, acting on their own or under pressure from others, would probably take steps to tone down his message or suppress it altogether; and they did. But "unseemly" though it may have been in the eyes of some, he was determined to persist in his efforts to get his fellow Christians to see that "*total war* must be condemned not only as immoral but also as impractical and self-defeating." And he did.

III: "The Bomb" and Nuclear Deterrence

The underlined reference to "total" war provides the key by which the apparent inconsistency in Merton's position on peace and pacifism can best be resolved. Although he continued to subscribe in theory to the traditional just war doctrines—even, as already noted, to allowing at one point for the possibility of a justifiable nuclear war of defense—he was a pacifist in that he rejected the legitimacy of war in the actuality. He was convinced that total war, and specifically nuclear war, would have to be immoral in the fact; and he was equally convinced that any war would necessarily escalate to the level of nuclear war. "The Bomb" was the eschatological weapon, its introduction having brought man and his world to the threshold of complete and final destruction. Not only *possible* destruction, he took care to note, but *probable* destruction, for "the possibility of destruction becomes a probability in proportion as the world's leaders commit themselves more and more irrevocably to policies which rely more or less exclusively on the threat to use these agents of extermination." There was not the slightest doubt in his mind but that both the United States and the Soviet Union were committed to such policies.

This essentially pessimistic assessment of the future prospects for the human race came to dominate his many writings on nuclear war and deterrence. His *Original Child Bomb* (New Directions, 1961), consisting of little more than the news reports of the Alamogordo test and the subsequent bombings of Hiroshima and Nagasaki, set forth in free verse or "easy essay" style, was subtitled "points for meditation to be scratched on the walls of a cave." The "original child" designation was a literal translation of one of the poetic names the Japanese found for the Hiroshima bomb, a term referring to its unique and unprecedented character. But his use of symbolic references went beyond this to the code names chosen for the various phases of the total event, names which seemed to take on their own reflection of the eschatological implications he sought to stress. The choice of "Trinity" for the desert test and "Papacy" for Tinian, the bomber's base, combined to produce the supreme irony of the report of the successful destruction of an entire city taking the form of a message reading, "Visible effects greater than Trinity. . . . Proceeding to Papacy." If the bombings were for Merton the sign of the end to come, he found a saving symbol in their victims. In a moving letter to the mayor of the rebuilt city, he wrote, "The people of Hiroshima stand today as a symbol of the hopes of humanity. It is good that such a symbol should exist. The events of August 6, 1945, give you the most solemn right to be heard and respected by the whole world." But it was at best a faint promise that he saw and a fleeting hope; almost immediately the pessimism breaks through again. The world, he felt, "only pretends to respect your witness. In reality it cannot face the truth which you represent." In an arresting image he spoke of everyone walking backwards toward a precipice they know is there, insisting all the while that they are going forward, and this because "the world in its madness is guided by military men, who are the blindest of the blind."

This reference to "madness" as a condition of the world takes on added importance in other contexts. Merton was troubled by the fact that so much of the fear surrounding the potential for total destruction was allowed to center upon the danger that some madman might come to power or have access to the bomb. The real threat, as he saw it, was far more serious. It lay precisely in the "sane" men, the "well-adapted" men, who will have "*perfectly good reasons*, logical well-adapted reasons" for ringing down the curtain on the history of man when the time comes. Like Eichmann, the men who will one day unleash doomsday will merely be following orders handed down by their better-informed legitimate superiors, and they will have no qualms whatever about doing so. "When the missiles take off, then, *it will be no mistake*."

Ample verification of this chilling thought was provided by the development of a new profession of nuclear strategists with its own pretensions to expertise and an impressive new language to match them. Characteristically enough, Merton made it his business to keep abreast of the various theories and the increasingly complicated concepts by which these experts justified the policy of nuclear deterrence and plotted its strategies on their banks of computers. The "nuclear mandarins," Herman Kahn and an assortment of Catholic "realists" who followed his lead, presented a special threat not only because of their close proximity to actual centers of power but by the persuasiveness and apparent reasonableness of their argumentation. Kahn's "technological puckishness," his "sly understatement of the inhuman, the apocalyptic enormity," and the "coolness of his tone" won for him Merton's designation as the "classic of this genre." But this note of admiration heightened rather than lessened the severity of his critique. "The language of escalation is the language of naked power, a language which is all the more persuasive because it is proud of being ethically illiterate and because it accepts, as realistic, the basic irrationality of its own tactics. The language of escalation, in its superb mixture of banality and apocalypse, science and unreason, is the expression of a massive death wish. We can only hope that this death wish is only that of a decaying Western civilization, and that it is not common to the entire race."

Death wish or not, one evident effect of the language of escalation once it was taken up by the mass media was that it tended to "contaminate" the thinking of everybody. Once the unthinkable was made thinkable it became discussable as a rational, even prudent, option until the point was reached where the "benefits" of the balanced terror of nuclear deterrence with its obscene calculations of megadeaths and overkill entered even the moral equations of professional theologians and responsible religious leaders. One example of the way this thinking filtered down until it began to pervade the quality of life of the individual citizen was the shelter frenzy that gripped much of the nation in the early 1960s. Reason and common sense should have made it clear that any shelter program could at best be counted on to save an inconsequential proportion of the population in the event of a major nuclear attack—and, at its worst, could be misread by our nuclear rivals as a provocative cover for a "first strike" policy, thereby increasing rather than mitigating the threat it was supposedly designed to overcome. Instead the program became for many a test of one's patriotism; failure to comply, or criticism that was too outspoken, verged on treason. Merton's attitude toward all this has already been noted in his support for the peace demonstrators who chose to defy the New York law requiring all to take cover during mock air-raid tests.

But an even more distressing episode reveals how far this frenzy had gone. An article in a reputable Catholic journal, written by a priest, addressed itself to a hypothetical problem in what we might term "shelter morality." The argument was advanced that in a case where the foresighted possessor of a backyard shelter was confronted by a less provident neighbor and his family once the bombs started to fall, it would be licit for him to defend his shelter against such intrusion at the point of a gun. It was not the correctness or the error of the theology that troubled Merton but, rather, the horrifying picture of Christian fighting Christian in the last days. He was perfectly willing to grant that a man did have the right to kill someone else if there was no other way to protect his family and himself; but he felt it was wrong to see the issue completely in these terms. By so doing "we run the risk of creating a very dangerous mentality and opening the way to moral chaos if we give the impression that from here on out it is just every man for himself, and the devil take the hindmost. This is not only fundamentally unchristian, but it is immoral on the purely natural level and is finally disastrous even to the political interests of our nation."

No advocate of unilateralism, at times even ready to give half-hearted assent to the possibility of a just nuclear war of defense, Merton wanted to do all he could to bring about the elimination of these weapons and the excessive reliance placed upon them and their threat to putative enemies. Efforts being launched by Catholic pacifists to have the Second Vatican Council condemn the bomb did not impress him as having much point. For one thing, he insisted, it was already condemned in many ways by its very nature; for another, it was doubtful whether that much attention would be paid to what the bishops of the world might have to say, even in the unlikely event that they could be persuaded to take such a stand. Nevertheless he did welcome the condemnation of total war (and, by inference, the Bomb) which was included in the Council's *Constitution on the Church in the Modern World.*

Perhaps because of his insistence that the issues of war and peace must be seen in eschatological terms, Merton's predictions of the nuclear holocaust made it more imminent than the event has justified. He simply could not believe that the balance of terror could remain balanced much longer; calling to mind Napoleon's famous aphorism that the one thing you cannot do with bayonets is sit on them, Merton warned that this was a thousand times more true of nuclear weapons. They, unlike the bayonet, had a built-in incitement in that they offer a first-strike possibility of the total destruction of an enemy before he has a chance to react. He did not have much confidence that either or both of the major nuclear powers would find the strength to ward off temptation over the long haul.

As a prophet of doom Merton might seem to be a failure. The first strike has not been struck, and both sides seem to be aware that there is not much chance that it could have the total success it would require. After years of talk, a treaty providing for a nonproliferation of nuclear weapons was concluded and has been signed by most of the nations of the world—unfortunately, however, *not* including all the nuclear powers. There is even now in prospect another treaty to provide for the limitation of nuclear strategic weapons and behind that the faintest glimmer of hope that this could even lead to the beginnings of nuclear disarmament. These are all encouraging signs, but they must be seen in the context of a weapons technology that has multiplied the original threat of mutual destruction many times over; and billions continue to be spent for new and greater advances in that technology. Merton, then, might still be much more right than we realize. As the reader of this volume reviews what appears to be his exaggerated anxiety over the Bomb and its threat to mankind, it would be well to put those dire warnings in the context of current debates involving ABM, MIRV, and all the other alphabetical sign-posts to doom. And it might be well, too, to bear in mind the sly line from *Die Fledermaus: "aufgeschoben ist nicht aufgehoben."* ("A threat which it but postponed is a threat that may yet come true.")

IV: Vietnam

If Merton's expectations of a global holocaust were premature, most of the elements on which they were predicated were to find expression in the "conventional" war in Southeast Asia which proved to be next on the agenda. This disgusting affair saw the most powerful nation, the self-proclaimed guardian of what it liked to call "the free world," engaged in a campaign of merciless destruction directed against a small and artificially divided country whose people had already known a decade and more of war in their efforts to win freedom from colonial domination. Predictably enough, this American adventure provoked Merton's sharpest disapproval and some of his bitterest writings. He was not alone in this, of course; all over the world intellectual and literary leaders joined in strong and concerted protest against this nation's policies and military excesses. Although he stopped short of joining Sartre in his explicit and public charges of genocide, Merton came to somewhat similar conclusions by drawing parallels between the Vietnam war and earlier wars of extermination conducted against the American Indian. In both he found "the same myths and misunderstandings, the same obsession with 'completely wiping out' an enemy regarded as diabolical. . . ."

Vietnam was but another sign that this nation had become a warfare state, one in which national policy was dominated and determined by a consortium of big-business interests, the military, and fear-ridden political extremists. Long before Vietnam had taken center stage he had been concerned about this trend; indeed, it was to combat this that he had compiled and circulated the mimeographed volume of "cold war letters" in 1962. Before Vietnam there had been the emergence of Fidel Castro in Cuba, and the questions that event, together with the ultimate American reaction, raised concerning relationships with the people of the Third World. Writing to one of his Latin American friends, Merton revealed a breadth of perception and understanding that would not have marked the opinions of the majority of Americans, Catholic or otherwise, in or out of positions of influence. This was not, he felt, just another case of some Latin American tyrant gaining power; the Cuban revolution had to be seen as symptomatic of much deeper currents that had to be recognized and taken into account. "Yes," he wrote, "we should try to understand Castro together. This is a significant and portentous phenomenon, and it has many aspects. Not the least, of course, is the fact that Castro is now about to become a figure with a hundred heads all over Latin America. [The letter, though undated, was written in 1961 or 1962.] One aspect of it that I can see is the embitterment and disillusionment of this well-intentioned man who was weak and passionate and easily abused. The man who like all of us wanted to find a third way, and was immediately swallowed up by one of the two giants that stand over all of us. The United States could have helped him and could perhaps have saved him, but missed its chance."

Vietnam, like Cuba, was a victim of the struggle between the giants and, if anything, an even more disastrous failure on the part of the United States to recognize the potential and the needs of the Third World. "Far from weakening Communism in Asia by our war policy, we are only strengthening it. The Vietnamese are no lovers of China, but by the ruthlessness of our war for 'total victory' we are driving them into the arms of the Red Chinese." This assessment, like much of his subsequent opposition to the war, reveals an interesting shift in emphasis. The spiritual and theological arguments which so completely dominated most of his discussions of war in general, the Bomb and deterrence, and, as we shall see below, Christian non-violence seemed to give way at times to stress on practical, even pragmatic, political considerations. Some of his strongest protests are prefaced with a phrase like "quite apart from moral considerations" or "quite apart from questions of conscience." To some extent, I suspect, this reflects Merton's extensive knowledge of, and affinity to, the cultures of the Far East. On matters concerning differences in values, outlook and modes of action between West and East he was an expert and, as such, could bring to his analysis of the tragic conflict and its probable consequences a "practical" perspective denied to others.

This is not to say, of course, that his customary spiritual and theological perspective was lacking or abandoned. Quite the contrary. His awareness of the "folly, brutality and massive stupidity" of American policy and the inability on the part of the nation's leaders to understand "that millions of people in Asia do not quite see things their way and do not have the same respect for brute force which they have" merely served to heighten and intensify his moral rejection of the excesses which were endangering an entire population and its culture. It was, in a sense, a sharing on his part of the crime being done to people he understood so well which sparked his determination to oppose the war. His moving plea on behalf of a Vietnamese poet-monk[7] is evidence of this. Claiming his Buddhist counterpart as a brother—more truly a brother, he noted, than many with whom he was bound by ties of common race and nationality—he declared that they saw things exactly the same way. "He and I deplore the war that is ravaging his country. We deplore it for exactly the same

7. Thich Nhat Hanh, author of *Lotus in a Sea of Fire,* was about to return to his native South Vietnam after an extensive American tour arranged by the pacifist and nondenominational Fellowship of Reconciliation. Merton, with apparently good reason, feared for the safety of his "brother" at the hands of the military authorities in his homeland.

reasons: human reasons, reasons of sanity, justice and love. We deplore the needless destruction, the fantastic and callous ravaging of human life, the rape of the culture and spirit of an exhausted people."

Merton's comments on the war (and on those persons he considered most responsible for the war and the conduct of the war) were sometimes so severe as to stretch the limits of charity. It was a completely poisonous situation without a shred of justification, and those responsible for it were described as men devoid of imagination, insight and moral sense who were sacrificing countless Vietnamese and American lives in a completely unnecessary power play for the benefit of an advantaged minority. Nor was he above personalizing his charges. In the Goldwater-Johnson election, he confessed giving reluctant support to the latter, the reluctance arising from the fact that LBJ was "as much a fire-eater on Vietnam" as his opponent. Later he was to express his regret for having voted for the man in a letter to a United States senator.

Despite the weight he placed upon the sheer inexpediency of the war in his opposition and protest, he did not abandon the Christian mission and witness theme that infused all of his writings on war and peace. His notes for a statement to be issued on behalf of civilian victims of the war called for a series of admissions "as Christians and quite apart from any political considerations." Among them was the recognition of a "grave moral responsibility before God" to give aid to the victims of our military activities by providing medical supplies and assistance and doing everything possible to remove all obstacles to the sending of such assistance. Strictly speaking, this was an incitement to violate the law since any such aid to the North Vietnamese (who were, of course, to be included) would constitute "trading with the enemy." Several attempts by such groups as the American Friends Service Committee, the Fellowship of Reconciliation, the Catholic Peace Fellowship, and Clergy and Laymen Concerned About Vietnam to provide medical supplies to North Vietnam were systematically blocked by the Treasury and other official agencies. Nevertheless in what Merton described as "this situation of utter shame for our nation" he saw such a program of aid as "an opportunity to salvage at least a vestige of our Christian decency by acts of humanity which, in any case, are demanded by the moral law."

The issue of Vietnam and its deeper meaning for the nation and the entire world extended beyond the threatened persecution of a fellow poet and monk who had dared to take a stand for peace; even beyond the tens, perhaps hundreds, of thousands of innocents scorched and maimed by American air power. The essential evil was the total commitment to violence in utter disregard for the rights of individuals the war had come to represent. With that same chilling accuracy of foresight we have noted before, he translated this ready willingness to rationalize and excuse acts of large-scale terrorism and what he termed a policy of nihilism into terms of what they could portend for America's own future. "We need not be surprised if we wake up one day to find fire and violence in our own front yards here in America. If the fire of hatred and violent anarchy happen to break out in some of our cities (as it can surely be expected to sooner or later) we will simply be getting a taste—perhaps only a very slight taste—of our own medicine."

We have gotten that taste and more. The ugly events of the months since those lines were written in February, 1967, need no elaboration: the debacle of the Democratic convention in Chicago; the war being waged in the ghetto streets; the violence and the fires, and more recently the deaths on our college campuses; the mobilization of the "hard hats" in New York City and elsewhere. And even these may be but the beginnings of our sorrows. Certainly it would be foolish beyond measure to assume the climax has been passed.

Vietnam, to Merton, was not just a matter of soldiers fighting and men killing one another, though that was evil enough. It was a symbol, a terrible foreshadowing, again, of the eschatological moment. "The war in Vietnam," he wrote in his Preface to the Vietnamese edition of *No Man Is an Island,* 'is a bell tolling for the whole world, warning the whole world that war may spread everywhere, and violent death may sweep over the entire earth."

V: Nonviolence

The importance of Merton's contribution to the peace movement, even were we to limit our evaluation to the themes already discussed, should be self-evident. He brought to it the "respectability" of his name and reputation as priest and contemplative and as one of the major Catholic spiritual writers of his time. He won for the peace-mongering element within his Church a hearing they might otherwise not have enjoyed, though it would be too much to say that this element, even with Merton's help, has even yet received the hearing it deserves. John XXIII and the Second Vatican Council notwithstanding, the majority of American Catholics remain completely unaware of the pacifist implications of their faith. But even granting that unfortunate truth, the fact that the peacemongering minority is as large and as vocal as it has become in recent years is largely due to Merton and his writings on peace.

Be that as it may, his major and probably most lasting contribution remains to be discussed. Up to this point our review of his exposition of the nature of Christian responsibility and witness as it relates to war has been predominantly negative: the rejection of war and the dismissal of the just war theology as no longer relevant; the call for renunciation of nuclear weaponry and national policies based on their prospective use; the outright condemnation of the American involvement in Vietnam. For Merton, however, Christianity had something much more positive and creative to say. He was not the only or even the first modern Catholic writer to take up the cause of nonviolence as the Christian alternative to war,[8] but he did succeed better than any other in bringing it to the attention of an American Catholic audience which, had it given any thought at all to the subject, would have dismissed it as an exotic but altogether impractical notion to be associated with fakirs on their beds of nails or similar manifestations of Eastern religious mysticism.

There would have been a kernel of truth to this, of course. There is much in the practice, if not the theory, of nonviolence which is not entirely compatible with Western values as we know them today. The fact that the most widely known application of nonviolence on any major scale was Gandhi's struggle for Indian freedom reinforces that alien image. But "Western values as we know them today" is the governing phrase. It is generally overlooked that the original teachings of Christianity, presumably the dominant religion of the Occident, centered upon the kind of approach Gandhi was to adopt and put into practice. "Surely," Merton wrote, "it is curious that in the twentieth century the one great political figure who has made a conscious and systematic use of the Gospel principles for nonviolent political action was not a Christian but a Hindu. Even more curious is the fact that so many Christians thought Gandhi was some kind of eccentric and that his nonviolence was an impractical and sensational fad." And where nonviolence has been employed in specific Western contexts—in Denmark, the heroic and successful resistance to the Nazis; in the United States, in labor disputes and the civil rights movement led by Martin Luther King—the tendency is to treat them solely as tactical maneuvers, as something applicable only to cases where violent resistance is not possible or not yet required.

Merton's nonviolence was ideological and not tactical; and it was a rigorous nonviolence he preached, much more rigorous in fact than King's. It had to be "the nonviolence of the strong" and not the passive acquiescence of the weak that so many took it to be. Indeed, like Gandhi himself, Merton expressed a preference for violent resistance to expedient surrender in a situation where one's basic rights are at stake; and, surprisingly enough, he granted this as a possibility in connection with the controversy over the fallout shelter. At this

8. Among others who have written on the subject from a Catholic perspective are P.-R. Regamey (*Non-Violence and the Christian Conscience,* Herder and Herder, 1966) and James W. Douglass (*The Non-Violent Cross,* Macmillan, 1967). Merton did a preface for the former in its American edition and was in close consultation with Douglass as his book was being prepared. Bede Griffiths and Hervé Chaigne are two others who have contributed understanding of the subject based largely upon their personal experiences in India.

point, of course, he parts company with the more absolutist pacifist, though obviously both are committed to nonviolence in principle and practice. This distinction between the nonviolence of the strong and the weak answers the objection so often raised in terms of the experience of the Jews in Nazi Germany: that dreadful program of extermination made possible at least in part by the docility, if not the active cooperation, of the victims would be for him a prime example of the passive nonresistance he rejected.

The "nonviolence of the weak" had another even more significant meaning in Merton's formulation. It would be the kind of nonviolence that presumes to measure its successes in terms of power, political or other, gained over others. In his rigorous definition this would be a spurious nonviolence. "Nonviolence is not for power but for truth. It is not aimed at immediate political results, but at the manifestation of fundamental and crucially important truth. Nonviolence is not primarily the language of efficacy, but the language of *kairos*. It does not say 'We shall overcome' so much as 'This is the day of the Lord, and whatever may happen to us, *He* shall overcome.' "

Putting the stress on the objective of attaining truth rather than tangible results obliges the practitioner of nonviolence to be more concerned about his opponent than might otherwise be the case, more concerned about him in fact than about one's own self and objectives. This is not just a matter of not killing him or causing him bodily harm; care must be taken to avoid humiliating him or causing him psychological harm as well. "Nonviolence, ideally speaking, does not try to overcome the adversary by winning over him, but to turn him from an adversary into a collaborator by winning him over." It is safe to say that much, perhaps most, of the organized nonviolence that has been employed in the peace movement and before that in the civil rights crusade would fall short of the Merton standard in this respect. To the extent that they included deliberate attempts to shame the opposition or to "break them down" by provoking them to the point where they commit excesses that disturb their own consciences, this would constitute the kind of "moral aggression" of which he disapproved. The basis for that disapproval was that such provocations could just as easily, perhaps more easily, lead the adversary away from the truth one was supposedly trying to help him discover.

Another fundamental of classic nonviolence stressed by Merton is the respect for law and the acceptance of punishment under the law. Civil disobedience if it is to achieve its ends, requires that the disobedient make it crystal clear precisely which law, or which aspect of the law, they are refusing to obey as well as their equally explicit reasons for their disobedience. This formulation has little in common with many of the nonviolent demonstrations of recent years which seem to manifest a generalized resistance to law itself and to the political order it sustains, sometimes reducing itself to a free-floating disobedience that seeks out and exploits any and all occasions to express itself. As for the acceptance of punishment, at the most superficial level this is merely another way of affirming support for law even while one persists in disobeying a specific law one considers unjust. But there is another and much more profound aspect to be considered. Acceptance of punishment becomes a continuation of the witness, not only in the sense that the protest goes on but, rather, that it takes on a new dimension, an intensely spiritual dimension. By undergoing punishment for disobedience in the cause of a greater truth, "you undergo redemptive suffering for religious—or anyway ethical—motives. You are 'doing penance' for the sin against which you have protested."

Nonviolence has its pitfalls too. Because the objective is proclaiming the truth and helping the adversary to discover that truth for himself, there is always present the temptation of self-righteousness and an unwillingness on the part of the practitioner of nonviolence, convinced as he is that he knows the truth, to listen to the other. Merton was forever emphasizing the need to keep open a two-way communication process and to avoid overly dramatic and extreme vehicles of protest that were likely to produce a backlash effect that would make such communication difficult if not impossible. His misgivings concerning the Berrigan-style draft board raids rested in part upon his feelings that much of the growing opposition to the draft was "oriented to the affirmation of the rightness, the determination and the conviction of the protesters, and not to the injustice of the law itself." Although he stopped short of applying this critical judgment to the Berrigan actions, he left little dobut that he was increasingly troubled by the search for ever more bizarre forms of civil disobedience as a means of winning the attention of the mass media. He realized that his cautions against the dangers of opportunism and improvisation might go unheard. A large proportion of the people involved in protests against the war were young and lacked perspective, whereas nonviolence to be fully effective had to be mature, well-prepared, and disciplined. It was all too easy under the circumstances to give way to the "resentment, immature rebelliousness, beatnik nonconformism and so on [which] may be taken automatically to be charismatic just because they are opposed to what is obviously stuffy and inert."

This observation was written in relatively quiet times, well before campus dissent and confrontations reached crisis proportions, but there were some signs already as to what was to come. The issues around which the demonstrations he questioned were organized were earlier versions of the issues that were to spark our more recent disturbances: peace and racial justice. In the case of the former, the objects of the demonstrators' attention were the Atomic Energy Commission and the various Civil Defense agencies—the agitation against the draft, campus recruitment, ROTC, and the like had not yet begun. On the race issue, the emphasis was still on integration and equal rights—militant separatism would have found little or no support. However dubious he may have been about some of the more aggressive tactics employed, Merton gave his full blessing to the objectives of both.

Although for obvious reasons he was unable to participate in them, he did support "direct action" demonstrations that did not cross the line separating creative experimentation from the more extreme forms of protest he considered self-defeating. He endorsed the two "Everyman" projects under which sailing vessels manned by pacifist crews were to enter the restricted area in the Pacific in an attempt to disrupt scheduled nuclear tests. Similarly he was so attracted to the "peace hostage" idea—which would have exchanged citizens of different countries making them potential victims of any nuclear attack their own country might unleash—that he tried to think of some way in which he could take part in the venture. He did not, of course, think that either project would have much chance of succeeding, but both did serve to demonstrate an important truth and both proposed to put their participants' lives and well-being on the line. His support for the New York demonstrators in their protests against the civil defense tests—protests which ultimately were successful—has already been noted.

It goes without saying that he gave full support to the nonviolent civil rights campaigns in the American South. The lunch-counter sit-ins, the freedom riders, and, of course, the mass demonstrations at Selma and Birmingham clearly fit his formulation of classic nonviolence. Although Merton's extensive writings on the subject of racial justice must be left for another volume, this issue cannot be ignored completely in any discussion of the nonviolence theme. In Martin Luther King, the charismatic activist, and Merton, the cloistered contemplative, we find two thoroughly committed Christians who found inspiration in the life and acts of Gandhi; and they were alike, too, in their determination to make Gandhi's way relevant to the American scene and situation. In both we find the same sensitivity to the underlying unity that made what appeared to be two separate social issues, racial justice and world peace, really one. King's nonviolent struggle against discrimination and poverty forced him into open opposition to the war in Vietnam against the wishes and advice of many who felt that such opposition might split or weaken the movement he headed. Merton, of course, had no such problem. With no activist movement dependent upon him for leadership, he was free to give equal weight to the search for peace and for justice to all men in his exposition of the fullness of Christian witness and responsibilities.

This does not mean, however, that he was not alert to the problems faced by the civil rights leaders and the probable future course the movement was likely to take. Much of what he wrote anticipated statements and programs since enunciated by the more articulate black militants who have come to the fore. In 1963 he was describing the purpose of the civil rights demonstrations as an attempt to awaken the white man and his conscience to the fact that "the Negro problem is really a *white* problem: that the cancer of injustice and hate which is eating white society and is only partly manifested in racial segregation with all its consequences *is rooted in the heart of the white man himself.*" Nor did his personal commitment to nonviolence blind him to the evidence of its decline and the reasons behind that decline. In the aftermath of the urban troubles of the summer of 1967, he noted the limited involvement of both Negroes and whites in the nonviolent movement, a clear sign to him that its message had never been clear for the majority of either race. As far as the Negro was concerned, except for an exceptionally gifted and spiritually committed few, they were suffering a severe identity crisis as "morally mutilated non-persons" and "could not be expected to grasp the full meaning of nonviolence." To the penniless and helpless Black, nonviolence "merely reinforced the feelings of helpless passivity and despair which were his. On the other hand, an appeal to violence, an assurance that he could burn houses and loot stores with relative impunity, proved an outlet to explosive suppressed hate—more satisfying to him than just being beaten over the head for the ten-thousandth time by a Southern cop, without recourse to anyone on this earth."

If he did not endorse the trend toward violence on the part of the disadvantaged Blacks, he could understand it in the context of their needs and objectives. Theoretically there would seem to be no comparable counter-strain to account for the similar shift in emphasis on the part of the peace movement. One might take it for granted that its declared objectives and any resort to violence would be mutually exclusive. But such assumed incompatibility has not been justified by the fact. Even before the 1967 Pentagon march, voices could be heard proclaiming a readiness to use any means available to bring the war to an end, and this morally dubious stance has since been adopted in the public rhetoric of the New Left segments of the "Movement." The April 1970 anti-war rally in Boston featured a series of speakers who went out of their way to ridicule pacifism, the ultimate being reached by one young man who challenged the tens of thousands assembled on the Common to "take up the gun" if they really wanted peace.

One can say with certainty that Merton would have opposed this new trend. Even though he did not consider himself a pacifist in the strictest sense and it might be possible to recognize a kind of adaptation of "just war" teachings (now applied to the cause of long oppressed minorities and populations) in the rhetoric of violence, there is nothing to suggest that he would have been swayed from his position that nonviolence is "per se and ideally *the only really effective resistance to injustice and evil.*" It was of no small concern to him that "the peace movement may be escalating beyond peaceful protest. In which case it would also be escalating into self-contradiction."

The militancy of the peace activists, like that of the new breed of civil rights activists, was not at issue. In Merton's conceptualization of the Christian witness, resistance to unjust authority and even, when necessary, revolution held an honored place. But the resistance, and the revolution, had to be nonviolent. To take this from the level of theory, or ideology, and put it into actual practice presented problems of which he was aware but which because of his state in life he did not have to resolve himself. This did not mean that he remained completely aloof from questions of tactics and the like. Instead he was always available—to PAX and the Catholic Peace Fellowship as well as to personal friends and correspondents—for whatever counsel or encouragement they might seek. Even in those cases where he may not have been completely in accord with an action taken, he would stand ready to support an individual for following what he believed to be the dictates of his conscience.

And there were specific actions and programs of which he did not entirely approve. The ceremonial burning of draft cards struck him as being little more than a symbolic statement of despair, a denial of hope that the political process could bring about an end to the war. This was not a judgment he was ready to accept, at least not at that relatively early stage. He felt, too, that the act was too steeped in ambiguity and would do more harm than good to the Christian peace effort. It is characteristic of the man that he changed his position on this issue once the rationale of the burnings was explained to him. Informed that (for some of the burners, if not perhaps for all) this was not just a dramatic show of opposition to the draft but, rather, a personal protest against the requirement that every registrant carry his card with him at all times, he withdrew his opposition. The ambiguity had been resolved and the act of burning the card became an affirmation, actually a response to a direct challenge. The law itself was now seen to be at fault; in making so unnecessary and, for some, so morally offensive a demand, it represented a provocative misuse of authority, repressive in nature and subtly aimed at silencing protest. It is significant, however, that even after he changed his mind on this, he modified his acceptance of the burnings by suggesting that the action should be limited to one or two reasonable people and not be allowed to degenerate into an irresponsible mass display on the part of young people merely out to prove themselves in a contest with public authority.

A far more dramatic and tragic form of protest caused Merton to overreact to the point of almost dissociating himself from organized peace activity. In November, 1965, a young member of the *Catholic Worker* staff immolated himself by fire in front of the United Nations headquarters in New York, offering himself as a sacrificial witness for peace. Eight days earlier a Quaker had done the same at the Pentagon in Washington. The first event had troubled Merton greatly, and he wrote a letter to another advocate of nonviolence in which he expressed his concern. Admitting that the act had to be taken as an incontestable statement against the war and, to this extent, was effective, he pointed to the danger of the "pathological attraction" this kind of incontestability might hold for others. The second case, coming less than a week later, must have been a brutal confirmation of his worst fears and a clear warning that others might follow suit. He immediately wired a request that his name be removed from the list of Catholic Peace Fellowship sponsors, explaining that the two suicides were but the latest evidence that the peace movement in its search for results and its passion for improvisation was "fanning up the war fever rather than abating it." He did not wish to give the impression that he was encouraging or endorsing actions of this kind, hence his desire to dissociate himself from organizational activity. An extensive exchange of correspondence ended with him agreeing to continue as a Fellowship sponsor after issuance of a formal statement clarifying the nature of his relationship with the Fellowship he expressed his continued confidence that "this dedicated group is sincerely striving to spread the teachings of the Gospel and the Church on war, peace, and the brotherhood of man"; at the same time it was to be understood that his position as sponsor did not "imply automatic approval of any and every move made by this group, still less of individual actions on the part of its members, acting on their own responsibility." [9] From that point forward, it should be noted, his association with the Fellowship remained as close as ever, and in some respects closer than it had been before.

This immediate and intense response to the tragic event must be seen as an emotional response to the sacrifice of a young life already marked by great idealism and deep religious commitment. But it was more than that. It reflected Merton's intellectual judgment that such actions, if allowed to multiply, would create a disastrous backlash and bring lasting discredit upon all forms of protest directed against a war he considered to be unjust and immoral. What was needed most, and what he looked to the Catholic peace movement in particular to provide, was "patient, constructive and pastoral work rather than acts of defiance which antagonize the average person without enlightening him."

We come, finally, to the series of raids upon draft board offices initiated by the Berrigan brothers and their associates in October, 1967, and emulated since by other raiding parties. Since most of the participants in these raids have been Catholic, it is entirely appropriate to consider them in the context of the Merton formulation of the Christian witness and nonviolence. The first thing that must be said is that Merton had a close and continuing personal relationship with the Berrigans and others involved in them. One might even refer back

9. Statement and press notice released by the Catholic Peace Fellowship, December 22, 1965.

to the 1964 retreat at Gethsemani as one of the sources of the later actions. Not only were both Dan and Phil Berrigan present, but James Forest and Robert Cunnane (of the Milwaukee Fourteen) were also included among the very select group of participants. Merton's 1968 volume, *Faith and Violence,* is dedicated to Forest and Philip Berrigan. There is no question but that Merton would have supported and honored those who took part in these raids in that they were following their consciences and had acted in a manner that avoided intentional physical violence to others or to themselves.

This does not mean, however, that he would have approved of the actions in themselves or recommended them to others as models to follow. His published evaluation of the Catonsville raid, originally published in *Ave Maria* and reprinted in the March, 1969, issue of *Fellowship,* was inconclusive. It was in this article that he voiced his concern about the peace movement escalating itself into self-contradiction, but he followed this gloomy observation with the assurance that he was not accusing Berrigan *et al.* of having reached that point. Their action had "bordered" on violence, but by intentionally violating a law and accepting the fact of punishment, the raiders had remained true to the traditions of nonviolence. But this seemingly favorable judgment was diminished by references to the "evident desperation" of the Catonsville Nine and the impact the action was likely to have. If, indeed, it had "frightened more than it has edified," this would be a confession of failure; for, again, it is the task of the nonviolent to edify, to open the adversary to the discovery and acceptance of the truth that is presumably being served—in this case, of course, the raiders' conviction that the war was immoral and the conscription system grossly unjust. Such a failure would be crucial in Merton's eyes.

As indicated, the article did not come to a definite conclusion one way or the other, though on balance it seemed to be more critical than approving. It remains a matter of pure speculation, but one that can scarcely be avoided, how he would have reacted to the proliferation of these raids until by 1970 they numbered at least a dozen in major cities all over the nation. My own opinion, based on my reading of Merton, is that his disapproval would have grown more outspoken once it had passed beyond the "one or two reasonable" test he suggested for the draft card burnings. A quite contrary opinion has been expressed by one of the participants in the Milwaukee action; it was his impression that Merton's attitude had shifted to the more favorable side following the appearance of the *Ave Maria* article. Unfortunately, there is nothing in the later Merton writings to confirm either point of view; most of the raids took place after his departure for Asia and his death there.

If this question must remain open and unresolved, an even more intriguing problem is presented by the decision of the Berrigans and some of their colleagues to refuse to submit willingly to the prison sentences passed upon them and subsequently upheld in the appeals process. In one of his messages from the "underground," Daniel Berrigan, then a fugitive, explained his change of heart as a new realization that the "chain of crime and punishment" was one of the "accidentals" that were to be separated from "the essentials of nonviolence."[10] Clearly this is a challenge to the traditional notion of nonviolence and one which Merton, assuming he was consistent with his past writings, would have had to reject. For one thing, Berrigan's justification of the decision to "go underground" stressed the failure of the raiders' hopes to use the judicial processes to put their case against the war before the public. But it is precisely such concern with immediate and measurable results that Merton would have placed among the "accidentals." For him, any act of civil disobedience that meets the test of being direct and unambiguous speaks for itself; the trial procedure would merely offer the opportunity to make a formal record of something that had already been adequately expressed. There is no doubt that he would have shared the raiders' frustration with legal maneuvers and court decision which refused to take full account of their witness, but it is unlikely that he would have agreed that such frustration would justify the avoidance of punishment.

If, as has been noted, the punishment is really the essential witness continued and extended into the spiritual dimension of penance and redemptive suffering, it cannot be dismissed so lightly as an accidental. To Merton the acceptance of the punishment is what distinguishes the nonviolent resister from "the mere revolutionary."[11] This is a distinction, incidentally, which has found confirmation, possibly unintentional, in a statement issued by Nicholas Riddell, a priest-member of the Chicago Fifteen who went underground before their trial was completed. He framed his explanation in frankly revolutionary terms: "In the future I shall continue my role in the revolution, but from a hidden and secure position. My energies shall be in unison with other revolutionaries; working together we shall bring about the type of change the oppressed are demanding."[12]

Merton for his part may well have supported the objectives of the revolution embraced by Fr. Riddell, but it is most likely that he would have considered it somewhat premature. To the extent that it implies a repudiation of traditional means of protest and an insistence upon a total commitment to more aggressive modes of action (as Riddell's statement does),[13] he may even have rejected it outright as a mis-

10. *The New Yorker* (July 25, 1970), pp. 20–23.
11. *Fellowship* (March 1969), p. 8. Interestingly enough, in the published version the sentence reads, "In this way you are distinguished from the mere seditious revolutionary." Whether Merton added the "seditious" to his final version or whether this was an editorial clarification is not clear.
12. *The Milwaukee Journal* (July 8, 1970), 2:2.
13. *Ibid.* Fr. Riddell's statement explains, "Protest, demonstrations and legal channels have all failed. The administration shows itself adamant in regards to war, racism, exploitation and the needs of the poor throughout the world.

guided distortion of the Christian mission. In his "Ulysses" note—one of his last, possibly the very last, writings on peace—he warned against the "half-truth" that only force works and suggested that this "may turn out to be one of the most dangerous illusions of our time." His concern for those to whom the message is to be directed and the possibility of backlash enters in: "It may do more than anything else to promote an irresponsible and meaningless use of force in a pseudo-revolution that will only consolidate the power of the police state. Never was it more necessary to understand the importance of genuine nonviolence as a power for real change because it is aimed not so much at revolution as at conversion." Then he went on to add one of his pessimistic observations that might seem to validate the very arguments the fugitives had advanced against this position: "Unfortunately, mere words about peace, love and civilization have completely lost all power to change anything."

Of course it does no such thing. Acts of civil disobedience, complete with the willingness to accept punishment, are much more than "mere words." For Merton they were the means by which the truth that can save us is to be achieved if it is to be achieved at all. The great need is to discover the form of civil disobedience that is most appropriate to a given place and time. Taken in this context, the Berrigan "improvisation" deserves further consideration. What Dan Berrigan in particular has accomplished—and I am confident that Merton would have been the first to recognize it—is to extend the disobedience while postponing, rather than seeking to evade, the punishment. His periodic "surfacings" before he was finally apprehended became a continuing witness. In published "notes from the underground," secret interviews with the press and even on television, and spontaneous "live" appearances at rallies or before religious congregations, he continued to give expression to the truth the courts had tried to silence. And, of course, every day he successfully evaded capture was an additional act of disobedience, clearly nonviolent in nature, and not in any sense a selfish attempt to evade the personal discomfort and inconvenience of prison. He made it very clear that when he was caught, he would not resist arrest, but until that moment he intended to use his "freedom" to alert his fellow Americans—and especially the Christians among them—to the total immorality of their nation's policies at home and throughout the world. The chase is over and he is now behind bars, but in those months as a fugitive Berrigan was already undergoing punishment, in many ways a more severe punishment than prison might have been. He spent his days under the constant psychological pressure of knowing he was being hunted down and knowing, too, that his friends and relatives were being subjected to observation and harassment on his account. He had reason to believe that his brother and

---

Our work is cut out for us; there will be no more begging and pleading for what is rightfully ours."

others of their "criminal" circle already in prison were being dealt with as hostages and suffering extra restrictions and penalties because he was still at large. And with it all there was the certain knowledge that when it was over, as it now is, he would still have the full prison term ahead to serve with little or no prospect of any reduction or mitigation of the sentence.

On balance I believe Merton would have supported and endorsed the Berrigan innovation. He would have opposed certain aspects of it: the overly pragmatic emphasis on the justification for going underground in the first place; the note of hopelessness in the conviction that "all solutions based on the sanity and health and recoverability of current structures are quickly proven wrong, untimely, unmanageable, bureaucratically infected; the same old kettle of fish, stinking worse than ever in the boiling juices of change." [14] He would have been concerned, too, over the likelihood that the crucial point would have been lost upon those who needed it most. Middle America's explanation of the efforts to evade arrest would almost certainly not be the fugitive's. For himself, then, Merton would probably have held to the classic form of nonviolence as practiced by Gandhi and King. I think, too, he may have been unhappy about the self-righteous overtones of some of the Berrigan statements and the tendency to make sport of the hunters, a kind of "moral aggression" he would have deplored. However that may be, the essential witness and Berrigan's continued commitment to the ideal of nonviolence would have been more than enough to guarantee that his old friend and fellow priest would have had the benefit of Merton's most fervent prayers and blessings—and, had the occasion presented itself, safe haven at his hermitage as well.

Even in the unlikely event that Merton would have disapproved altogether, he would have known where to put the blame. In an invited memorandum to the Kerner Commission he pointed to the rise in violence as evidence that people who once had been—or, at least, could have been—attracted to nonviolent solutions had become "disillusioned not only with the established structure but also (more tragically) with the whole civilized tradition of religious humanism." For such as these, and the Riddells of the peace movement testify to the fact, revolution and the revolutionary mystique are likely to take its place. To Merton this was both tragic and futile and an invitation to a totalitarian backlash. But, as he was quick to point out, the answer, assuming there is one, lay not with the new revolutionaries but with the commission itself and the social structure it had been established to advise and serve. In its hands lay the choice between looking for the villains among rioting students and peace demonstrators or daring to probe more deeply into the nature of American culture. The causes of American violence, he told the commission, lay "not in esoteric groups

14. Daniel Berrigan, "How to Make a Difference," *Commonweal* (August 7, 1970), p. 385.

but in the very culture itself, its mass media, its extreme individualism and competitiveness, its inflated myths of virility and toughness, and its overwhelming preoccupation with the power of nuclear, chemical, bacteriological, and psychological overkill." His recommendation closes on a note of pessimism comparable to Berrigan's: "If we live in what is essentially a culture of overkill, how can we be surprised at finding there is violence in it? Can we get to the root of the trouble? In my opinion, the best way to do it would have been the classic way of religious humanism and nonviolence exemplified by Gandhi. That way seems now to have been closed. I do not find the future reassuring."

VI: End and Continuation

That future is much darker today than when those lines were written. The "folly, brutality and massive stupidity" of the Vietnamese war continues and even expands, but the Christian community has not yet found it possible to unite in effective opposition to it. New revelations of unspeakable horrors—most notably, of course, the atrocity at My Lai and other similar, though more routine, episodes—may occasionally spark a momentary surge of protest only to have it subside into the complacency and complicity that have characterized the behavior of America's Christians for more than a decade. The relatively few who somehow do manage to persist in efforts to awaken the Church to its responsibility to voice the prophetic message the world so sorely needs and perhaps to go further and actually disrupt the well-oiled machinery of war soon learn that the most bitter criticism and condemnation of such efforts is likely to come from the very religious community they are trying to reach. Scandals abound, not the least of which involve bishops who have never found it within themselves to express public concern over the napalming of innocent civilians but who are quick to publish fervent denunciations of the napalming of Selective Service records.

Breaking under the pressure of frustration and futility, certain elements of the peace movement have confirmed Merton's gloomy prediction and have escalated into self-contradiction. On campuses throughout the nation, the peaceful pickets and sit-ins at ROTC headquarters and other buildings housing war-related activities have given way, first, to broken windows and Molotov cocktails, then to threats of bombings, and now, as at the University of Wisconsin, to actual bombings with loss of life. The rumors and threats of full-scale organized and violent revolution as the next stage in anti-war activity are too insistent to be dismissed as empty rhetoric.

The Berrigans are in jail.

Thomas Merton is dead.

Because 1968, a year of blood and fire, of riots and assassinations, had already been in so many ways a spiritual disaster for this nation and the entire world, the news of Merton's death in Bangkok, as that year drew to its close, was for many of us the fitting final touch. The sense of almost insurmountable tragedy was made all the greater by the high expectations we had held for his Asian pilgrimage. His travels and his discussions with the spiritual leaders of the East, we were sure, would make it easier for him to continue building the bridges of faith he had already begun to erect in his writings and correspondence. Certainly it would make him more effective than ever as a teacher of nonviolence and a spokesman for the nonviolent way of life.

Now he is gone, and all those hopes go unfulfilled. We can take pride and solace in the knowing that he was with us for a time and gave us a start, much more of a start than we had any right to expect from someone in his state of life. He was as much aware as anyone, of course, of what some regarded as an apparent incongruity and seemed to feel it called for some explanation. Thus, in one of his cold war letters we find him writing to Alceu Amorosa Lima, ". . . When speech is in danger of perishing or being perverted in the amplified noise of beasts, perhaps it becomes obligatory for a monk to try to speak." That he tried and succeeded so well was, and remains, no small blessing.

Who is to measure the extent and the worth of that blessing and by what standards? In a very real sense Merton was unique and without precedent, every bit as much an "original child" in his way as was the bomb that brought mankind to the threshold of total self-annihilation. This volume can provide at best a partial testimony to the contribution he made. The writings it contains are, needless to say, valuable in their own right, lending themselves to the kind of analysis and interpretation I have attempted here. But their true value extends far beyond the insights they provide and the effectiveness of their argumentation to the spiritual and practical impact they have had. Readers of this volume are to be warned that they are in danger, that many who were exposed to these writings on war, peace, and nonviolence at their first appearance were persuaded and have not found it possible since to be entirely comfortable in a world and a nation in which ordered injustice and violence are taken for granted. It is not too much to expect that others will now experience the same almost traumatic shock of awakening to the full implications of the Christianity they have dared to profess and find themselves drawn irresistibly along the path leading to dissent, perhaps even to disobedience and the prison cells that have housed some of the earlier discoverers of Merton. To the extent that this is so, we will be able to say with joy that his work continues: "he lives."

Of course, there is another sense (and one which he undoubtedly would have preferred us to stress) in which Merton lives and may be counted on for continued sponsorship and support in our efforts to win Christians to the cause of peace and nonviolence. We have only to accept as our own his unwavering focus upon the supernatural dimensions of peace action to have every confidence that the inspiration and guidance he gave us when he was physically in our midst will continue at another level and in a different mode. In the unity of spirit, too, he lives.

If knowing this does not relieve us of our sense of loss; if, indeed, the amplified noise of beasts is much louder now that his voice has been stilled, this means only that each of us who heard that voice and his message and loved and honored this monk and prophet must do all he possibly can to fill the void. That same letter to Lima contained a passage that reads today like a kind of instruction from beyond the grave, reminding us of the continuing task, the sacrifices it will require, and the reward it will bring: "We are all nearing the end of our work. The night is falling upon us, and we find ourselves without the serenity and fulfillment that were the lot of our fathers. I do not think that this is necessarily a sign that anything is lacking, but rather is to be taken as a greater incentive to trust more fully in the mercy of God, and to advance further into His mystery. Our faith can no longer serve merely as a happiness pill. It has to be the Cross and the Resurrection of Christ. And this will be, for all of us who so desire."

Gordon C. Zahn
Professor of Sociology
University of Massachusetts at Boston

I

PRINCIPLES OF PEACE

Original Child Bomb

Points for meditation to be scratched on the walls of a cave

1: In the year 1945 an Original Child was born. The name Original Child was given to it by the Japanese people, who recognized that it was the first of its kind.

2: On April 12th, 1945, Mr. Harry Truman became the President of the United States, which was then fighting the Second World War. Mr. Truman was a vice president who became President by accident when his predecessor died of a cerebral hemorrhage. He did not know as much about the war as the President before him did. He knew a lot less about the war than many people did.

About one hour after Mr. Truman became President, his aides told him about a new bomb which was being developed by atomic scientists. They called it the "atomic bomb." They said scientists had been working on it for six years and that it had so far cost two billion dollars. They added that its power was equal to that of twenty thousand tons of TNT. A single bomb could destroy a city. One of those present added, in a reverent tone, that the new explosive might eventually destroy the whole world.

But Admiral Leahy told the President the
bomb would never work.

3: President Truman formed a committee of
men to tell him if this bomb would work, and if
so, what he should do with it. Some
members of this committee felt that the bomb
would jeopardize the future of civilization.
They were against its use. Others wanted it to
be used in demonstration on a forest of
cryptomeria trees, but not against a civil or
military target. Many atomic scientists warned
that the use of atomic power in war would
be difficult and even impossible to control. The
danger would be very great. Finally, there
were others who believed that if the bomb were
used just once or twice, on one or two Japanese
cities, there would be no more war. They
believed the new bomb would produce eternal
peace.

4: In June 1945 the Japanese government
was taking steps to negotiate for peace. On one
hand the Japanese ambassador tried to
interest the Russian government in acting as a
go-between with the United States. On the
other hand, an unofficial approach was made
secretly through Mr. Allen Dulles in Switzerland.
The Russians said they were not interested
and that they would not negotiate. Nothing was
done about the other proposal, which was
not official. The Japanese High Command was
not in favor of asking for peace, but wanted
to continue the war, even if the Japanese
mainland were invaded. The generals believed
that the war should continue until everybody
was dead. The Japanese generals were
professional soldiers.

5: In the same month of June, the President's
committee decided that the new bomb
should be dropped on a Japanese city. This
would be a demonstration of the bomb on a
civil and military target. As "demonstration" it
would be a kind of a "show." "Civilians"
all over the world love a good "show." The

"destructive" aspect of the bomb would
be "military."

6: The same committee also asked if America's
friendly ally, the Soviet Union, should be
informed of the atomic bomb. Someone
suggested that this information would make the
Soviet Union even more friendly than it was
already. But all finally agreed that the
Soviet Union was now friendly enough.

7: There was discussion about which city
should be selected as the first target. Some
wanted it to be Kyoto, an ancient capital
of Japan and a center of the Buddhist religion.
Others said no, this would cause bitterness.
As a result of a chance conversation, Mr.
Stimson, the Secretary of War, had recently
read up on the history and beauties of Kyoto. He
insisted that this city should be left untouched.
Some wanted Tokyo to be the first target,
but others argued that Tokyo had already been
practically destroyed by fire raids and
could no longer be considered a "target." So
it was decided Hiroshima was the most
opportune target, as it had not yet been bombed
at all. Lucky Hiroshima! What others had
experienced over a period of four years
would happen to Hiroshima in a single day!
Much time would be saved, and "time is
money!"

8: When they bombed Hiroshima they would
put the following out of business: the
Ube Nitrogen Fertilizer Company; the Ube Soda
Company; the Nippon Motor Oil Company;
the Sumitoma Chemical Company; the
Sumitoma Aluminum Company, and most of
the inhabitants.

9: At this time some atomic scientists
protested again, warning that the use of the
bomb in war would tend to make the
United States unpopular. But the President's
committee was by now fully convinced that the
bomb had to be used. Its use would arouse

the attention of the Japanese military class
and give them food for thought.

10: Admiral Leahy renewed his declaration that
the bomb would not explode.

11: On the 4th of July, when the United States
in displays of fireworks celebrates its
independence from British rule, the British and
Americans agreed together that the bomb
ought to be used against Japan.

12: On July 7th the Emperor of Japan
pleaded with the Soviet Government to act as
mediator for peace between Japan and the
Allies. Molotov said the question would
be "studied." In order to facilitate this "study"
Soviet troops in Siberia prepared to attack
the Japanese. The Allies had, in any case, been
urging Russia to join the war against Japan.
However, now that the atomic bomb was
nearly ready, some thought it would be better
if the Russians took a rest.

13: The time was coming for the new bomb to
be tested, in the New Mexico desert. A name
was chosen to designate this secret operation. It
was called "Trinity."

14: At 5:30 A.M. on July 16th, 1945, a
plutonium bomb was successfully exploded in
the desert at Alamogordo, New Mexico. It
was suspended from a hundred-foot steel tower
which evaporated. There was a fireball a
mile wide. The great flash could be seen for a
radius of 250 miles. A blind woman miles
away said she perceived light. There was a cloud
of smoke 40,000 feet high. It was shaped
like a toadstool.

15: Many who saw the experiment expressed
their satisfaction in religious terms. A
semi-official report even quoted a religious book
—the New Testament—"Lord, I believe, help
thou my unbelief." There was an atmosphere
of devotion. It was a great act of faith.

They believed the explosion was exceptionally powerful.

16: Admiral Leahy, still a "doubting Thomas," said that the bomb would not explode when dropped from a plane over a city. Others may have had "faith," but he had his own variety of "hope."

17: On July 21st a full written report of the explosion reached President Truman at Potsdam. The report was documented by pictures. President Truman read the report and looked at the pictures before starting out for the conference. When he left his mood was jaunty and his step was light.

18: That afternoon Mr. Stimson called on Mr. Churchill, and laid before him a sheet of paper bearing a code message about the successful test. The message read "Babies satisfactorily born." Mr. Churchill was quick to realize that there was more in this than met the eye. Mr. Stimson satisfied his legitimate curiosity.

19: On this same day sixty atomic scientists who knew of the test signed a petition that the bomb should not be used against Japan without a convincing warning and an opportunity to surrender.

At this time the U.S.S. *Indianapolis*, which had left San Francisco on the 18th, was sailing toward the Island of Tinian, with some U 235 in a lead bucket. The fissionable material was about the size of a softball, but there was enough for one atomic bomb. Instructions were that if the ship sank, the uranium was to be saved first, before any life. The mechanism of the bomb was on board the U.S.S. *Indianapolis*, but it was not yet assembled.

20: On July 26th the Potsdam declaration was issued. An ultimatum was given to Japan: "Surrender unconditionally or be destroyed."

Nothing was said about the new bomb. But
pamphlets dropped all over Japan
threatened "an enormous air bombardment"
if the army would not surrender. On July 26th
the U.S.S. *Indianapolis* arrived at Tinian and the
bomb was delivered.

21: On July 28th, since the Japanese High
Command wished to continue the war,
the ultimatum was rejected. A censored version
of the ultimatum appeared in the Japanese
press with the comment that it was "an
attempt to drive a wedge between the military
and the Japanese people." But the Emperor
continued to hope that the Russians, after
"studying" his proposal, would help to
negotiate a peace. On July 30th Mr. Stimson
revised a draft of the announcement that was to
be made after the bomb was dropped on the
Japanese target. The statement was much
better than the original draft.

22: On August 1st the bomb was assembled in an
airconditioned hut on Tinian. Those who
handled the bomb referred to it as "Little Boy."
Their care for the Original Child was devoted
and tender.

23: On August 2nd President Truman was
the guest of His Majesty King George VI
on board the H.M.S. *Renown* in Plymouth
Harbor. The atomic bomb was praised. Admiral
Leahy, who was present, declared that the
bomb would not work. His Majesty George VI
offered a small wager to the contrary.

24: On August 2nd a special message from the
Japanese Foreign Minister was sent to the
Japanese Ambassador in Moscow. "It is
requested that further efforts be exerted. . . .
Since the loss of one day may result in a
thousand years of regret, it is requested that you
immediately have a talk with Molotov."
But Molotov did not return from Potsdam until
the day the bomb fell.

25: On August 4th the bombing crew on Tinian
watched a movie of "Trinity" (the
Alamogordo Test). August 5th was a Sunday but
there was little time for formal worship.
They said a quick prayer that the war might end
"very soon." On that day, Col. Tibbetts,
who was in command of the B-29 that was to
drop the bomb, felt that his bomber ought
to have a name. He baptized it Enola Gay, after
his mother in Iowa. Col. Tibbetts was a well-
balanced man, and not sentimental. He did not
have a nervous breakdown after the bombing,
like some of the other members of the crew.

26: On Sunday afternoon "Little Boy"
was brought out in procession and devoutly
tucked away in the womb of Enola Gay.
That evening few were able to sleep. They were
as excited as little boys on Christmas Eve.

27: At 1:37 A.M. August 6th the weather scout
plane took off. It was named the Straight
Flush, in reference to the mechanical action of a
water closet. There was a picture of one,
to make this evident.

28: At the last minute before taking off, Col.
Tibbetts changed the secret radio call
sign from "Visitor" to "Dimples." The Bombing
Mission would be a kind of flying smile.

29: At 2:45 A.M. Enola Gay got off the ground
with difficulty. Over Iwo Jima she met her
escort, two more B-29s, one of which was called
the Great Artiste. Together they proceeded
to Japan.

30: At 6:40 they climbed to 31,000 feet, the
bombing altitude. The sky was clear. It was a
perfect morning.

31: At 3:09 they reached Hiroshima and
started the bomb run. The city was full of sun.
The fliers could see the green grass in
the gardens. No fighters rose up to meet them.

There was no flak. No one in the city
bothered to take cover.

32: The bomb exploded within 100 feet of the aiming point. The fireball was 18,000 feet across. The temperature at the center of the fireball was 100,000,000 degrees. The people who were near the center became nothing. The whole city was blown to bits and the ruins all caught fire instantly everywhere, burning briskly. 70,000 people were killed right away or died within a few hours. Those who did not die at once suffered great pain. Few of them were soldiers.

33: The men in the plane perceived that the raid had been successful, but they thought of the people in the city and they were not perfectly happy. Some felt they had done wrong. But in any case they had obeyed orders. "It was war."

34: Over the radio went the code message that the bomb had been successful: "Visible effects greater than Trinity. . . . Proceeding to Papacy." Papacy was the code name for Tinian.

35: It took a little while for the rest of Japan to find out what had happened to Hiroshima. Papers were forbidden to publish any news of the new bomb. A four-line item said that Hiroshima had been hit by incendiary bombs and added: "It seems that some damage was caused to the city and its vicinity."

36: Then the military governor of the Prefecture of Hiroshima issued a proclamation full of martial spirit. To all the people without hands, without feet, with their faces falling off, with their intestines hanging out, with their whole bodies full of radiation, he declared: "We must not rest a single day in our war effort. . . . We must bear in mind that the annihilation of the stubborn enemy is our road to revenge." He was a professional soldier.

37: On August 8th Molotov finally summoned the
Japanese Ambassador. At last neutral
Russia would give an answer to the Emperor's
inquiry. Molotov said coldly that the Soviet
Union was declaring war on Japan.

38: On August 9th another bomb was dropped
on Nagasaki, though Hiroshima was still
burning. On August 11th the Emperor
overruled his high command and accepted the
peace terms dictated at Potsdam. Yet for three
days discussion continued, until on August
14th the surrender was made public and final.

39: Even then the Soviet troops thought
they ought to fight in Manchuria "just a little
longer." They felt that even though they could
not, at this time, be of help in Japan, it
would be worthwhile if they displayed their
goodwill in Manchuria, or even in Korea.

40: As to the Original Child that was now born,
President Truman summed up the philosophy
of the situation in a few words. "We found
the bomb," he said, "and we used it."

41: Since that summer many other bombs have
been "found." What is going to happen?
At the time of writing, after a season of brisk
speculation, men seem to be fatigued by the
whole question.

Peace: Christian Duties and Perspectives[1]

It has been said so often that it has become a cliché, but it must be said again at the beginning of this brief article: the world and society of man now face destruction. *Possible* destruction: it is relatively easy, at the present time, to wipe out the entire human race either by nuclear, bacterial or chemical agents, separately or together. *Probable* destruction: the possibility of destruction becomes a probability in proportion as the world's leaders commit themselves more and more irrevocably to policies which rely more or less exclusively on the threat to use these agents of extermination. At the present moment, the United States and the Soviet bloc are committed to such policies. Not only are they committed to the use of these weapons for self-defense in case of attack, but even to their use as a *deterrent.* This means that the policies of the United States and Russia are now frankly built on the presumption that each one is able, willing and *ready* to completely destroy the other at a moment's notice by a "first strike"; that the one destroyed is capable of "post mortem retaliation" that would annihilate not only the attacker but all his allies and satellites, even though the defender were already wiped out himself. This is the main purpose of the Polaris submarine on which we are currently spending billions of dollars a year.

There is no need to insist that in a world where another Hitler is not only possible but likely the mere existence of such weapons constitutes the most tragic and serious problem that the human race has ever had to contend with.

1. The reader will find similarities of thought and language between this chapter and Chapter 12, "Peace: A Religious Responsibility." This is the original version written for magazine publication, which the author later developed much more fully into a section of *Breakthrough to Peace* (New York: New Directions, 1962). Since there are differences as well as similarities, it was thought useful to include both pieces. [Ed.]

It is no exaggeration to say that our times are apocalyptic, in the sense that we seem to have come to a point at which all the hidden, mysterious dynamism of the "history of salvation" revealed in the Bible has flowered into final and decisive crisis. The term "end of the world" may or may not be one that we are capable of understanding. But at any rate we seem to be assisting at the unwrapping of the mysteriously vivid symbols of the last book of the New Testament. In their nakedness, they reveal to us our own selves as the men whose lot it is to live in the time of a possibly ultimate decision. In a word, the end of the world is quite really and quite literally up to us and to our immediate descendents, if any. And this, I might venture to suggest, is more "apocalyptic" than anything our fathers discovered in the Revelations of Saint John.

We know that Christ came into the world as the Prince of Peace. We know that Christ Himself is our peace (Ephesians 2:14). We believe that God has chosen for Himself, in the Mystical Body of Christ, an elect people, regenerated by the Blood of the Savior, and committed by their baptismal promise to wage war with the great enemy of peace and salvation. As Pope John XXIII pointed out in his first encyclical, *Ad Petri Cathedram,* Christians are obliged to strive for peace "with all the means at their disposal" and yet, as he continues, this peace cannot compromise with error or make concessions to it. Therefore it is by no means a matter of passive acquiescence in injustice, since this does not produce peace. However, the Christian struggle for peace depends first of all upon a free response of man to "God's call to the service of His merciful designs." The lack of man's response to this call, says Pope John, is the "most terrible problem of human history" (Christmas message, 1958). Christ Our Lord did not come to bring peace to the world as a kind of spiritual tranquilizer. He brought to His disciples a vocation and a task, to struggle in the world of violence to establish His peace not only in their own hearts but in society itself.

The Christian is and must be by his very adoption as a son of God, in Christ, a peacemaker (Matthew 5:9). He is bound to imitate the Savior who, instead of defending Himself with twelve legions of angels (Matthew 26:53) allowed Himself to be nailed to the Cross and died praying for His executioners. The Christian is one whose life has sprung from a particular spiritual seed: the blood of the martyrs who, without offering forcible resistance, laid down their lives rather than submit to the unjust laws that demanded an official religious cult of the Emperor as God. That is to say, the Christian is bound, like the martyrs, to obey God rather than the state whenever the state tries to usurp powers that do not and cannot belong to it. We have repeatedly seen Christians in our time fulfilling this obligation in a heroic manner by their resistance to dictatorships that strove to interfere with the rights of their conscience and of their religion.

We are no longer living in a Christian world. The ages which we are pleased to call the "ages of faith" were certainly not ages of earthly paradise. To say that we are less Christian than our medieval forefathers is not to insist that their society was unfailingly just, honest or even at all times profoundly religious.

But at least they officially recognized and favored the Christian religion. They professed to be guided by Christian standards of morality and justice. They fought some very bloody and unchristian wars, and in doing so they also committed great crimes which remain in history as a permanent scandal. However, certain limits were recognized. Morality was at least allowed to exist, and was perhaps more than a matter of words. Today, a non-Christian world still retains a few vestiges of Christian morality, a few formulas and clichés, which serve on appropriate occasions to adorn indignant editorials and speeches. But otherwise we witness deliberate campaigns to oppose and eliminate all education in Christian truth and morality.

It is a great mistake to identify a nationalistic society that was once officially Christian with Christendom or Christianity. It is a serious error to imagine that because the West was once largely Christian, the cause of the Western nations is now to be identified, without further qualification, with the cause of God. The incentive to do this, and to proceed on this assumption to a nuclear crusade to wipe out Bolshevism, may well be one of the apocalyptic temptations of twentieth-century Christendom.

It is quite true that Communism is built on violence, and that the very essence of Communism is the violent overthrow of its enemies in what purports to be a class war, but is in reality a new form of the old nationalism which has produced all the European wars since the Reformation. Hence Christianity is not only opposed to Communism, but in a very real sense at war with it. But this warfare is spiritual and ideological. "Devoid of material weapons," says Pope John, "the Church is the trustee of the highest spiritual power." If the Church has no weapons of her own, it means that her wars are fought without any weapons at all and not that she intends to call upon the weapons of nations that were once Christian. There is no thought of the Church considering France, England or the U.S.A. as a kind of "secular arm" and there would be immediate indignant protest in all these countries at the very idea of it.

We must remember that the Church does not belong to any political power bloc. Christianity exists on both sides of the Iron Curtain and we should feel ourselves bound by very special bonds with those Christians who, living under Communism, often suffer heroically for their principles.

At the same time, one of the most disturbing things about the Western world of our time is that it is beginning to have much more in common with the Communist world than it has with the professedly Christian society of several centuries ago. On both sides of the Iron Curtain we find two profoundly disturbing varieties of the same moral sickness: both of them are rooted in the same basically materialist view of life. Both are basically opportunistic and pragmatic in their own way. And both have the following characteristics in common. On the level of *morality* they are blindly passive in their submission to a determinism which, in effect, leaves man completely irresponsible. Therefore moral obligations and decisions have become practically meaningless. At best they are only forms of words, rationalizations of pragmatic decisions that have already been dictated by the political needs of the moment.

Naturally, since not everyone is an unprincipled materialist even in Russia, there is bound to be some moral sense at work, even if only as a guilt feeling that produces uneasiness and hesitation, blocking the smooth efficiency of machinelike obedience to immoral commands. Yet the history of Nazi Germany shows us how appalling was the irresponsibility which would carry out even the most revolting of crimes under the protection of "obedience." This moral passivity is the most terrible danger of our time, as the American bishops pointed out in their joint letter of December, 1960.

On the level of political, economic and military activity, this moral passivity is balanced, or overbalanced, by a *demonic activism*, a frenzy of the most varied, versatile, complex and even utterly brilliant technological improvisations, following one upon the other with an ever more bewildering and uncontrollable proliferation. Politics pretends to use all this force as its servant, to harness it for social purposes, for the "good of man." The intention is certainly good. The technological development of power in our time is certainly a challenge, but that does not make it essentially evil. On the contrary, it can be and should be a very great good. In actual fact, however, the furious speed with which our technological world is plunging toward disaster is evidence that no one is any longer fully in control—and this includes the political leaders.

A simple study of the steps which led to the dropping of the first A-bomb on Hiroshima is devastating evidence of the way well-meaning men, the scientists and leaders of a victorious nation, were guided step by step, without realizing it, by the inscrutable yet simple "logic of events" to fire the shot that was to make the cold war inevitable and prepare the way inexorably for World War III. This they did purely and simply because they thought in all sincerity that the bomb was the simplest and most merciful way of ending World War II and perhaps all wars, forever.

The tragedy of our time is then not so much the malice of the wicked as the helpless futility even of the best intentions of "the good." We have war-makers, war criminals, indeed. But we ourselves, in our very best efforts for peace, find ourselves maneuvered unconsciously into positions where we too can act as criminals. For there can be no doubt that Hiroshima and Nagasaki were, though not fully deliberate crimes, nevertheless crimes. And who was responsible? No one. Or "history." We cannot go on playing with nuclear fire and shrugging off the results as "history." We are the ones concerned. We are the ones responsible. History does not make us, we make it—or end it.

In plain words, in order to save ourselves from destruction we have to try to regain control of a world that is speeding downhill without brakes, because of the combination of factors I have just mentioned: almost total passivity and irresponsibility on the moral level, plus demonic activism in social, military and political life. The remedy would seem to be slow down our activity, especially all activity concerned with the production and testing of weapons of destruction, and indeed to backtrack by disarming and destroying all stockpiles of all such weapons everywhere in the world. This may be of some help, but it is only a palliative, not a solution. Yet *at least this* is perhaps feasible, and should at all costs be attempted, even at the cost of great sacrifice and greater risk. It is not morally licit for us as a nation to refuse the risk merely because our whole economy now depends on this war effort.

Equally important, and perhaps even more difficult, is the restoration of a sane moral sense and the resumption of genuine responsibility. Without this it is illusory for us to speak of freedom and "control." Unfortunately, even where moral principles are still regarded with some degree of respect, morality has lost touch with the realities of our situation. Moralists tend to discuss the problems of atomic war as if men still fought with bows and arrows. Modern warfare is fought as much by machines as by men. An entirely new dimension is opened up by the fantastic processes and techniques involved. An American President can speak of warfare in outer space and nobody bursts out laughing—he is perfectly serious. Science fiction and the comic strip have all suddenly come true. When a missile armed with an H-bomb warhead is fired by the pressing of a button and its target is a whole city, the number of its victims is estimated in hundreds of thousands "more or less." A thousand or ten thousand more here and there are not even matter for comment. Under such conditions can there be serious meaning left in the fine decisions that were elaborated by scholastic theologians in the day of hand-to-hand combat? Can we as readily assume that in atomic war the conditions which make double effect legitimate will be realized?

In atomic war, there is no longer question of simply permitting an evil, the destruction of a few civilian dwellings, in order to attain a legitimate end: the destruction of a military target. It is well understood on both sides that atomic war is purely and simply massive and indiscriminate destruction of targets chosen not for their military significance alone, but for their importance in a calculated project of terror and annihilation. Often the selection of the target is determined by some quite secondary and accidental circumstance that has not the remotest reference to a morality. Hiroshima was selected for atomic attack, among other reasons, because it had never undergone any notable air bombing and was suitable, as an intact target, to give a good idea of the effectiveness of the bomb.

It must frankly be admitted that some of the military commanders of both sides in World War II simply disregarded all the traditional standards that were still effective. The Germans threw these standards overboard with the bombs they unloaded on Warsaw, Rotterdam, Coventry and London. The allies replied in kind over Hamburg, Cologne, Dresden and Berlin. Spokesmen were not wanting on either side to justify these crimes against humanity. And today, while "experts" calmly discuss the possibility of the United States being able to survive a war if *"only fifty millions"* (!) of the population are killed; when the Chinese speak of being able to *spare* "three hundred million" and "still get along," it is obvious that we are no longer in the realm where moral truth is conceivable.

The only sane course that remains is to work frankly and without compromise for the total abolition of war. The pronouncements of the Holy See all point to this as the only ultimate solution. The first duty of the Christian is to help clarify thought on this point by taking the stand that all-out nuclear, bacterial or chemical warfare is absolutely forbidden by all standards of natural and divine morality, because it means the destruction of the world. There is simply no "good end" that renders such a risk permissible or even thinkable on the level of ordinary common sense.

It might be possible to get people to admit this in theory, but it is going to be very difficult in practice. They will admit the theory because they will say that they "certainly do not want a war" in which nuclear agents will be used on an all-out scale. Obviously no one wants the destruction of man. But they will not admit it in practice because foreign policy entirely depends on wielding the threat of nuclear destruction. But in an issue of such desperate seriousness, we have to face the fact that the calculated use of nuclear weapons as a political threat is almost certain to lead eventually to a hot war. Every time another hydrogen bomb is exploded in a test, every time a political leader boasts his readiness to use the same bomb on the cities of his enemy, we get closer to the day when the missiles armed with nuclear warheads will start winging their way across the seas and the polar ice cap. The danger must be faced. Whoever finds convenient excuses for this adventurous kind of policy, who rationalizes every decision dictated by political opportunism and finds it justified, must stop to consider that he is perhaps himself cooperating in the evil. On the contrary, our duty is to help emphasize with all the force at our disposal that the Church earnestly seeks the abolition of war, we must underscore declarations like those of Pope John XXIII pleading with world leaders to renounce force in the settlement of international disputes and confine themselves to negotiation.

Let us suppose that the political leaders of the world, supported by the mass media in their various countries, and carried onward by a tidal wave of ever greater and greater war preparations, see themselves swept inexorably into a war of disastrous proportions. Let us suppose that it becomes morally certain that these leaders are helpless to arrest the blind force of the process that has been irresponsibly set in motion. What then? Are the masses of the world, including you and me, to resign ourselves to our fate and march on to global suicide without resistance, simply bowing our heads and obeying our leaders as showing us the "will of God"? I think it should be evident to everyone that this can no longer, in the present situation, be accepted unequivocally as Christian obedience and civic duty.

On the contrary, this brings us face to face with the greatest and most agonizing moral issue of our time. This issue is not merely nuclear war, not merely the possible destruction of the human race by a sudden explosion of violence. It is something more subtle and more demonic. If we continue to be morally passive and irresponsible, if we continue to yield to the theoretically irresistible determinism and to vague "historic forces" without striving to resist and to control them, if we let these forces drive us to demonic activism in the realm of politics and technology, we face something more than the material evil of universal destruction. We face the *moral responsibility of global suicide*. Much more than that, we are going to find ourselves gradually moving into a situation in which we are practically compelled by the "logic of circumstances" deliberately *to choose the course that leads to destruction.*

We all know the logic of temptation. We all know the confused, vague, hesitant irresponsibility which leads us into the situation where it is no longer possible to turn back, and how, arrived in that situation, we have a moment of clear-sighted desperation in which we freely commit ourselves to the course that we recognize to be evil. That may well be what is happening now to the whole world. The actual destruction of the human race is an enormous evil, but it is still, in itself, only a physical evil. Yet the free choice of global suicide, made in desperation by the world's leaders and ratified by the consent and cooperation of all their citizens, would be a moral evil second only to the Crucifixion. The fact that such a choice might be made with the highest motives and the most urgent purpose would do nothing whatever to mitigate it. The fact that it might be made as a gamble, in the hope that some might escape, would not excuse it. After all, the purposes of Caiphas were, in his own eyes, perfectly noble. He thought it was necessary to let "one man die for the people."

The most urgent necessity of our time is therefore not merely to prevent the destruction of the human race by nuclear war. Even if it should happen to be no longer possible to prevent the disaster, (which God forbid) there is still a greater evil that can and must be prevented. It must be possible for every free man to refuse his consent and deny his cooperation to this greatest of crimes.

Here we are met with a truly frightening problem. In what does this effective and manifest refusal of consent consist? How does one "resist"? How are the conscientious objectors to mass suicide going to register their objection and their refusal to cooperate? I do not know. I am merely saying that this is an urgent problem that we have to consider and study with all our attention. Ideally speaking, in the imaginary case where all-out nuclear war seemed inevitable and the world's leaders seemed morally incapable of preventing it, it would become legitimate and even obligatory for all sane and conscientious men everywhere in the world to lay down their weapons and their tools and starve and be shot rather than cooperate in the war effort. If such a mass movement should spontaneously arise in all parts of the world, in Russia and America, in China and France, in Africa and Germany, the human race could be saved from extinction. This is, of course, a purely imaginary case. Innumerable complex problems would be involved in its actualization. How such a thing could ever be brought about is beyond conceiving. It would be a miracle. However, Christians believe in miracles. They also, on occasion, pray for them.

All this is very nice on paper, but it is pure speculation. Perhaps it raises more problems than it solves. On a more practical level, it is certainly necessary that we study and clarify *the great question of responsibility.* We have to make up our minds and form our conscience in regard to participation in the effort that threatens to lead us to universal destruction. We have to be convinced that there are certain things already clearly forbidden to all men, such as the use of torture, the killing of hostages, genocide (or the mass extermination of racial, national or other groups for no reason than that they belong to an "undesirable" category). We have to become aware of the poisonous effect of the mass media that keep violence, cruelty and sadism constantly present to the minds of unformed and irresponsible people. We have to recognize the danger to the whole world in the fact that today the economic life of the more highly developed nations is centered largely on the production of weapons, missiles and other engines of destruction. We have to consider that hate propaganda, and the consistent nagging and baiting of one government by another, have always inevitably led to violent conflict. These are activities which, in view of their possible consequences, are so dangerous and absurd as to be morally intolerable. We have still time to do something about it, but the time is rapidly running out.

The Christian in World Crisis:

Reflections on the Moral Climate of the 1960s

> We feel it our duty to beseech men, especially those who have the responsibility of public affairs, to spare no pain or effort until world events follow a course in keeping with man's destiny and dignity. . . . Nevertheless, unfortunately the law of fear still reigns among peoples. . . . There is reason to hope, however, that by meeting and negotiating men may come to discover that one of the most profound requirements of their nature is this: between them and their respective peoples it is not fear that should reign, but love—a love that tends to express itself in collaboration."
>
> JOHN XXIII, *Pacem in Terris.*

---

1. Can We Choose Peace?

A man is said to be "responsible" in so far as he is able to give a rational and humanly satisfactory answer, or "response," concerning his acts and the motives behind them. Cain, for instance, after the murder of Abel, was asked where Abel was—a question of primordial and typological importance. Cain's answer was not clear.

In discussing the fateful problems of violence, hatred and power politics in terms of Christian responsibility, we must first discover what question is being asked of us, and by whom. If we are willing to face the question along with the questioner, we may eventually become able to give a true and clear answer.

The question is not merely, "Where is our violent and overstimulated culture leading us?" or "Can total war be avoided?" or "Will the

Communists take over the West?" or "Will the West win the cold war?" or "Will the survivors of a nuclear war envy the dead?" From the standpoint of the present essay, such questions are irrelevant. Not that the issues they raise may not be vitally important, but the surmises and conjectures which might be offered as answers to such questions are really not answers to anything. They are beguiling guesses which seek to allay anxiety and which may well threaten to misdirect our best efforts if not to justify actions of which we ought to be ashamed.

The more important question is not "What is going to happen to us?" but "What are we going to do?" or more cogently, "*What are our real intentions?*" This last question is probably seldom asked with sufficient seriousness. Let us suppose it is not simply something we ask ourselves. Let us hear it as a question that is proposed to us by the Lord and Judge of life and death. Let us bear in mind another such question: "Friend, whereto art thou come?" (Matthew 26:50). Judas, somewhat subtler and far unhappier than Cain, having learned some fundamental truths, happened to know that the acceptable answer to such crucial questions had something to do with love. So he kissed Christ. But his kiss was a sign of betrayal.

We are being asked the very same question, if not directly and openly by Christ, at least by history of which we, as Christians, believe Him to be the Lord. I do not say that our love of Christ, desperate and confused as it is, is little more than a gesture of betrayal. But let us be sincere about facing the question, and hope, through God's grace, to answer it better than Judas.

Quite apart from what the Communists may or may not do, what are we, the dwindling and confused Christian minority in the West, going to do? Or at least, what do we *really want to do?* Do we intend to settle our problems peacefully or by force? Have we anything left to say about it at all? Have not the decisions been taken, to a great extent, out of our hands? Not yet. Among our leaders, some are Christians. Others cling to humanitarian principles which should be relevant here. These leaders will (we hope) take kindly to suggestions and to pleas that are based on Christian ethical norms. We have been very close to nuclear war, more than once, in the past five years. Has disaster been avoided merely by a healthy fear of the bomb, or have more humane and rational motives come to our aid?

The Christian is not only bound to avoid certain evils, but he is responsible for very great goods. This is often forgotten. The doctrine of the Incarnation leaves the Christian obligated at once to God and to man. If God has become man, then no Christian is ever allowed to be indifferent to man's fate. Whoever believes that Christ is the Word made flesh believes that every man must in some sense be regarded as Christ. For all are at least potentially members of the Mystical Christ. Who can say with absolute certainty of any other man that Christ does not live in him? Consequently in all our dealings with other men we must realize ourselves to be often, if not always, facing the questions that were asked of Cain and Judas.

If we are disciples of Christ we are necessarily our brother's keepers. And the question that is being asked of us concerns all men. It concerns, at the present moment, the entire human race. We cannot ignore this question. We cannot give an irresponsible and unchristian consent to the demonic use of power for the destruction of a whole nation, a whole continent, or possibly even the whole human race. Or can we? The question is now being asked.

This is the question that forms the subject of the present essay.

In this most critical moment of history we have a twofold task. It is a task in which the whole race is to some degree involved. But the greatest responsibility of all rests upon the citizens of the great power blocs which hold the fate of other nations in their hands.

On one hand we have to defend and foster the highest human values: the right of man to live freely and develop his life in a way worthy of his moral greatness. On the other hand we have to protect man against the criminal abuse of the enormous destructive power which he has acquired. To the American and Western European, this twofold task seems reducible in practice to a struggle against totalitarian dictatorship and against war.

Our very first obligation is to interpret the situation accurately, and this means resisting the temptation to oversimplify and generalize. The struggle against totalitarianism is directed not only against an external enemy—Communism—but also against our own hidden tendencies towards fascist or totalist aberrations. The struggle against war is directed not only against the bellicosity of the Communist powers, but against our own violence, fanaticism and greed. Of course, this kind of thinking will not be popular in the tensions of the cold war. No one is encouraged to be too clear-sighted, because conscience can make cowards, by diluting the strong conviction that our side is fully right and the other side is fully wrong. Yet the Christian responsibility is not to one side or to the other in the power struggle: it is to God and truth, and to the whole of mankind.

This is not a political study. But the moral options of our times are necessarily involved in various interpretations of political reality. The different views of the situation prevailing in the West react upon each other, and all together they combine to create extreme difficulties and complexities. The question arises then whether man is really capable of choosing peace rather than nuclear war, whether the choices are ineluctably made for him by the interplay of social forces. The answer to this question must depend on many factors beyond the control of any individual or any one group. But the fact remains that we cannot face the moral issue as free and rational beings unless we can still assume that our freedom and rationality have a meaning. If we are not able to choose to survive, then all discussion of the present crisis is pointless. If we are still free, then this essay can be considered as a very imperfect contribution to the work of moral renewal which is absolutely necessary if we are to make significant use of our freedom.

Freedom does not operate in a void. It is guided, or should be guided, by the light of intelligence. It should conform to a rational estimate of reality. It should not be simply an arbitrary exercise of choice. Blind affirmation of will is irrational and tends to destroy freedom. In any case, however, whether rational or not, freedom depends necessarily on man's concept of himself and of the situation in which he finds himself. If he is able to grasp clearly and realistically the truth of his plight, even though that plight may be desperate or extremely perilous, he can make good use of his freedom and can transcend even the most tragic injustices and be more truly a man because of them. He can turn defeat into victory. On the other hand, the will that is obsessed with power can refuse to see and to assess vitally important realities. It can remain obdurate and closed in the presence of human facts that contradict its obsessions. It is often precisely the will to power that is most stubborn in refusing to accept evidence of goodness and of hope. The blind drive to self-assertion rejects indications that love might be more meaningful and more powerful than force.

One of our most important tasks today is to clear the atmosphere so that men can understand their plight without hatred, without fury, without desperation, and with the minimum of good will. A humble and objective seriousness is necessary for the long task of restoring mutual confidence and preparing the way for the necessary work of collaboration in building world peace. This restoration of a climate of relative sanity is perhaps more important than specific decisions regarding the morality of this or that strategy, this or that pragmatic policy.

And so this essay will concern itself with the climate of opinion and thought in the years of crisis in which we live. Public opinion is intimately concerned with the decisions of authority, decisions which may affect the life and death of millions of people. It is therefore in the general climate of thought (or of thoughtlessness) that moral and sociological epidemics—of panic, hatred, destruction—take their origin. There are certain "climates" of opinion which make it practically impossible to solve civil or international problems except by resort to violence. When such a climate exists, certainly the fact ought to be recognized and something ought to be done about it. And that explains Pope John's encyclical *Pacem in Terris.* In a document devoted to the question of war and peace in the nuclear age, relatively little is said about war itself. The greater part of the encyclical concentrates on basic principles: the dignity of the human person and the primacy of the universal common good over the particular good of the political unit. Above all, Pope John realized that his main job was one of "clearing the air" morally, psychologically and spiritually. To a world lost in a pea-soup fog of exhausting and half-comprehended technicalities about law, economics, politics, weaponry, technology, etc., the Pope did not offer a series of casuistic solutions to complex and detailed questions. He recalled the minds of men to the fundamental ideas on which peace among nations and races must always depend. In other words, he tried to re-create for them the climate of thought in which they could *see* their objectives in a human and even a hopeful light, and he invited them at least for a moment to emerge from the obscurity and smog of arguments that are without issue. The world was grateful for this moment of fresh air, and in political life, especially on the international level, the smallest gestures and advances toward peace should be accepted with gratitude. Many such gestures followed the publication of *Pacem in Terris* on Holy Thursday of 1963. So many in fact that there has been a significant relaxation of tensions, at least between the U.S. and the USSR.

Without flattering ourselves that we are on the way to a quick solution of our problems, or even that the world at large has fully committed itself to implementing Pope John's Encyclical of Peace, we can at least recognize that such things are possible. We are not utterly condemned to think our way into an impasse from which the only issue is destructive violence. Human and reasonable solutions are still open to us. But they depend on our climate of thought, that is to say, on our ability to hope in peaceful solutions.

A weather map is necessarily very superficial. The storm areas in thought and opinion are not all concentrated on one side or the other of the iron curtain. On both sides extremists, characterized by negativism, distrust of the other side, suspicion, fear, hate and the willingness to resort to force, are very outspoken and have access to the mass media so that their opinions often take on the appearance of quasi-dogmatic finality and are uncritically accepted, with a few unspoken reservations, perhaps, by the majority of the population. Not that most men want war, or even willingly face the possibility that certain trends might lead suddenly to war, but they assume, in a guarded and more or less resigned silence, that the most menacing voices are probably right and that what is printed in most of the papers and shouted from most of the house-tops must quite probably represent a more or less coherent interpretation of political reality. They know that total war is always possible, yet they blindly and confusedly hope that what they refuse to think about is so "unthinkable" that it will never occur, and so they busy themselves with the absorbing rush of life and unconsciously withdraw from any kind of dissenting commitment that would leave them exposed to ostracism. They submit and conform, and trust to the protective coloring that conformity provides in a mass society.

The current moral climate is one of more or less resigned compliance with the world view popularized by the mass media.

Apart from a very small minority who demand uncompromising unilateral initiatives toward peace, the necessity of force and military strength seems unquestionable to the majority. But there are of course considerable differences of attitude, and many gradations in the opinions of statesmen, strategists and dictators of opinion. Indeed, reflection on strategy in the nuclear age has at times assumed the appearance of an esoteric cult to which only the expert with access to a computer can really consider himself initiated. There is unquestionably a sincere desire for peace, or at least an earnest desire to avoid total war, in the minds of most policy-makers. But the legacy of recent history and the frustrating ambiguities of the international situation seem to make really effective steps toward peace impossible. In the minds of the world leaders a continued stalemate is accepted, in practice, as "peace," and the power struggle continues under the constant menace of accidental global war.

Therefore, though there are many good minds earnestly concerned with the technical problem of peace, and many plans have been proposed and even initiated, the details of this peace-thinking do not reach and illuminate the mind of the common man. For him there remains only the confused apprehension of a perilous situation in which force or the threat of force is a practical necessity, war a proximate danger, and peace at best a fond hope.

Pope John reflects on this climate of confusion and practical despair. "How strongly does the turmoil of individual men and peoples contrast with the perfect order of the universe! *It is as if the relationships which bind them together could only be controlled by force!*" (*Pacem in Terris,* n.4). And he adds: *"The fickleness of opinion often produces this error, that many think that the relationships between men and states can be governed by the same laws as the forces and irrational elements of the universe"* (n.6).

While praising and fully accepting science, Pope John protests against the common opinion which deifies pseudo-science and leaves man's freedom subject to a vague determinism of laws and forces, thus failing to see that man's freedom and intelligence are the instruments by which he elevates himself above his material surroundings and controls his own destiny by living according to truth, justice and love.

Pope John's message of freedom calls man, first of all, to liberate himself from the climate of confusion and desperation in which he finds himself because he passively accepts and follows a mindless determinism.

Though there are significant differences in ideology in the different power blocs, nevertheless the stratification of opinion is more or less the same everywhere. The extremists on both sides are mirror images of each other.

The thought that is obsessed with war puts aside other considerations and concentrates on the fact that one is threatened with attack, indeed with destruction. This type of thinker is convinced that only the strongest measures are of any use. He distrusts negotiation because he is sure that the adversary is an arch deceiver, and because he is so sure of this he thinks that he himself has to resort to deception whenever possible, so as not to be deceived. He is convinced that the enemy will attack him violently as soon as he thinks he can get away with it. In this climate of thought, strategy tends to work around to the idea of "hitting the enemy before he hits me first."

The crude simplicity of this view tends to recommend it to the average man who does not have time to do a great deal of thinking and who, in any case, does not have access to the more selective and thoughtful sources of information which might enable him to form a more sophisticated judgment. It is clear, and its sweeping ruthlessness gives it an appearance of realism. But unfortunately it maintains a moral and political atmosphere of fear and hatred in which it is more difficult even for "experts" to view things with objective detachment. Who is to say to what extent the statesmen themselves are influenced, in practice, by the horrendous mythology of the mass man? The leaders help to make a myth by their own pronouncements and slogans, and because the myth is so willingly believed by the common man they themselves assume that this is a kind of divine ratification. *Vox populi vox Dei.*

That there are large numbers of Christians who live somewhat easily in this climate of opinion is clear from the popular religious press. This is not surprising if we reflect that most Christians belong to the rank and file of common humanity and that the Catholic press has a tendency to follow accepted and prevalent opinions in matters of world politics. It is also possible that a certain negativism and pessimism which has been widespread in both Catholic and Protestant spirituality since the Renaissance and the Reformation may account for the willingness with which believers accept the idea of a crusade against nations that can quite easily be caricatured as essentially wicked and perverse: made up of beings hardly human, never deserving of trust, always worthy of being destroyed.

This was what prompted Pope John to speak out against the abuse of the mass media, both in *Mater et Magistra* and *Pacem in Terris.* A falsely informed public with a distorted view of political reality and an oversimplified, negative attitude toward other races and peoples cannot be expected to react in any other way than with irrational and violent responses. Therefore the Pope condemned the dissemination of prejudice and hate by the mass media and said: "Truth demands that the various media of social communication . . . be used with serene objectivity. . . . Methods of information which fall short of the truth and by that very token impair the reputation of this or that people, must be discarded" (*Pacem in Terris,* n.90).

An important element in *Pacem in Terris* is Pope John's repeated insistence that one of the basic rights of free men is "the right to be informed truthfully about public events" (n.12), along with the right both to basic and higher education (n.13), the right to form associations to defend their just aims (ns. 23,24), and to take an active (not passive) part in public affairs (n.25). One who merely echoes the opinions in the newspaper is not taking an "active" part in the life of his nation. Hence Pope John's paragraphs on human rights imply not only the privilege but also at times the obligation of dissent from a prevailing and passively accepted viewpoint. And this is extremely important when we consider the context of war and peace, since in a time of crisis and mass emotionalism the dissenter who maintains his insistence on the rights of peace is easily regarded as a traitor. Nevertheless such dissent may acquire a decisive importance, and it should always be protected by law against arbitrary attack and suppression (n.27). Rights also imply obligations, and the "right to investigate the truth freely [is correlative with] the duty of seeking it ever more completely and profoundly" (n.29). It is unfortunate that the advantages of freedom in a democratic society have been so little appreciated and that men have abdicated their right and neglected their opportunity in order to remain passive, confused and hopeless, not using the sources of information and dissenting opinions to which they might have access.

Cardinal Suenens speaking to the United Nations on May 13, 1963, and explaining the encyclical *Pacem in Terris,* compared it to a symphony with the leitmotif: "Peace among all peoples requires: Truth as its foundation, justice as its rule, love as its driving force, liberty as its atmosphere."

But in the moral climate of mass opinion, engineered by publicists, "truth" tends to mean a sensational revelation of some new inquiry on the part of the enemy. And the misfortune is that on both sides there is enough real iniquity around to make the concoction of sensational news items quite easy. Justice, in this climate, operates on a double standard: one for one's own side and another for the enemy, so that what in him is criminal is, in us, simple "realism." Love is assuredly not the driving force of peace policies which are inert and firmly rooted in inveterate distrust. Liberty is not exactly the mark of relationships in which big powers reduce smaller ones to the status of political or economic satellites. Yet, says Cardinal Suenens, these four are "the rules of the road which lead to peace, rules which must be respected in the relations between various political communities."

Perhaps the chief reason why these rules are neglected are that the most basic principles of human social life are not respected. *Pacem in Terris* reminds us that mankind is one family in which all nations, groups and individuals must cooperate, on the basis of truth, justice, love and liberty in attaining the universal common good which is also at the same time the good of the individual person in his individuality, in his dignity and in his basic rights. If man does not seek, by reasonable collaboration, to attain these ends, there is no alternative but the arbitrary exercise of the will to power, in which case the law of reason, of nature and of God is usurped by the law of the jungle. A theologian commenting on *Pacem in Terris* says:

> If owing to antiphilosophic prejudice, universal truths dictated by reason are rejected and only the manifestations of the changing will of nations are revered, whatever these may be, it would be absurd to attempt the construction of a juridical organization of the human race.
>
> (P. Riga, "Peace on Earth," p. 33)

The climate of irrationality, confusion and violence which is characteristic of such times as ours is after all nothing new. The circumstances are different, but in the end we can find in our world much that is analogous to the classic description of Athens after the Peloponnesian War. Thucydides masterfully outlines the political situation of a rich society that is in a crisis of decline and change:

> War destroys the comfortable routine of life, trains us in violence and shapes our character according to the new conditions. . . . The cause of all these evils was imperialism, whose fundamental motives are ambition and greed, and from which arises the fanaticism of class conflict. The politicians on each side were armed with high-sounding slogans. . . . Both boasted that they were servants of the community and both made the community the prize of war. The only purpose of their policy was the extermination of their opponents, and to achieve this they stopped at nothing. Even worse were the reprisals which they perpetuated in total disregard of morality or of the common good. The only standard which they recognized was party caprice and so they were prepared, either by the perversion of justice or by revolutionary action, to satisfy the passing passions begotten by the struggle. . . . Society was divided into warring camps suspicious of one another. Where no contract or obligation was binding, nothing could heal the conflict, and since security was only to be found in the assumption that nothing was secure, everyone took steps to preserve himself and no one could afford to trust his neighbor. On the whole the baser types survived best. Aware of their own deficiencies and their opponents' abilities, they resorted boldly to violence, before they were defeated in debate, and struck down, by conspiracy, minds more versatile than their own.
>
> (Thucydides, *Peloponnesian War*, iii, 82)

In such a situation, Plato, who hoped that a return to reason could be brought about by the participation of the philosopher in public life, also recognized that intelligent men would be tempted to withdraw from a situation they regarded as "hopeless." The lover of justice, Plato wrote, seeing himself as though thrown into a "den of beasts" and unable to change the jungle law around him;

> Will remain quietly at his own work like a traveller caught in a storm who retreats behind a wall to shelter from the driving gusts of dust and hail. Seeing the rest of the world full of iniquity, he will be content to keep his own life on earth untainted by wickedness and impious actions, so that he may leave this world with a fair hope of the next, at peace with himself and God.
>
> (*Republic,* 496)

It is perhaps true that sometimes individuals may be forced into this position, but to view it as normal and to accept it as preferable to the risks and conflicts of public life is an admission of defeat, an abdication of responsibility. This secession into individualistic concern with one's own salvation alone may in fact leave the way all the more open for unscrupulous men and groups to gain and wield unjust power.

The example of Taoism in China in the chaotic period of the third to the first centuries B.C. is there to show how an other-worldly spiritualism in public life can end in the worst kind of arbitrary tyranny. The intellectual and the spiritual man cannot therefore justify themselves in abandoning society to the rule of an irrational will to power.

If sheer arbitrary will and brute force are not to take command of everything, reason must seek more solid and more harmonious solutions to problems by arbitration and discussion. Men must collaborate sincerely in solving their difficulties. This is a basic Christian obligation.

But rational collaboration is manifestly impossible without mutual trust and this in turn is out of the question where there is no basis for sure communication. Not only is communication lacking: it is blocked. It is fiercely resisted by groups and nations which close themselves in upon themselves and refuse to communicate with one another except by ultimatums and threats of destruction. Not only that, but esoteric thought systems and complex vocabularies erect barriers that only a specialist can penetrate. Thus the failure of communication between the great powers leads to resentment, distrust and disillusionment among the others.

A pervasive climate of boredom, exasperation and indifference tends to prevail where the grosser moods of bellicism and fanaticism are seen for what they are. A reviewer in *Commentary,* summarizing the argument of a book on this subject, gives us in a readable paragraph the picture of liberal and neo-conservative discontent in Europe and the "emerging nations."

> The cold war from being a necessary defensive operation against the armed threat emanating from the USSR in 1948 has

> turned into an endless struggle for global hegemony: a struggle that neither side can (and perhaps no longer wants to) win. Meanwhile the neutrals are getting restive: Asia, Africa and Latin America want to break out of this straitjacket. Industrialization—whether capitalist or socialist—has become *the* preoccupation of elites who speak for two-thirds of mankind: the hungry two-thirds. Yet all the while Washington and Moscow exchange verbal brickbats amidst growing boredom and indifference, and latterly to the accompaniment of catcalls from Peking. . . .
> ("The Cold War in Perspective," by George Lichtheim, *Commentary*, June 1964, p. 25.)

So, while the policies of force continue to invoke traditional notions of justice, rights, international law, etc., the repetition of these formulas makes them sound more and more hollow and absurd to everyone. This climate of disillusionment and disgust is dangerous because it implies a growing contempt for reason and for the basic human powers without which man cannot organize his life in a free and orderly fashion. This engenders a deeper pessimism, a more tenacious hopelessness, and communication becomes more and more precarious.

Pacem in Terris certainly recognized that Catholics themselves were to a great extent out of contact with the rest of the world, enclosed in their own spiritual and religious ghetto. One of the chief contributions of Pope John's brief pontificate was that he opened the ghetto and told Catholics to go out and talk to other people, to Protestants, to Jews, to Hindus, and even to Communists. He realized that without this climate of openness, the communication which was essential for mutual trust would be out of the question. He insisted on making a "clear distinction between false philosophical teachings . . . and movements which have a direct bearing either on economic or social questions or cultural matters . . ." (*Pacem in Terris*, n.159). It is necessary to communicate with those who hold different ideologies when we are confronting common problems that can only be solved in collaboration. If we speak different languages we must nevertheless attempt to find the essential points of agreement without which there is, as Cardinal Suenens says, a permanent risk of disaster. We must therefore either decide to continue in a fatal rivalry or begin to trust one another in progressive negotiations in which peace may eventually be stabilized and guaranteed.

It is the attitude of openness prescribed by *Pacem in Terris* that must form our thinking as Christians in time of crisis, and not the closed and fanatical myths of nationalistic or racial paranoia. Only if we remain open, detached, humble in the presence of objective truth and of our fellow man, will we be able to choose peace.

2. *The Christian as Peacemaker*

Like his predecessor in the papacy, like all deeply religious and indeed all truly rational men, Pope John XXIII deplored the gigantic stockpiles of weapons, the arms race and the cold war. He asked the leaders of the great powers to bring the arms race to an end and come "to an agreement on a fitting program of disarmament, employing mutual and effective controls" (*Pacem in Terris,* n.122). This and other passages of the Peace Encyclical, where Pope John speaks of disarmament and modern warfare, have often been quoted and need not be repeated here. But it is more important to observe that Pope John did not merely call for the reduction of weapons and the easing of international tensions. He asserted that there was really no hope of this being done effectively unless it was prompted by deep inner conviction. Such conviction demands that "everyone sincerely cooperates to banish the fear and anxious expectation of war with which men are oppressed."

Once again we see that Pope John was chiefly concerned with the general climate of thought and the current outlook of mankind. It would be of little use for one side or the other, or both, to disarm, if men continued in the same state of confusion, suspicion, hostility and aggressiveness.

Therefore, if a climate favorable to peace is to be produced, Pope John continues, "the fundamental principle upon which our present peace depends must be replaced by another, which declares that the true and solid peace of nations consists not in equality of arms but in mutual trust alone. We believe that this can be brought to pass, and we consider that, since it concerns a matter not only demanded by right reason but also eminently desirable in itself, it will prove the source of many benefits" (n.113).

But it would be sentimental to ask men to awaken feelings of optimism and trust in their hearts without laying that firm foundation of order which *Pacem in Terris* repeatedly demands as the essential condition for true peace on earth.

"Peace will be an empty-sounding word unless it is founded on the order which this present document has outlined in confident hope: an order founded on truth, built according to justice, vivified and integrated by charity, and put into practice in freedom" (n.168). The duty of working together for peace in this sense binds not only public authority but all those to whom the Encyclical is addressed: that is to say *everybody.* But of course it is a special obligation of the Christian who, as a follower of Christ, must be a peacemaker.

Pope John understood and clearly stated that being a "peacemaker" meant more, not less, than being a "pacifist." It is not only a matter of protesting against the bomb, but also of working tirelessly and constructively at the "most exalted task of bringing about true peace in the order established by God . . . [by establishing] *new methods of relationships in human society*" (n.163). Pope John publicly and emphatically praises the few who have devoted themselves to this work, and hopes "that their number will increase, especially among those who believe" (n.164).

Let us reflect on the emphasis with which Pope John called Christians, in the name of Christ their Head, to this work of peace based on truth, justice, love and liberty in human relations. This summons to fight in the ranks of an army of peace is of course traditionally Christian, and yet it is also new because it occurs in a context so new that Cardinal Suenens called it "unprecedented in history."

Pope John's call to peace was based not on distrust of man and denunciation of his wickedness, but on the assertion of man's fundamental goodness. Not only the material world, not only technological society, but even the society built by unbelievers and enemies of the Church with the aim of raising man to a better temporal state is regarded by Pope John with eyes of friendly concern. Not only does he tolerate the presence of a non-Christian society, but he embraces it in the love of Christ. The context of Christian peacemaking is then something other than that even of so-called Christian pacifism. This must be brought out, because there are certain ambiguities in the term "pacifist" which lay it open to manipulation and misinterpretation by those for whom world peace is not a seriously credible option, except on a basis of overwhelming force.

No need to mention the facile caricature of the "pacifist" as a maladjusted creature lost in impractical ideals, sentimentally hoping that prayer and demonstrations can convert men to the ways of peace. It is routine for the mass media to treat even the most eminent and reasonable defenders of peace, men with a worldwide reputation as scientists, as if they were slightly addled egg-heads as well as Communist sympathizers, or indeed undercover agents of Moscow. I refer rather to fundamental religious ambiguities in the term "pacifism." Actually it is often hard to pin these ambiguities down with precision. They depend in each case on the implicit spiritual bases of the pacifism in question, and these are not easy to find.

Often "pacifism" in the religious sense is rooted in a world-denying and individualistic asceticism, or it is found in the context of a small eschatological community (like that of the Shakers, for instance) which also may have other beliefs, rejecting marriage, the use of flesh meat, etc., which in their turn may be justified by a kind of manichaean theology. In other words a pacifism that regards war as an inevitable and intolerable evil, as intolerable as the unregenerate world from which it cannot be separated, and which the individual believer must renounce, by that very fact tends to rejoin the pessimism of the belligerent crusader who implicitly carries his denial of the world to the point of wishing it to be destroyed.

Probably no one has ever accused *Pacem in Terris* of being "pacifist," and there is good reason not to do so. There is in this document nothing of the world-hating rejection that identifies war with the city of man. Pope John's optimism was really something new in Christian thought because he expressed the unequivocal hope that a world of ordinary men, a world in which many men were not Christians or even believers in God, might still be a world of peace if men would deal with one another on the basis of their God-given reason and with respect for their inalienable human rights. Note that *Pacem in Terris* is the first encyclical in which the language of human rights has been so clearly espoused.

The religious ambiguities in the term "pacifism" give it implications that are somewhat less than Catholic. I do not here refer to the inaccurate and perverse generalization that "a Catholic cannot be a conscientious objector," but to the fact that "pacifism" tends, as a cause, to take on the air of a quasi-religion, as though it were a kind of faith in its own right. A pacifist is then regarded as one who "believes in peace" so to speak as an article of faith, and hence puts himself in the position of being absolutely unable to countenance any form of war, since for him to accept any war in theory or in practice would be to deny his faith. A Christian pacifist then becomes one who compounds this ambiguity by insisting, or at least by implying, that pacifism is an integral part of Christianity, with the evident conclusion that Christians who are not pacifists have, by that fact, apostatized from Christianity.

This unfortunate emphasis gains support from the way conscientious objection is in fact treated by the selective service laws of the United States. An objector who is a religious "pacifist" is considered as one who for subjective and personal reasons of conscience and belief refuses to go to war, and whose "conscientious objection" is tolerated and even recognized by the government. There is of course something valuable and edifying in this recognition of the personal conscience, but there is also an implication that any minority stand against war on grounds of conscience is ipso facto a kind of deviant and morally eccentric position, to be tolerated only because there are always a few religious half-wits around in any case, and one has to humor them in order to preserve the nation's reputation for respecting individual liberty.

In other words, this sanctions the popular myth that all pacifism is based on religious emotion rather than on reason, and that it has no objective ethical validity, but is allowed to exist because of the possibility of harmless and mystical obsessions with peace on the part of a few enthusiasts. It also sanctions another myth, to which some forms of pacifism give support, that pacifists are people who simply prefer to yield to violence and evil rather than resist it in any way. They are fundamentally indifferent to reasonable, moral or patriotic ideals and prefer to sink into their religious apathy and let the enemy overrun the country unresisted.

To sum it all up in a word, this caricature of pacifism which reduces it to a purely eccentric individualism of conscience declares that the pacifist is willing to let everyone be destroyed merely because he himself does not have a taste for war. It is not hard to imagine what capital can be made out of this distortion by copy writers for, say, *Time* magazine or the New York *Daily News.* It is also easy to see how the Catholic clergy might be profoundly suspicious of any kind of conscientious objection to war when myths like these have helped them to form their judgment.

Speaking in the name of Christ and of the Church to all mankind, Pope John was not issuing a pacifist document in this sense. He was not simply saying that if a few cranks did not like the bomb they were free to entertain their opinion. He was saying, on the contrary, that we had reached a point in history where it was clearly no longer reasonable to make use of war in the settlement of international disputes, and that the important thing was not merely protest against the latest war technology, but the construction of permanent world peace on a basis of truth, justice, love and liberty. This is not a matter for a few individual consciences, it urgently binds the conscience of every living man. It is not an individual refinement of spirituality, a luxury of the soul, but a collective obligation of the highest urgency, a universal and immediate need which can no longer be ignored.

He is not saying that a few Christians may and ought to be pacifists (i.e., to protest against war) but that all Christians and all reasonable men are bound by their very rationality to work to establish a real and lasting peace.

Already in his first encyclical, *Ad Petri Cathedram,* Pope John had said that Christians were obliged to strive "with all the means at their disposal" for peace. Yet he warned that peace cannot compromise with error or make concessions to injustice. Passive acquiescence in injustice, submission to brute force are not the way to genuine peace. There is some truth in Machiavelli's contention that mere weakness and confusion lead in the long run to greater disasters than a firm and even intransigent policy. But the Christian program for peace does not depend on human astuteness, ruthlessness or force. Power can never be the keystone of a Christian policy. Yet our work for peace must be energetic, enlightened and fully purposeful. Its purpose is defined by our religious belief that God has called us "to the service of His merciful designs" (John XXIII, Christmas Message, 1958). If we are now in possession of atomic power, we have the moral obligation to make a good and peaceful use of it, rather than turning it to our own destruction. But we will not be able to do this without an interior revolution that abandons the quest for brute power and submits to the wisdom of love and of the Cross.

It must however be stated quite clearly and without compromise that the duty of the Christian as a peacemaker is not to be confused with a kind of quietistic inertia that is indifferent to injustice, accepts any kind of disorder, compromises with error and with evil, and gives in to every pressure in order to maintain "peace at any price." The Christian knows well, or should know well, that peace is not possible on such terms. Peace demands the most heroic labor and the most difficult sacrifice. It demands greater heroism than war. It demands greater fidelity to the truth and a much more perfect purity of conscience. The Christian fight for peace is not to be confused with defeatism.

What is the traditional attitude of the Christian peacemaker? Let us glance back over a few sources and briefly examine some traditional witnesses to the Christian concern for peace on earth.

Christians believe that Christ came into this world as a Prince of Peace. We believe that Christ Himself is our peace (Ephesians 2:14). We believe that God has chosen for Himself, in the Mystical Body of Christ, an elect people, regenerated by the Blood of the Savior, and committed by their baptismal promise to wage war upon the evil and hatred that are in man, and help to establish the Kingdom of God and of peace, in truth and love.

Indeed for centuries the Old Testament prophets had been looking forward to the coming of the Messiah as the "Prince of Peace" (Isaias 9:6). The Messianic Kingdom was to be a kingdom of peace because first of all man would be completely reconciled with God and with the hostile forces of nature (Osee 2:18–20), the whole world would be full of the manifest knowledge of the divine mercy (Isaias 11:9) and hence men, the sons of God and objects of His mercy, would live at peace with one another (Isaias 54:13). The early Christians were filled with the conviction that since the Risen Christ had received Lordship over the whole cosmos and sent His Spirit to dwell in men (Acts 2:17) the kingdom of peace was already established in the Church.

This meant a recognition that human nature, identical in all men, was assumed by the Logos in the Incarnation, and that Christ died out of love for all men, in order to live in all men. All were henceforth "one in Christ" (Galatians 3:28) and Christ Himself was their peace, since His Spirit kept them united in supernatural love (Ephesians 4:3). The Christian therefore has the obligation to treat every other man as Christ Himself, respecting his neighbor's life as if it were the life of Christ, his rights as if they were the rights of Christ. Even if that neighbor shows himself to be unjust, wicked and odious to us, the Christian cannot take upon himself a final and definite judgment in his case. The Christian still has an obligation to be patient, and to seek his enemy's highest spiritual interests and indeed his temporal good in so far as that may be compatible with the universal common good of man.

The Christian commandment to love our enemies was not regarded by the first Christians merely as a summons to higher moral perfection than was possible under the Old Law. The New Law did not compete with the Old, but on the contrary fulfilled it, at the same time abolishing the conflicts between various forms of obligation and perfection.

The love of enemies was not therefore the expression of a Christian moral ideal, in contrast with Stoic, Epicurean or Jewish ideals. It was much more an expression of eschatological faith in the realization of the messianic promises and hence a witness to an entirely new dimension in man's life.

Christian peace was therefore not considered at first to be simply a religious and spiritual consecration of the Pax Romana. It was an eschatological gift of the Risen Christ (John 20:19). It could not be achieved by any ethical or political program. It was given with the supreme gift of the Holy Spirit, making men spiritual and uniting them to the "mystical" Body of·Christ. Christian peace is in fact a fruit of the Spirit (Galatians 5:22) and a sign of the Divine Presence in the world.

Division, conflict, strife, schism, hatreds and wars are then evidence of the "old life," the unregenerate sinful existence that has not been transformed in the mystery of Christ (I Corinthians 1:10; James 3:16). When Christ told Peter to "put away his sword" (John 18:11) and warned him that those who struck with the sword would perish by it, He was not simply forbidding war. War was neither blessed nor forbidden by Christ. He simply stated that war belonged to the world outside the Kingdom, the world outside the mystery and the Spirit of Christ and that therefore for one who was seriously living in Christ, war belonged to a realm that no longer had a decisive meaning, for though the Christian was "in the world" he was not "of the world." He could not avoid implication in its concerns, but he belonged to a kingdom of peace "that was not of this world" (John 18:36).

The Christian is and must be by his very adoption as a son of God, In Christ, a peacemaker (Matthew 5:9). He is bound to imitate the Savior who, instead of defending Himself with twelve legions of angels (Matthew 26:55), allowed Himself to be nailed to the Cross and died praying for His executioners. The Christian is one whose life has sprung from a particular spiritual seed: the blood of the martyrs who, without offering forcible resistance, laid down their lives rather than submit to the unjust laws that demanded an official religious cult of the Emperor as God. One verse in Saint John's account of the Passion of Christ makes clear the underlying principles of war and peace in the Gospel (John 18:36). Questioned by Pilate as to whether He is a King, Jesus replies "My Kingdom is not of this world" and explains that if he were a worldly king his followers would be fighting for him. In other words, the Christian attitude to war and peace is fundamentally eschatological. The Christian does not need to fight and indeed it is better that he should not fight, for in so far as he imitates his Lord and Master, he proclaims that the Messianic kingdom has come and bears witness to the presence of the *Kyrios Pantocrator* in mystery, even in the midst of the conflicts and turmoil of the world. The book of the New Testament that definitely canonizes this eschatological view of peace in the midst of spiritual combat is the Apocalypse, which sets forth in mysterious and symbolic language the critical struggle of the nascent Church with the powers of the world, as typified by the Roman Empire.

This struggle, which is definitive and marks the last age of the world, is the final preparation for the manifestation of Christ as Lord of the Universe (the *Parousia*) (Apocalypse 11:15–18). The Kingdom is already present in the world, since Christ has overcome the world and risen from the dead. But the Kingdom is still not fully manifested and remains outwardly powerless. It is a kingdom of saints and martyrs, priests and witnesses, whose main function is to bide their time in faith, loving one another and the truth, suffering persecution in the furious cataclysm which marks the final testing of earthly society. They will take no direct part in the struggles of earthly kingdoms. Their life is one of faith, gentleness, meekness, patience, purity. They depend on no power other than the power of God, and it is God they obey rather than the state, which tends to usurp the powers of God and to blaspheme Him, setting itself up in His stead as an idol and drawing to itself the adoration and worship that are due to Him alone (Apocalypse 13:3–9).

The Apocalypse describes the final stage of the history of the world as a total and ruthless power struggle in which all the Kings of the earth are engaged, but which has an inner, spiritual dimension these kings are incapable of seeing and understanding. The wars, cataclysms and plagues which convulse worldly society are in reality the outward projection and manifestation of a hidden, spiritual battle. Two dimensions, spiritual and material, cut across one another. To be consciously and willingly committed to the worldly power struggle, in politics, business and wars, is to founder in darkness, confusion, and sin. The saints are "in the world" and doubtless suffer from its murderous conflicts like everybody else. Indeed they seem at first to be defeated and destroyed (13:7). But they see the inner meaning of these struggles and are patient. They trust in God to work out their destiny and rescue them from the final destruction, the accidents of which are not subject to their control. Hence they pay no attention to the details of the power struggle as such and do not try to influence it or to engage in it, one way or another, even for their own apparent benefit and survival. For they realize that their survival has nothing to do with the exercise of force or ingenuity.

The ever recurrent theme of the Apocalypse is then that the typical power-structured empire of Babylon (Rome) cannot but be "drunk with the blood of the martyrs of Jesus" (17:6) and that therefore the saints must "go out from her" and break off all relations with her and her sinful concerns (18:4 ff) for "in one hour" is her judgment decided and the smoke of the disaster "shall go up forever and ever" (19:3). Yet the author of the Apocalypse does not counsel flight, as there is no geographical escape from Babylon: the one escape is into a spiritual realm by martyrdom, to lay down one's life in fidelity to God and in protest against the impurity, the magic, the fictitiousness and the murderous fury of the city whose god is force (21:4–8).

What is the place of war in all this? War is the "rider of the red horse" who is sent to prepare the destruction of the power structure (6:4) for "he has received power to take away peace from the earth and to make them all kill one another, and he has received a great sword." The four horsemen (war, hunger, death and pestilence) are sent as signs and precursors of the final consummation of history. Those who have led the saints captive will themselves be made captive, those who have killed the saints will themselves be killed in war: and the saints in their time will be rescued from the cataclysm by their patience (13:10).

Translated into historical terms, these mysterious symbols of the Apocalypse show us the early Christian attitude toward war, injustice and the persecutions of the Roman empire, even though that empire was clearly understood to possess a demonic power. The battle was nonviolent and spiritual, and its success depended on the clear understanding of the totally new and unexpected dimensions in which it was to be fought. On the other hand, there is no indication whatever in the Apocalypse that the Christian would be willing to fight and die to maintain the "power of the beast," in other words to engage in a power struggle for the benefit of the Emperor and of his power.

Nevertheless, it must not be stated without qualification that all the early Christians were purely and simply pacifists and that they had a clear, systematic policy of pacifism which obliged them to refuse military service whenever it was demanded of them. This would be too sweeping an assertion. There were Christians in the armies of Rome, but they were doubtless exceptional. Many of them had been converted while they were soldiers and remained in "the state in which they had been called" (I Corinthians 7–10). They were free to do so because the Imperial army was considered as a police force, maintaining the *Pax Romana,* and the peace of the empire as Origen said (*Contra Celsum* II, 30) was something the early Church was able to appreciate as in some sense providential. However, the military life was not considered ideal for a Christian. The problem of official idolatry was inescapable. Many Christian soldiers suffered martyrdom for refusing to participate in the sacrifices. Nevertheless, some soldiers, like Saint Maximilian, were martyred explicitly for refusal to serve in the army. Others, like Saint Martin of Tours, remained in service until they were called upon to kill in battle, and then refused to do so. Martin, according to the office in the monastic Breviary, declared that "because he was a soldier of Christ it was not licit for him to kill." Christians were the first to lay down their lives rather than fight in war.

The early Christian apologists tend to condemn military service. Clement of Alexandria again takes up the theme of the Christian as a "soldier of peace" whose only weapons are the word of God and the Christian virtues (*Protreptic* XI, 116). Justin Martyr declares in his *Apology* (I, 39), "We who formerly murdered one another [he is a convert from paganism] now not only do not make war upon our enemies, but that we may not lie or deceive our judges, we gladly die confessing Christ." Saint Cyprian remarked shrewdly that while the killing of one individual by another was recognized as a crime, when homicide is carried out publicly on a large scale by the state it turns into a virtue! (*Ad Donatum*, VI, 10). Tertullian declared that when Christ took away Peter's sword, "he disarmed every soldier" (*De Idololatria*, XIX).

3. War in Origen and Saint Augustine

It is interesting to examine in some detail the attack on Christianity written by a pagan traditionalist, Celsus, who is refuted in Origen's *Contra Celsum* (third century A.D.). Celsus is a conservative who is deeply disturbed by the decay of the Roman Empire, and he agrees with many of his contemporaries in ascribing that decay to the nefarious revolutionary influence of the secret society called Christians. The anxiety which Celsus, a cultivated pagan, feels over the imminent downfall of the society to which he belongs discharges itself in a mixture of contempt and hatred upon Jews and above all the new sect of Jews who worship Christ. For though he despises the Jews, Celsus can tolerate them because their worship and customs are "at least traditional." But Christianity is completely subversive of the old religious and social order which Celsus conceives to be more or less universal and cosmopolitan. His chief grievance against the Christians is their claim to exclusiveness, to the possession of a special revealed truth which forms no part of the socio-religious heritage of the various nations, but contradicts all known religions, rejecting them along with the traditional norms of culture and civilization. Abandoning the reasonable and universal norms of polytheism, Christianity, he says, worships a crucified Jew. Christians are rebels who deliberately cut themselves off from the rest of mankind. They are undermining the whole fabric of society with their insidious doctrines. Above all, they are irresponsible and selfish, indeed antisocial. Instead of returning to the customs of their fathers and living content like the rest of men with the *status quo*, they refuse to take part in public life, they do not carry out their duties as citizens, and in particular they *refuse to fight in the army*. In a word, they remain callously indifferent to the service of the threatened empire, and have no concern with peace and order, or with the common good. It is the familiar condemnation of the pacifist: "Just because he perversely refuses to fight, everyone else is threatened with destruction!"

In a word, Celsus reflects the profound insecurity of one who is totally attached to decaying social forms, and who thinks he beholds in some of his contemporaries a complete indifference towards the survival of all that is meaningful to him. Christians, it seemed, not only believed that Celsus' Roman world was meaningless, but that it was under judgment and doomed to destruction. He interpreted the other-worldly Christian spirit as a concrete, immediate physical threat. There was doubtless no other way in which he was capable of understanding it.

Origen replies first of all by vigorously denying that the Christians are violent revolutionaries, or that they have any intention of preparing the overthrow of the empire by force. He says:

> Christians have been taught not to defend themselves against their enemies; and because they have kept the laws which command gentleness and love to man, on this account they have received from God that which they would not have succeeded in doing if they had been given the right to make war, even though they may have been quite able to do so. He always fought for them and from time to time stopped the opponents of the Christians and the people who wanted to kill them.
> (*Contra Celsum*, III, Chadwick, translation, p. 133)

After this Origen takes issue with the basic contention of Celsus that there have to be wars, because men cannot live together in unity. Origen announces the Christian claim that a time will come for all men to be united in the Logos, though this fulfillment is most probably eschatological (realized only after the end and fulfillment of world history). Nevertheless, Christians are *not totally unconcerned* with the peace, fortunes and survival of the Empire. Origen does not take the categorically unworldly view of the Apocalypse. He has a great respect for Greek and Roman civilization at least in its more spiritual and humane aspects. The unified Roman world is the providentially appointed scene for the Gospel *kerygma.*

Origen as a matter of fact was far from antisocial, still less anti-intellectual. A man who united in himself profound learning, philosophical culture and Christian holiness, Origen took an urbane, optimistic view of classical thought and of Greco-Roman civilization. Indeed his arguments against Celsus are drawn in large measure from classical philosophy and demonstrate, by implication, that a Christian was not necessarily an illiterate boor. The chief value of Origen's apologetic lay in his capacity to meet Celsus on the common ground of classical learning.

Notice that Origen and Celsus have radically different notions of society. For Celsus, the social life of men is a complex of accepted traditions and customs which are "given" by the gods of the various nations and have simply to be accepted, for, as Pindar said, "Custom is the king of all." Indeed it is impious to question them or to try to change them. The cults of the gods, the rites and practices associated with those cults, are all good in their own ways, and must be preserved. The Christians who discard all this are plainly subversive and dangerous.

Origen on the other hand sees that human society has been racially transformed by the Incarnation of the Logos. The presence in the world of the Risen Savior, in and through His Church, has destroyed the seeming validity of all that was in reality arbitrary, tyrannical or absurd in the fictions of social life. He has introduced worship and communal life of an entirely new kind, "in spirit and in truth."

The opening lines of the *Contra Celsum* openly declare that it is not only right but obligatory to disobey human laws and ignore human customs when these are contrary to the law of God:

> Suppose that a man were living among the Scythians (cannibals) whose laws are contrary to the Divine law, who had no opportunity to go elsewhere and was compelled to live among them; such a man for the sake of the true law, though illegal among the Scythians, would rightly form associations with like-minded people contrary to the laws of the Scythians. . . . It is not wrong to form associations against the errors for the sake of truth.
>
> (*Contra Celsum,* I, 1)

But among other things, the Christians are united against war, in obedience to Christ. This is one of their chief differences with the rest of society.

> No longer do we take the sword against any nations nor do we learn war any more since we have become the sons of peace through Jesus who is our author instead of following the traditional customs by which we were strangers to the covenant.
>
> (*Ibid.,* V, 33)

Origen argues, then, that if Christians refuse military service it does not mean that they do not bear their fair share in the common life and responsibilities. They play their part in the life of the *Polis.* But this role is spiritual and transcendent. Christians help the Emperor by their prayers, not by force of arms. "The more pious a man is the more effective he is in helping the emperors—more so than the soldiers who go out into the lines and kill all the enemy troops that they can" (III, 73, Chadwick, p. 509).

This should not be totally unfamiliar to Celsus. After all pagan priests were officially exempted from military service so that they might be able to offer sacrifices "with hands unstained from blood and pure from murders." Christians both laity and clergy were a "royal priesthood," and did more by their prayers to preserve peace than the army could do by threats of force.

"We who by our prayers destroy all demons which stir up wars, violate oaths and disturb the peace, are of more help to the Emperors than those who seem to be doing the fighting" (*Ibid.*, p. 509).

If at first Origen's claim that the Christians "helped the Emperor" by their prayers may have seemed naïve, we see here more clearly what he is driving at. He does not mean that the prayers of the Church enable the Emperor to pursue successfully some policy or other of worldly ambition and power. He does not claim for the prayers of the Church a magic efficacy. He means that prayers are weapons in a more hidden and yet more crucial type of warfare, and one in which the peace of the Empire more truly and certainly depends. In a word, if peace is the objective, spiritual weapons will preserve it more effectively than those which kill the enemy in battle. For the weapon of prayer is not directed against other men, but against the evil forces which divide men into warring camps. If these evil forces are overcome by prayer, then both sides are benefitted, war is avoided and all are united in peace. In other words, the Christian does not help the war effort of one particular nation, but he fights against war itself with spiritual weapons.

This basic principle, that love, or the desire of the good of all men, must underlie all Christian action, reappears even more forcefully in Saint Augustine. But now we find it incorporated into a defense of the "just war," and the perspective has been completely altered.

Roughly two hundred years separate the two greatest apologetic works of early Christians against the classical world: Origen's *Contra Celsum* and Saint Augustine's *City of God*. During these two hundred years a crucially important change has taken place in the Christian attitude to war. Origen took for granted that the Christian is a peacemaker and does not indulge in warfare. Augustine, on the contrary, pleads with the soldier, Boniface, not to retire to the monastery but to remain in the army and do his duty, defending the North African cities menaced by barbarian hordes.

In these two hundred years, there have been two events of outstanding importance: the Battle of Milvian Bridge in 312, leading to the conversion of Constantine and his official recognition of Christianity, and then, in 411, the fall of Rome before the onslaught of Alaric the Goth. When Augustine laid the foundation for Christian theories of the "just war," the barbarians were at the gates of the city of Hippo, where he was bishop.

This is not the place to go into the crucially important question of Saint Augustine's ideas of the human commonwealth, the earthly City, and its relations with the City of God. Suffice it to say that the question had become far more complex for him than it had ever been for the tranquil and optimistic Origen.

For Augustine, the essence of all society is union in common love for a common end. There are two kinds of love in man—an earthly and selfish love (*amor concupiscentiae*) and a heavenly, spiritual, disinterested love (*caritas*). Hence there are two "cities" based on these two kinds of love: the earthly city of selfish and temporal love for power and gain, and the heavenly city of spiritual charity. It will be seen at once that this distinction throws the followers of Augustine's theology of war in contemporary America into a radically ambivalent position, for the pessimistic Augustinian concept of society directly contradicts the optimistic American ethos. Indeed, the current American concept is that love of earthly and temporal ends is automatically self-regulating and leads to progress and happiness. Our city is frankly built on *concupiscentia*.

Every society, according to Augustine, seeks peace, and if it wages war, it does so for the sake of peace. Peace is the "tranquility of order." But the notion of order in any given society depends on the love which keeps that society together. The earthly society, in its common pursuit of power and gain, has only an apparent order—it is the order of a band of robbers, cooperating for evil ends. Yet in so far as it is an order at all, it is good. It is better than complete disorder. And yet it is fundamentally a disorder, and the peace of the wicked city is not true peace at all.

Cain is the founder of the earthly city (Genesis 4:17). Abel founded no city at all, but lived on earth as a pilgrim, a member of the only true city, the heavenly Jerusalem, the city of true peace. For Augustine, as for the Apocalypse and Origen, all history tends towards the definitive victory of the heavenly city of peace. Yet on earth, citizens of heaven live *among* the citizens of earth, though not *like* them.

This creates a problem. In so far as the Christian lives in the earthly city and participates in its benefits, he is bound to share its responsibilities though they are quite different from those of the heavenly city. Hence he may possess property, he marries and brings up children although in heaven "no one marries or is given in marriage" (Luke 20:34). *And also he participates in the just wars of the earthly city*, unless he is exempted by dedication to a completely spiritual life in the priestly or monastic state.

A pagan, Volusianus, confronted Augustine with the same objection Celsus proposed to Origen. If Christians did not help defend the state, they were antisocial. Augustine replied not that they simply pray for the earthly city, but that they do in all truth participate in its defense by military action, but the war must be a just war and its conduct must be just. In a word, for the earthly city war is sometimes an unavoidable necessity. Christians may participate in the war, or may abstain from participation. But their *motives* will be different from the motives of the pagan soldier. They are not really defending the earthly city, they are waging war to establish peace, since peace is willed by God. So now the attention of the Christian is focused on the interior motive which justifies war: the love of peace to be safeguarded by force.

It is no accident that the Protestant thinkers of our own day who rate as nuclear "realists" and defend war as a practical and unavoidable necessity owe much to Augustine. But this is not a distinction belonging to Protestants alone. All Catholics who defend the just war theory are implicitly following Augustine. *Saint Augustine is, for better or for worse, the Father of all modern Christian thought on war.*

Can we not say that if there are to be significant new developments in Christian thought on nuclear war, it may well be that these developments will depend on our ability to get free from the overpowering influence of Augustinian assumptions and take a new view of man, of society and of war itself? This may perhaps be attained by a renewed emphasis on the earlier, more mystical and more eschatological doctrine of the New Testament and the early Fathers, though not necessarily a return to an imaginary ideal of pure primitive pacifism. It will also require a more optimistic view of man. Certainly Pope John XXIII has done more than anyone else to give us a new perspective.

What are the basic assumptions underlying Augustine's thought on war? First of all, there is one which Celsus the pagan proposed, and Origen rejected: that it is impossible for man to live without getting into violent conflict with other men. Augustine agrees with Celsus. Universal peace in practice is inconceivable. In the early days of the Church this principle might perhaps have been accepted as logical, but then discarded as irrelevant. The eschatological perspectives of the early Church were real, literal and immediate. The end was believed to be very near. There would not be time for an indefinite series of future wars.

But Augustine saw the shattered and collapsing Empire attacked on all sides by barbarian armies. War could not be avoided. The question was, then, to find out some way to fight that did not violate the Law of Love. And in order to reconcile war with Christian love, Augustine had recourse to pre-Christian, Classical notions of justice. His ideas on the conduct of the just war were drawn to a considerable extent from Cicero.

How does Augustine justify the use of force, even for a just cause? The external act may be one of violence. War is regrettable indeed. But if one's interior motive is purely directed to a just cause and to love of the enemy, then the use of force is not unjust. This distinction between the external act and the interior intention is entirely characteristic of Augustine. "Love," he says, "does not exclude wars of mercy waged by the good" (Letter 138).

But here we come upon a further, most significant development in Augustine's thought. The Christian may join the non-Christian in fighting to preserve peace in the earthly city. But suppose that the earthly city itself is almost totally made up of Christians. Then cooperation between the "two cities" takes on a new aspect, and we arrive at the conclusion that a "secular arm" of military force can be called into action against heretics, to preserve not only civil peace but the purity of faith. Thus Augustine becomes also the remote forefather of the Crusades and of the Inquisition.

"Love does not exclude wars of mercy waged by the good!" The history of the Middle Ages, of the Crusades, of the religious wars has taught us what strange consequences can flow from this noble principle. Augustine, for all his pessimism about human nature, did not foresee the logical results of his thought, and in the original context, his "wars of mercy" to defend civilized order make a certain amount of sense. Always his idea is that the Church and the Christians, whatever they may do, are aiming at ultimate peace. The deficiency of Augustinian thought lies therefore not in the good intentions it prescribes but in an excessive naïveté with regard to the good that can be attained by violent means which cannot help but call forth all that is worst in man. And so, alas, for centuries we have heard kings, princes, bishops, priests, ministers, and the Lord alone knows what variety of unctuous beadles and sacrists, earnestly urging all men to take up arms out of love and mercifully slay their enemies (including other Christians) without omitting to purify their interior intention.

Of course when we read Augustine himself, and when we see that he imposes such limits upon the Christian soldier and traces out such a strict line of conduct for him, we can see that the theory of the just war was not altogether absurd, and that it was capable of working in ages less destructive than our own. But one wonders at the modern Augustinians and at their desperate maneuvers to preserve the doctrine of the just war from the museum or the junk pile. In the name of "realism" (preserving, that is to say, a suitable dash of Augustinian pessimism about fallen man) they plunge into ambivalence from which Augustine was fortunately preserved by the technological ignorance of his dark age.

Augustine kept a place in his doctrine for a certain vestige of the eschatological tradition. There were some Christians who would not be permitted to fight: these were the monks, first of all, the men who had totally left the world and abandoned its concerns to live in the Kingdom of God, and then the clergy who preached the Gospel of Peace—or at least the Gospel of the merciful war. Yet as Christianity spread over Europe and the ancient Roman strain was vivified and restored by the addition of vigorous barbarian blood from the north, even monks and clerics were sometimes hard to restrain from rushing to arms and loving exuberantly with the sword. Do we not read that when a Frankish ship loaded with Crusaders ran into the Byzantine fleet in the first Crusade, the Byzantines were shocked at a Latin priest who stood on the stern covered with blood and furiously discharged arrows at them, clad in vestments, too: and he even went on shooting after the declaration of a truce.[1]

Still, there were recognized limits. Councils sternly restricted warfare. In tenth-century England a forty-day fast was prescribed as penance for anyone who killed an enemy in war—even in a just war. Killing was regarded as an evil to be atoned for even if it could not be avoided (see Migne, P.L., vol. 79, col. 407). However, later theologians of the Middle Ages (see Migne, P.L., vol. 125, col. 841) made clear that killing in a just war was not a sin and intimated that the soldier who did this required no penance, as he had done a work pleasing to God. We were then close to the time of the Crusades. But even then, especially in wars among Christians themselves, severe limitations were prescribed. War might be virtuous under certain conditions, but in any case, good or bad, one must sometimes abstain from it at any cost. The truce of God in the tenth century forbade fighting on holy days and in holy seasons. The hesitation and ambivalence of the Christian warrior are reflected in a curious oath of Robert the Pious (tenth century) who wrote: "I will not take a mule or a horse . . . in pasture from any man from the kalends of March to the Feast of All Saints, unless to recover a debt. I will not burn houses or destroy them unless there is a knight inside. I will not root up vines. I will not attack noble ladies traveling without husband, nor their maids, nor widows or nuns unless it is their fault. From the beginnings of Lent to the end of Easter, I will not attack an armed knight."[2]

It is easy to find texts like these which bring out the ridiculous inner inconsistencies that are inseparable from this view of war and the constant temptation to evade and rationalize the demands of the just war theory. The twofold weakness of the Augustinian theory is its stress on a subjective purity of intention which can be doctored and manipulated with apparent "sincerity" and the tendency to pessimism about human nature and the world, now used as a *justification* for recourse to violence. Robert the Pious is characteristically naïve when he blandly assumes that traveling nuns might at any moment be "at fault" and give a knight such utterly intolerable provocation that he would "have to attack them"—with full justice. Expanded to the megatonic scale, and viewing as licit the destruction of whole cities which are suddenly wicked and "at fault," this reasoning is no longer amusing.

We are told that Hitler, viewing the terrible conflagration of Warsaw when it had been bombed by the Luftwaffe, wept and said: "How wicked those people were to make me do this to them!"

1. This was in the First Crusade. Quoted from the Alexiad of Anna Comnena, in Bainton, R.H., *Christian Attitudes to War and Peace* (New York and Nashville: Abingdon Press, 1960), p. 114.
2. Quoted in Bainton, op. cit., p. 110.

4. *The Legacy of Machiavelli*

It seems likely that the doctrine of the just war and the moral inhibitions it implied did, at times, restrain barbarity in medieval war. We know that when the crossbow was invented it was at first banned by the Church as an immoral and cruel weapon.

However, in the Renaissance we find Machiavelli, one of the Fathers of *Realpolitik,* frankly disgusted with the half-heartedness and inefficiency with which wars were being carried on by certain Princes. It is instructive to read his grammar of power, *The Prince,* and to see how his pragmatic, not to say cynical, doctrine on the importance and the conduct of war are precisely those which are accepted in practice today in the international power struggle. It is difficult to say whether many of the more belligerent policy-makers of our time have read Machiavelli, but one feels that he would be a man after their own heart: one who tolerates no nonsense about a sentimental and half-hearted use of force.

As Machiavelli is indifferent to moral considerations, we can say that he implicitly discards the theory of the just war as irrelevant. And in a sense one can agree with his evident contempt for all the absurd mental convolutions that Robert the Pious had to go through to provide escape clauses for his belligerent needs. It is certainly more practical, if what you intend is war, simply to go ahead and wage war without first vowing not to fight and then creating exceptional cases in which your vow is no longer binding. Surely we can agree that this is a great waste of time and energy and it may lead to fatal errors and to defeat. In a world of power politics, there is no question that conscience is a nuisance. But it is also true that in *any situation,* a conscience that juggles with the law and seeks only to rationalize evasions, is not only a nuisance but a fatal handicap, because it is basically unreasonable.

One might almost say that the present power struggle presents man with two clear alternatives: we can be true to the logic of our situation in two ways—either by discarding conscience altogether and acting with pure ruthlessness, or else by purifying our conscience and sharpening it to the point of absolute fidelity to moral law and Christian love. In the first case we will probably destroy one another. In the second, we may stand a chance of survival. Such at least is the teaching of Pope John.

The Prince, says Machiavelli, should have "no other aim or thought but war." He should reflect that disarmament would only render him contemptible. And in order to guard against temptation to relax his vigilance and reconcile himself to peace, the Prince must learn not to be too good:

> A man who wishes to make profession of goodness in everything must necessarily come to grief among so many who are not good. Therefore it is necessary for a Prince who wishes to maintain himself to learn how not to be good, and to use this knowledge and not use it, according to the necessity of the case.
>
> (*The Prince,* Ricci-Vincent Trans. c. 15)

After all, the Prince must be practical. Not only must he create a suitable image of himself, as we would say today: not only must he be feared rather than loved (unless he is smart enough to be both loved and feared at the same time), but he must be feared with very good reason. He must not listen to conscience, or to humane feeling. He must not practice virtue when it is not expedient to do so, and he must not let himself be either too kind, too generous, or too trustworthy. Let him not waste time abiding by legalities or by his pledged word, unless it happens to be useful. Virtue, Machiavelli warns, has ruined many a prince. It it better to rely on force.

> There are two methods of fighting, the one by law and the other by force: The first method is that of men, the second of beasts; but as the first method is often insufficient, one must have recourse to the second. It is well then for a prince to know well how to use both the beast and the man.

This is the kind of practicality that is taken for granted but seldom stated so clearly in our age of power. It is refreshing to see it set forth with such primitive and pleasant frankness, free from all double-talk. Machiavelli goes on to justify this line of conduct, with reasons which constitute in their own way a kind of "humanism." Cruelty, he says, is after all more merciful than an indulgent softness which leads only to disorder and chaos in the long run. Better to be firm like Cesare Borgia. (Machiavelli has nothing but praise for the Borgias.)

> Cesare Borgia was considered cruel, but his cruelty had brought order to the Romagna, united it, and reduced it to peace and fealty. If this is considered evil, it will be seen that he was in reality much more merciful than the Florentine people who, to avoid the name of cruelty, allowed Pistoia to be destroyed.
>
> (*Id.* C. 17)

This is exactly the argument we hear today. The only hope of peace and order, according to "realists" is the toughest, hardest and most intransigent policy. This in the long run is "merciful" and peaceful.

Incidentally, Machiavelli was not praising simply the *appearance* of cruelty, although this is a necessary minimum. He thought that one of the chief qualities of Hannibal had been his genuine inhumanity. It really kept his army together!

While Saint Augustine transferred the question of war into the internal forum and concentrated on the intention of the Christian to wage a just war, Machiavelli ignores the forum of conscience as completely irrelevant. He is concerned with the brute objective facts of the power struggle—a struggle in which conscience generates only ambivalence and therefore leads to defeat. Morality interferes with efficiency, therefore it is absurd to concern oneself with moral questions which in any case are practically meaningless, since the vicissitudes of the power struggle may demand at any moment that they be thrown aside as useless baggage.

For Machiavelli power is an end in itself. Persons and policies are means to that end. And the chief means is war, not a "just" war but a *victorious* war. For Machiavelli the important thing was to *win*. As Clausewitz was to say in our modern age of *Realpolitik: "To introduce into the philosophy of war a principle of moderation would be absurd. War is an act of violence pursued to the uttermost."*

And this of course was a philosophy which guided the policies of Hitler. The rest of the world, for all its good intentions, was forced to learn it from Hitler in order to beat him.

With modern technology the principles of unlimited destruction and violence have become in practice axiomatic. Deputy Defense Secretary of the U.S. Roswell Gilpatric declared in 1961: "We are not going to reduce our nuclear capability. Personally I have never believed in a limited nuclear war. I do not know how you would build a limit into it when you use any kind of a nuclear bang."

Yet Machiavelli was not altogether typical of the Renaissance. Leonardo da Vinci, the exemplar of Renaissance genius, developed a plan for a submarine but destroyed the plan without making it known because he saw that the only serious purpose of an underwater craft would be treacherous and hidden attack in naval war. In his mind, this was immoral.

While *The Prince* is a clear and articulate expression of the principles of power politics, we must be careful not to assume that the present power struggle is purely and simply Machiavelli. This would be a grave error.

On the contrary, it is reasonable to suppose that in our day Machiavelli would have proceeded on different and more original assumptions, for this is no longer an age of warring princes of Italian city-states. He would doubtless be able to see through the romantic mythology with which the power struggle has been invested (for instance the ideas of proletarian, nationalist or racist messianism) and he would certainly recognize the importance of rational control over the vast technological developments which, in fact, dominate our policies.

Machiavelli wrote his advice for the individual monarch, in a day when men believed in the divine right of kings. But after Machiavelli, political thought underwent considerable evolution. The "Prince" was replaced by the "Sovereign State," and the revolutions which sought to liberate man from the tyranny of absolute monarchs brought them under the more subtle and more absolute tyranny of an abstraction. Just as mathematics, business and technology needed the discovery of zero in order to develop, so too political and economic power needed the faceless abstractions of state and corporation, with their unlimited irresponsibility, to attain to unlimited sovereignty. Hence the paradox that in the past ages usually regarded as times of slavery the individual actually counted for much more than he does in the alienation of modern economic, military and political totalism. At the same time it is the modern, irresponsible, faceless, alienated man, the man whose thinking and decisions are the work of an anonymous organization, who becomes the perfect instrument of the power process. Under such conditions, the process itself becomes totally self-sufficient and all absorbing. As a result the life and death not only of individual persons, families and cities, but of entire nations and civilizations must submit to the blind force of amoral and inhuman forces. The "freedom" and "autonomy" of a certain minority may still seem to exist: it consists in little more than understanding the direction of the historically predetermined current and rowing with the stream instead of against it. There should be no need to point out the demonic potentialities of such a situation.

These summary notes on Machiavelli are of course oversimplified to the point of being naïve. They are not intended as a critical or historical evaluation of his political philosophy, but only as a typology of popular notions about "Machiavellianism." This is a philosophy which England and America have traditionally regarded as villainous, and hence it would not be fair to blame even a Machiavellian typology for moral eccentricities that have other formal causes.

Machiavelli, who wanted to be ruthless, was actually leading a dull and rather innocuous life, and wrote his wicked book in the hope that it would get him a steady job under a powerful protector. In the atmosphere of a more northern morality, it sometimes happens that the same practical ruthlessness has been propounded with the air of greater respectability. Certainly the radical naturalism and secularism of Hobbes is just as uncompromising in its rejection of the possible ambiguities and sentimentalities of the too tender conscience. For Hobbes, the root of morality is obedience to the all-powerful despotic state and to the law of self-preservation and pleasure. The selfish interests of the individual are regulated by the power of the state. The Law of Nature, for Hobbes, is simply the "primitive and brutish" law of battle in which the strong overwhelm the weak, and this is kept under control by the force of that despotic Leviathan, the state, maintaining order by force. This confusion between the natural law considered as rooted in the essence of man as a free and rational being, and natural law as an empirical and primitive state of fact, interpreted moreover in crude and pessimistic terms, has had very serious consequences (see Maritain, *Moral Philosophy*, p. 94). It has undoubtedly exercised some effect on Christian moralists in America, without their realizing it perhaps, since Hobbes has contributed something to our national moral climate of rugged individualism.

So, too, of course, have Bentham and Mill. Here again the concept of nature as the basis of morality becomes more and more statistical, secularist and hedonistic. Mercantile calculation of the "greatest happiness of the greatest number" finally eroded away the traces of the good as what was right and just in itself, and substituted for it the concept of the good as the advantageous. Justice was then replaced by "good business," and though the image of good business had and retains a specious folksiness, it is certainly no less ruthless and no less cynical in its roots than the political thought of Machiavelli. When it is optimistic, it remains a thoroughly inferior and jejune morality. When pessimistic, it legitimates any injustice as long as you don't get caught, or as long as you can get the courts on your side. In either event it represents a rather degraded concept of man, for all its seemingly humanistic slogans.

Kant's effort to put morality back on a firm basis of pure duty did not in fact restore a healthy climate of moral thought. The Kantian ethic easily degenerates into pietistic sentimentalities or moral platitudes. And after Kant came confusion: Hegel's emphasis on the power of the state in the face of the "prodigious power of the Negative," and other implicit philosophies of force. The Marxian dialectic of historical determinism, its humanism without the human person, leaves man powerless to transcend the forces of the social process in which he is immersed. Positivism is, once again, and even more than Bentham and Mill, statistical, amoral, a pointless and vapid sociologism. But it has had a profound effect in shaping "moral" thought in the climate of "free enterprise." One wonders how Christian thinkers, who are outraged by the Kinsey Report's approach to sexual morality, are so eager to accept a no less amoral and statistical approach to other crucial problems when it is made by Herman Kahn and the men with computers.

5. *The Reply of "Pacem in Terris"*

Machiavelli devotes an extraordinary intelligence to the service of the Prince's will to power, and is concerned with the inner dynamics of the struggle to subdue all rivals without concern for the means used except in so far as they obey the pragmatic laws of the struggle itself. His advice is certainly "rational," "intelligent" and even in a certain sense "scientific" and yet when it is considered on a deeper level it is seen to be utterly without rationality. It leads to ruinous consequences. The moralist who would seek, by accepting the moral climate and the premises of Machiavelli, to find a basis for distinctions between right and wrong within this program of power and to outline a morally licit use of the means and techniques suggested by the author of The Prince, might perhaps succeed, if he had sufficient casuistical ingenuity. If he were concerned only with the individual spiritual guidance of the Prince, his project might be viewed with tolerance and even with a certain sympathy. But we must consider that the actions of the Prince in obtaining power for himself do not concern himself alone, they affect the whole of society. And while the Prince may be cleverly reconciling his ascent to power with the demands of a rather relaxed morality, others may be paying with their fortunes and with their lives for the luxury of his "good conscience."

The encyclical *Pacem in Terris* is not concerned with casuistry because it is not laying down norms merely for the individual "case." In fact the perspectives of individualism are not those of Pope John. It is true that the basis of the whole argument in *Pacem in Terris* is to be sought in the rights and dignity of the human person, but we must distinguish between *person* and *individual*. The individual can be considered as an isolated human unit functioning and acting for himself and by himself. The person can never be properly understood outside the framework of social relationships and obligations, for the person exists not merely in order to fight for survival: not only to function efficiently, and overcome others in competition for the goods of this earth which are thought to guarantee happiness. The person finds his reason for existence in the realm of truth, justice, love and liberty. He fulfills himself not by closing himself within the narrow confines of his own individual interests and those of his family, but by his openness to other men, to the civil society in which he lives and to the society of nations in which he is called to collaborate with others in building a world of security and peace.

If the person is to function rationally as a member of society, he must meet others on a common ground of reason. Common decisions and efforts must be oriented toward the universal common good. This raises the question of arbitration when differences and disagreements arise. Hence one of the most important aspects of *Pacem in Terris* is its discussion of authority, its open criticism of the current failures of authority in the national and international sphere, and its demand for the formation of a valid supranational authority with real power to arbitrate between nations and to deal fairly with the problems and needs of all.

Authority in Machiavelli rests on force and ruse, ruthlessness and cruelty, the ability to seize power and hold on to it against all contenders. This viewpoint, which is in practice quite commonly shared today, is not as "realistic" as it seems. It is actually a very unreal concept of authority. The authority of the strongest is no authority at all because it has no power to elicit the intelligent submission of man's inmost personal being. Authority cannot be properly understood if it is confused with mere external compulsion, supported by force.

Authority in *Pacem in Terris* rests on the objective reality of man, on the natural law, that is on the inner orientation of man to freedom, and on the obligations which this entails. The Legislator "is never allowed to depart from natural law" (*Pacem in Terris*, ns. 81, 85. For the rest of this chapter, numbers otherwise not identified refer simply to paragraphs of *Pacem in Terris*).

The Legislator, in Pope John's eyes, should not be a ruthless and clever operator with unlimited power at his disposal, justified in taking any decision that serves him and his party or nation in the power struggle. He must be a "man of great equilibrium and integrity" (71) competent and courageous, prompt to take decisions which respond to the situation and of the principles that are at stake. And he must not evade his basic moral obligations for "reasons of state." On the contrary, statesmen and governments which put their own interests before everything else, including justice and the natural law, are no better than bandits.

> As men in their private enterprises cannot pursue their own interests to the detriment of others, so too states cannot lawfully seek that development of their own resources which brings harm to other states and unjustly oppresses them. This statement of Saint Augustine seems to be very apt in this regard: What are kingdoms without justice but large bands of robbers? (92).

At the same time, the Pope condemns all isolationism and nationalist individualism which might prompt a government to seek its own interests, ignoring and condemning the rest of the world. At the present time all the countries in the world are in fact so closely interrelated that no one nation can simply turn in upon itself and seek its own advantage without affecting the others. Hence "it is obvious that individual countries cannot seek their own interests and development in isolation from the rest" (131).

Pope John tirelessly repeats the principle that *force is not and cannot be a valid basis of public authority:*

> A civil authority that uses as its only or chief means either threats and fear of punishment or promises of rewards cannot effectively move men to promote the common good of all. (48)
>
> For that reason [both men and nations] are right in not easily yielding obedience to authority imposed by force or to an

> authority in whose creation they had no part, and to which they themselves did not decide to submit by their own free choice. (138)

If force is not the basis of authority, then what is? Reason and conscience. The "free choice" made by men in accepting authority is of course something more than a whim of fashion. Men do not necessarily accept authority because they are pleased by all its manifestations. But it is right and just to accept a rule of authority that obeys truth, guarantees men's rights, and recommends itself to free men by its respect for liberty. "Civil authority must appeal primarily to the conscience of individual citizens, that is to each one's duty to collaborate readily for the common good of all" (48). Authority can exercise a rightful appeal to the consciences of men in so far as it offers them some convincing indication that it can provide them with an ordered and productive life, with liberty and the advantages of a peaceful culture. But ultimately this pragmatic assurance which may be deduced from the successful working of authority is only a sign of the moral order from which it derives its obligatory force (47). The "ultimate source and final end of all authority" is God Himself (47).

Incidentally, this shows why Pope John is so intent on preserving the independent authority of the small and struggling nation, so that it may settle its own internal affairs without interference from more powerful neighbors.

> No country may unjustly oppress others or unduly meddle in their affairs. On the contrary all should help to develop in others a sense of responsibility, a spirit of enterprise, and an earnest desire to be the first to promote their own advancement in every field (120).

Since all authority ultimately rests on God Himself, a civil or international authority which promotes policies contrary to the moral order thereby renounces its right to be obeyed, for "God is to be obeyed rather than men" (51) (cf. Acts 5:29). *Pacem in Terris* declares frankly and clearly that "those therefore who have authority in the State may oblige men in conscience only if their authority is intrinsically related to the authority of God and shares in it" (49).

> It follows that if civil authorities pass laws or command anything opposed to the moral order and consequently contrary to the will of God, neither the laws made nor the authorization granted can be binding on the consciences of the citizens. [The Pope then quotes Saint Thomas, after referring to Acts 5:29.] "In so far as it falls short of right reason a law is said to be a wicked law; and so lacking the true nature of law it is rather a kind of violence." (I II Q. 93, a.3, ad.2) (51)

It should, by the way, be clear from the context of the encyclical that when the Pope speaks of civil authority being "intrinsically related to the authority of God" he is in no way saying that a quasi-religious and clerical form of society has more authority than any other. *Pacem in Terris,* as everyone well knows who understands the language of John XXIII and its background in Saint Thomas, is by no means a tract in favor of theocracy. The Pope takes pains to point out that he is speaking of "any truly democratic regime" (52) chosen by the people themselves in a free and just manner. There is even some basis for respecting the claims of a government which represents "men of no Christian faith whatever but who are endowed with reason and adorned with a natural uprightness of conduct" (157). This does not imply that false ideologies are approved, but if men following these ideologies are justly and sincerely striving to improve the lot of their people, they retain certain rights in the eyes of the natural law and of God. Their legitimate efforts to improve their living conditions should be aided, not hindered, by other nations.

This principle is very important when we come to consider the revolutions that mark the emergence of new nations and new societies, and will continue to do so especially in Latin America, Africa and Asia. Pope John warns that superior strength does not warrant interference in the affairs of small states even though the "revolutionary" character of the social ferment may not be acceptable to those more advanced and more highly civilized powers. "This superiority, far from permitting [an advanced nation] to rule others unjustly, imposes the obligation to make a greater contribution to the general development of the people" (88). In this context, Pope John condemns all forms of racism (86, 94, 95) and explicitly points to genocide as a flagrant crime against humanity (95).

To sum this all up in one word: Pope John teaches that when authority ignores natural law, human dignity, human rights and the moral order established by God, it undermines its own foundations and loses its claim to be obeyed because it no longer speaks seriously to the conscience of free man. One very serious consequence flows from this teaching: one of the great collective questions of conscience of our time is, according to Pope John, the failure of authority to cope with the critical needs and desperate problems of man on a world scale. A truly international authority is the only answer, and the establishment of a genuine world community is "urgently demanded today by the requirements of the universal common good" (7).

> Today the universal common good poses problems of worldwide dimensions which cannot be adequately tackled or solved except by the efforts of public authority . . . on a worldwide basis. The moral order itself demands that such a form of authority be established. (137)

What is the reason? The Pope does not hesitate to tell us:

> Under the present circumstances of humanity both the structure and form of governments as well as the power which public authority wields in all the nations of the world MUST BE CONSIDERED INADEQUATE TO PROMOTE THE UNIVERSAL COMMON GOOD. (135)

If we understand the nature of this document and its profound seriousness, we can see that certain deeply Christian obligations begin to emerge from the world crisis in which we live. The obligation to work for collaboration and harmony among nations, to respect the rights of small and emergent nations and of racial minorities, to collaborate actively and generously in helping these nations and races to attain their full development and to enjoy their full rights as members of the human race. The obligation to work for peace and the need for a clear and forthright protest of the Christian conscience against the abuse of authority which marshals men more and more under the command of those who explicitly announce their intention to make use of brute force in order to gain or to maintain a position of power for themselves or for the social and political system which they represent.

All this implies a willing and intelligent participation of the Christian in civil and public life, to the extent that it fits in with his other duties (7, 137).

To say that authority has its source in God is then to say that it begins and ends in liberty. It exists for the sake of liberty. It is the servant of liberty, and when it ceases to be the servant of liberty in the highest sense it loses its power to command the obedience of the free conscience. For man is made free in the image and likeness of God and social authority exists only to help him use his freedom in truth, love and justice as a child of God. This is all new and strange, no doubt, to those who have become accustomed to exhortations to obedience in a quite other context, where authority seems to be rooted only in the *power to compel obedience by external force* or by the law of fear. But that concept of authority, Pope John reminds us, is not the Christian concept. It is in fact closer to Machiavelli than it is to the Gospel because it fits into the framework of a power structure dominated by arbitrary will, rather than an intelligent order tending toward the full development of freedom in justice and love.

We can now begin to see why an Encyclical of Peace on Earth actually devotes so much thought to the true nature of authority within the order of justice and love, which is the order of freedom into which we are called by the very fact that we are persons created in the image and likeness of God. And we see that the real difference between the authority of love and truth, taught by Pope

John, and the authority of brute force implies totally different concepts of man and of the world. And when we grasp this difference we see how it happens that so many "right thinking men" often end up with an ideology of authority based on force (analogous to that of Machiavelli) and fail to grasp the Christian need for an authority of freedom and love.

The difference of course is this: the totalitarian and absolute concept of authority based on force implies a completely pessimistic view of man and of the world. It is for one reason or another implicitly closed to human values, distrustful or openly contemptuous of reason, fearful of liberty which it cannot distinguish from licence and rebellion. It seeks security in force because it cannot believe that the powers of nature, if left to grow spontaneously, can develop in a sane and healthy fashion. Nature must be controlled with an iron hand because it is evil, or prone to evil: man is perhaps capable of good behavior, but only if he is forced into it by implacable authority. We find this idea cropping up in all kinds of contexts, religious or otherwise, from Calvin to Stalin, from Port Royal to Hitler; there are traces of it in Plato and in Saint Augustine; we see it in Fathers of the Church like Tertullian; it provides specious reasons for the Inquisition as well as for Auschwitz. It is in Machiavelli, of course, in a slightly different form (Machiavelli is not concerned over anyone being "good," but his philosophy of ruthlessness implies that the law of fear is the only one that can be relied upon to keep men under control).

Pope John was opposed, and passionately opposed, to this kind of pessimism which he diagnosed as a sickness akin to despair, masking as strength and rectitude, but in reality refusing a generous response to the grace and the call of God to twentieth-century Christians. Against the triumphalist hopes which exalt the Church by placing an authoritarian heel on the neck of prostrate man, Pope John dared to hope in the goodness placed in human nature by God the Creator. Only if human nature is radically good can a concept of authority based on the natural law and on human liberty be conceived as also at the same time rooted in the will of God. If human nature is evil, then obviously all God-given authority has no other function than to take up arms against it, to restrict it, punish it and imprison it in blind and disciplined servitude.

Indeed, if human nature is evil, the question of peace and war and the authority of nations and of the Church comes to be seen in a different light. If man is evil, then it is obvious that he will tend to destroy himself by fighting greedily for his own advantage. War is therefore inevitable, because the struggle for power is inescapable. *This* indeed is the law of nature! The supernatural authority of the Church must then save man in spite of himself by making him obey the authority of "the right side" in this blind conflict for power. And fortunately the Church still has enough power to demand his submission! She must preserve her power so that wicked man may have a supernatural authority to which he may submit. . . .

This is not Pope John's conception of authority, of man or of the order of salvation!

It is easy to see that Pope John's ideas go back to the optimism of Saint Paul and of the Gospels. Saint Paul in moving passages outlines the great mystery of the whole cosmos redeemed in Christ, the new creation.

> For the eager longing of creation awaits the revelation of the sons of God. For creation was made subject to vanity—not by its own will but by reason of him who made it subject—in hope, because creation itself also will be delivered from its slavery to corruption into the freedom of the glory of the sons of God. For we know that all creation groans and travails in pain until now. And not only it, but we ourselves also who have the first-fruits of the Spirit—we ourselves groan within ourselves, waiting for the adoption as sons, the redemption of our body.
>
> (Romans 8:19–23)

> He is the image of the invisible God, the firstborn of every creature. For in him were created all things in the heavens and on the earth, things visible and things invisible, whether Thrones, or Dominations, or Principalities, or Powers. All things have been created through and unto him, and he is before all creatures, and in him all things hold together. Again, he is the head of his body, the Church; he, who is the beginning, the firstborn from the dead, that in all things he may have the first place. For it has pleased God the Father that in him all his fullness should dwell, and that through him he should reconcile to himself all things, whether on earth or in the heavens, making peace through the blood of his cross.
>
> (Colossians 1:15–20)

Pope John also echoes the optimism of Saint Thomas Aquinas who was regarded as a revolutionary in the thirteenth century because of the bold scope of his vision which united the created and the uncreated, nature and grace, reason and faith in a vast unity. Saint Thomas gave the Church his great unified theology in a period when the division between earth and heaven, nature and supernature, philosophy and theology, reason and faith, had become so acute that they threatened to become irreconcilable. His task, as Joseph Pieper sees it, was this:

> A "legitimate union" would mean two things. First it would mean joining the two realms so that their distinctiveness and

> irreducibility, their relative autonomy, their intrinsic justification, were seen and recognized. Second it would mean making their unity, their compatibility, and the necessity for their conjunction apparent not from the point of view of either of the two members of the union—neither simply from the point of view of faith nor simply from the point of view of reason—*but by going back to a deeper root of both.*
>
> (*Guide to Thomas Aquinas,* p. 120)

Caught between radical Averroism (which was frankly rationalistic) and the conservative supernaturalism of those who could not accept Aristotle and so fell back on traditional positions, rejecting reason and "the world," Saint Thomas dared to transcend them both and to demonstrate the natural goodness of the world as something that could not be fully understood and vindicated except in the light of the revealed doctrine of creation.

> Things are good—*all* things. The most compelling proof of their goodness in the very act of being lies in their createdness; there is no more powerful argument for affirmation of natural reality of the world than the demonstration that the world is *creatura.* . . . Sin, whether on the part of the angels or on the part of men, cannot essentially have changed the structure of the world. Therefore, Thomas argues, I refuse to consider the present state of the world as a basically unnatural state, a state of denaturalization. What is, is good because it was created by God; whoever casts aspersions upon the perfections of created beings casts aspersions upon the perfection of the divine power.
>
> (Pieper, op. cit., p. 131)

The optimism of Pope John is not the vapid and sentimental cheerfulness of a pseudo naturalistic religiosity. Yet it embraces all the best hopes and intuitions of the modern world of science and technology, and unites them with the spiritual vision of Christianity. The union is reached, as was that of Saint Thomas's *Summa,* by going to a "deeper root."

Let us be perfectly clear about the optimism of *Mater et Magistra* and *Pacem in Terris.* Pope John is not *excusing* nature, or tolerantly *defending* nature. He is not saying that humanity is not so bad after all, and that there is a chance for it to act as if it were good, once it has been brought into line by the wisely applied will of an external power. As Pieper said of Saint Thomas, so we can say of Pope John: "to his mind it would be utterly ridiculous for man to undertake to defend the creation. Creation needs no justification. The order of creation is, on the contrary, precisely the standard which must govern man's every judgment of things and of himself" (*Id.* p. 122).

This truth rings out clearly in the very first line of *Pacem in Terris* where Pope John declares that all men desire peace and that "it can be established only if the order laid down by God be dutifully observed." That order is the law implanted in man's free nature as an intelligent being who is capable of desiring peace in justice and of being a peace-maker in the fulness of love. These very capacities implanted in his nature by God are the sign of man's radical goodness, the guarantee of his honest hopes, the challenge which his intelligence and love are summoned to meet, the "law" of his nature which is made in the image and likeness of a loving God. Pope John's optimism lies in this belief: that because man was made by God to seek peace and to achieve it, and because God has given man the abundant help of supernatural grace, then no matter how great man's confusion and servitude to evil may have become, he can still be liberated and fulfil his vocation in peace as a free, spiritual being redeemed in the blood of Christ.

The pessimist view, on the contrary, considers man's aspiration to peace to be at best a delusive hope which can be exploited by any kind of power: the evil power that enslaves him or the benevolent paternal power that leads him blindly, like a helpless child, and almost in spite of himself, to heaven.

The pessimistic view is closed, inattentive to man's desperate aspirations for peace, social justice, progress, change. It tells man that these are simply manifestations of pride and naturalism. Let him learn to be resigned to war on earth and peace in heaven! The optimism of Pope John is wide open to every legitimate hope of man for peace *on earth*! It is willing to listen to any reasonable plan, and to share any worthy human desire. It is willing to discuss possibilities of agreement even with those who do not believe in God and who reject the truths of faith and the world of the spirit, for the "acceptance of all natural reality necessarily involves the acceptance of valuable insights wherever they may be found—and therefore also in the pre-Christian and extra Christian worlds" (Pieper, op. cit., 125).

The great difference between Pope John and Machiavelli is not that the Pope believed in God and Machiavelli did not (as far as I know Machiavelli was, in his own way, a "practicing Catholic") but rather that Pope John believed *in man* and Machiavelli did not. Because he had confidence in man, Pope John believed in love and peace. Because he lacked this confidence, Machiavelli believed in force and in deceit.

The power for peace in this great encyclical resides then not in a casuistical treatment of the problem of nuclear war but in the profound and optimistic Christian spirit with which the Pope lays bare the deepest roots of peace, roots which are placed in man by God Himself and which man himself has the mission to cultivate. If the roots of peace are not in our hearts, it would be useless to condemn total war over and over again with ecclesiastical anathemas. But because the roots of peace are there, it makes sense for the Church to remind us of the fact in all simplicity and to tell us about them, adding at the same time:

> There can be, or at least there should be, no doubt that relations between states as between individuals should be regulated not by the force of arms but by the light of reason, by the rule that is of truth, of justice, and of active and sincere co-operation. (144)

> In an age such as ours which prides itself on its atomic energy it is contrary to reason to hold that war is now a suitable way to restore rights that have been violated. (127)

One last remark about the encyclical: without being in any sense a professional Thomist, the Pope reflects everywhere the principles and sanity of Aquinas. But the whole climate of the encyclical, in its love of man and of the world, and in its radiant hopefulness, is Franciscan. The optimism of Pope John is not logical only: it is spiritual, mystical, rooted in a deep and simple love for God which is also, love for His creation and for God's child: man.

Anyone familiar with the writings of Saint Francis and with his life is aware that the Saint was always urging his friars to be at peace with each other and to go among men as peacemakers. A remarkable chapter on missions among the Saracens (First Rule of Saint Francis, C. 16) anticipates the ecumenical ideas of our own time, even though it was written in the age of crusades:

> There are two ways in which the friars who go out (to the Saracens) can act with spiritual effect. The first is not to dispute or be contentious, but for love of the Lord to bow to every human authority and to acknowledge themselves Christians. The other way, whenever they think it to be God's will, is to proclaim the Word of God and then faith in God Almighty, the Father, the Son and the Holy Spirit. . . .

> All friars everywhere are to remember that they have given and surrendered themselves soul and body to our Lord Jesus Christ and for love of Him they must expose themselves to all enemies both visible and invisible, for our Lord says: "The man who loses his life for my sake shall save it in life everlasting."

And we know that Saint Francis, toward the end of his life, made peace between the Mayor and Bishop at Assisi by sending one of the friars to sing his wonderful hymn in praise of God in His creatures in their presence. He thought (as did Pope John) that the best way to turn men's minds to peace was to remind them of the goodness of life and of the world. The friar came, sang the "Song of Brother Sun," to which Saint Francis had added two lines, about peace. The mayor listened in tears. The bishop confessed his own haughtiness. And there was peace between them.

This is a charming story. No doubt we will need more than charming stories to bring peace to the world of our time. But the meaning is there: where there is a deep, simple, all-embracing love of man, of the created world of living and inanimate things, then there will be respect for life, for freedom, for truth, for justice and there will be humble love of God. But where there is no love of man, no love of life, then make all the laws you want, all the edicts and treaties, issue all the anathemas; set up all the safeguards and inspections, fill the air with spying satellites, and hang cameras on the moon. As long as you see your fellow man as a being essentially to be feared, mistrusted, hated, and destroyed, there cannot be peace on earth. And who knows if fear alone will suffice to prevent a war of total destruction? Pope John was not among those who believe that fear is enough.

June 1964.

Preface to Vietnamese Translation of No Man Is an Island

The expression "No man is an island," which is now almost proverbial in the English language, comes from the meditation of a seventeenth-century English Christian poet, John Donne. In the midst of the new optimistic individualism of the Renaissance he pointed out that it was an illusion for man to imagine himself perfectly and completely autonomous in himself, as if he were able to exist independently from his relation to other men and other living beings. This intuition was brought home to the poet by the fact of death. Hearing the bell toll for the funeral of a dead man, he reflected that there is one death for all and when the bell tolls "it tolls for thee."

Death is a silent yet eloquent teacher of truth. Death is a teacher that speaks openly and yet is easily heard. Death is very much present in our modern world: and yet it has become an enigma to that world. Instead of understanding death, it would seem that our world simply multiplies it. Death becomes a huge, inscrutable *quantity*. The mystery of death, more terrible and sometimes more cruel than ever, remains incomprehensible to men who, though they know they must die, retain a grim and total attachment to individual life as if they could be physically indestructible.

Perhaps it is this failure to understand and to face the fact of death that helps beget so many wars and so much violence. As if men, attached to individual bodily life, thought they could protect themselves against death by inflicting it on others.

Death cannot be understood without *compassion*. Compassion teaches me that when my brother dies, I too die. Compassion teaches me that my brother and I are one. That if I love my brother, then my love benefits my own life as well, and if I hate my brother and seek to destroy him, I destroy myself also. The desire to kill is like the desire to attack another with an ingot of red-hot iron: I have to pick up the incandescent metal and burn my own hand while burning the other. Hate itself is the seed of death in my own heart, while it seeks the death of the other. Love is the seed of life in my own heart when it seeks the good of the other.

When this book was written, the author had in mind the personal problems of men in a nation at peace. Now he is faced with the responsibility of introducing that same book to readers in a country that is burned, ravaged and torn to pieces by nearly twenty-five years of bitter war. What can be said in such a situation? It brings out as clearly as anything else the meaning of the title: "No man is an island." It is not difficult to sit in a quiet monastery and meditate on love, humility, mercy, inner silence, meditation and peace. But "no man is an island." A purely individualistic inner life, unconcerned for the sufferings of others, is unreal. Therefore my meditation on love and peace must be realistically and intimately related to the fury of war, bloodshed, burning, destruction, killing that takes place on the other side of the earth.

This raises the great problem of responsibility in a world which has now become a vast unity, and in which everyone is involved in the lives and in the joys and sorrows of everyone else. There is war in Vietnam. The power of my own country is engaged in the fight and in the destruction. Whatever may be the political issues, the rights and the wrongs, soldiers are fighting, men are killing each other, and their death tells me that "no man is an island." The war in Vietnam is a bell tolling for the whole world, warning the whole world that war may spread everywhere, and violent death may sweep over the entire earth. And then perhaps men will ask: Why? Is there really a reason for this? Could these problems not be solved peacefully? Is there not some other answer than the shedding of so much blood? The burning and destruction of so many innocent people?

It is true, statesmen are concerned about this problem: they are sincerely asking these questions. But there never seems to be any answer other than to increase the killing, to multiply the dead. Can that be the answer of love, peace, mercy? If the answer is always brutal and destructive, then perhaps the question is being asked in the wrong terms. Or perhaps both the question and the answer are fundamentally dishonest. How can we know?

Without true compassion for others, without the sincere intention of seeing others as ourselves and treating others as we would want to be treated ourselves, we cannot ask and answer such questions in a really peaceful and honest manner. Violence rests on the assumption that the enemy and I are entirely different: the enemy is evil and I am good. The enemy must be destroyed and I must be saved. But love sees things differently. It sees that even the enemy suffers from the same sorrows and limitations that I do. That we both have the same hopes, the same needs, the same aspiration for a peaceful and harmless human life. And that death is the same for both of us. Then love may perhaps show me that my brother is not really my enemy and that war is both his enemy and mine. War is *our* enemy. Then peace becomes possible.

It is true, political problems are not solved by love and mercy. But the world of politics is not the only world, and unless political decisions rest on a foundation of something better and higher than politics, they can never do any real good for men. When a country has to be rebuilt after war, the passions and energies of war are no longer enough. There must be a new force, the power of love, the power of understanding and human compassion, the strength of selflessness and cooperation, and the creative dynamism of *the will to live and to build, and the will to forgive. The will for reconciliation.*

The principles given in this book are simple and more or less traditional. They are the principles derived from religious wisdom which, in the present case, is Christian. But many of these principles run parallel to the ancient teachings of Buddhism. They are in fact in large part universal truths. They are truths with which, for centuries, man has slowly and with difficulty built a civilized world in the effort to make happiness possible, not merely by making life materially better, but by helping men *to understand and live their life more fruitfully.*

The key to this understanding is the truth that "no man is an island." A selfish life cannot be fruitful. It cannot be true. It contradicts the very nature of man. The dire effort of this contradiction cannot be avoided: where men live selfishly, in quest of brute power and lust and money, they destroy one another. The only way to change such a world is to change the thoughts and the desires of the men who live in it. The conditions of our world are simply an outward expression of our own thoughts and desires. The misfortune of Vietnam today is that the war there expresses not merely the thoughts and desires of the people of Vietnam but, unfortunately, the inner confusion of men in other nations in different parts of the earth. The sickness of the entire earth is now erupting in Vietnam. But perhaps also the sickness of the entire earth may be cured there. . . .

The pages of this book will not enable anyone to wage war and destroy other men. It was not written for that. But these pages may perhaps help some men to find peace even in the midst of war. Above all, they may help everyone who reads them to discover other ways of thinking, ways that will perhaps one day help them in building a world of peace. But for this to be possible, we must all believe in life and in peace. We must believe in the power of love. We must recognize that our being itself is grounded in love: that is to say that we come into being because we are loved and because we are meant to love others. The failure to believe this and to live accordingly creates instead a deep mistrust, a suspicion of others, a hatred of others, and a failure to love. When a man attempts to live by and for himself alone, he becomes a little "island" of hate, greed, suspicion, fear, desire. Then his whole outlook on life is falsified. All his judgments are affected by this untruth. In order to recover the true perspective, which is that of love and compassion, he must once again learn, in simplicity, trust and peace, that "no man is an island."

Peace and Protest:

A Statement

If a pacifist is one who believes that all war is always morally wrong and always has been wrong, then I am not a pacifist. Nevertheless I see war as an avoidable tragedy and I believe that the problem of solving international conflict without massive violence has become the number one problem of our time. As President Kennedy said, "If we do not end war, war is going to end us." Pope John XXIII, Pope Paul VI, have said this with all the solemn authority of their position. The task of man and of the Church is to end all wars, to provide a satisfactory international power to police the world and subdue violence while conflicts are settled by reason and negotiation. Therefore the entire human race has a most serious obligation to face this problem and to do something about it. Each one of us has to resist an ingrained tendency to violence and to destructive thinking. But every time we renounce reason and patience in order to solve a conflict by violence we are side-stepping this great obligation and putting it off. How long can we continue to do this? Our time is limited, and we are not taking advantage of our opportunities.

The human race today is like an alcoholic who knows that drink will destroy him and yet always has "good reasons" why he must continue drinking. Such is man in his fatal addiction to war. He is not really capable of seeing a constructive alternative to war.

If this task of building a peaceful world is the most important task of our time, it is also the most difficult. It will, in fact, require far more discipline, more sacrifice, more planning, more thought, more cooperation and more heroism than war ever demanded.

The task of ending war is in fact the greatest challenge to human courage and intelligence. Can we meet this challenge? Do we have the moral strength and the faith that are required? Sometimes the prospect seems almost hopeless, for man is more addicted to violence now than he ever has been before, and we are today spending more for war alone than we spent for everything, war included, thirty years ago. We also live in a crisis of faith in which to most men "God is dead" and even some Christians no longer accept Christ except as a symbol.

I do not advocate the burning of draft cards. It is not my opinion that the draft law is so unjust that it calls for civil disobedience. But nevertheless I believe that we must admit patriotic dissent and argument at a time like this. Such dissent must be responsible. It must give a clear and reasonable account of itself to the nation, and it must help sincere and concerned minds to accept alternatives to war without surrendering the genuine interests of our own national community. This dissent should not be ambiguous or threatening.

There is considerable danger of ambiguity in protests that seek mainly to capture the attention of the press and to gain publicity for a cause, being more concerned with their impact upon the public than with the meaning of that impact. Such dissent tends to be at once dramatic and superficial. It may cause a slight commotion, but in a week everything is forgotten—some new shock has occurred in some other area. What is needed is a constructive dissent that recalls people to their senses, makes them think deeply, plants in them a seed of change, and awakens in them the profound need for truth, reason and peace which is implanted in man's nature. Such dissent implies belief in openness of mind and in the possibility of mature exchange of ideas. When protest becomes desperate and seemingly extreme, then perhaps one reason for this is that the ones protesting have given up hope of a fair hearing, and therefore seek only to shock or to horrify. On the other hand, perhaps the public is too eager to be shocked and horrified, and to refuse a fair hearing. The reaction of shock seems to dispense us from serious thought. This is a problem for all of us now. We are Americans, and we have a duty to live up to our heritage of open-mindedness. We must always be tolerant and fair and never persecute others for their opinions. The way to silence error is by truth, not by violence. But we will always prefer violence to truth if our imaginations are at every moment overstimulated by frenzied and dangerous fantasies.

Therefore one of the most important tasks of the moment is to recognize the great problem of the *mental climate* in which we live. Our minds are filled with images which call for violent and erratic reactions. We can hardly recover our senses long enough to think calmly and make reasoned commitments. We are swept by alternate fears and hopes which have no relation to deep moral truth. A protest which merely compounds these fears and hopes with a new store of images can hardly help us become men of peace.

The great value of Pope Paul's visit to the United Nations was precisely this: it was a positive and constructive witness which, together with a clear and firm protest against war and injustice, reawakened a definite hope in peaceful alternatives to war. It was a most serious and highly credible reminder that instruments for peaceful conflict solution are at hand. These instruments are abused and discredited, but if men *want to* make serious and effective use of them, they are still free to do so.

All protest against war and all witness for peace should in some way or other strive to overcome the desperation and hopelessness with which man now, in fact, regards all his existing peace-making machinery as futile and beyond redemption. It is this practical despair of effective peace-making that drives man more and more to embrace the conclusion that only war is effective and that because violence seems to pay off, we must finally resort to it.

Is it perhaps this insatiable hunger for visible and quick returns that has driven the majority of Americans to accept the war in Vietnam as reasonable? Are we so psychologically constituted and determined that we find real comfort in a daily score of bombed bridges and burned villages, forgetting that the price of our psychological security is the burned flesh of women and children who have no guilt and no escape from the fury of our weapons?

One thing that gives such a drastic character to the protest against war is the realization which the peace people have of this unjust suffering inflicted on the innocent largely as a result of our curious inner psychological needs, fomented by the climate of our culture.

In order to resist this appeal to mercy, those who want and "need" the violence in Vietnam disregard the sufferings of "the enemy" and concentrate on the very real and desperate hardships of our own GIs in Vietnam.

Yet there remains a difference:

The sufferings of our own men are avoidable. There are alternatives. It is even possible that these alternatives would be more effective and would restore the honor of our country in the eyes of those nations that feel threatened by us and therefore hate us.

Can we not keep open in our minds the possibility of seeking these alternatives? Can our government not divert some of the money paid out for our overkill capacity, to investigate the chances of lasting and realistic peace? Or will we continue to abandon ourselves to the flow of immediate reactions and superficial events, with no plan and no hope for an intelligible future, content only to wring some practical and visible effect by the use of violence from a confused and unintelligible present?

Let there be no mistake about the end to which this road leads. It is man's ruin, degradation and dishonor.

Peace and Revolution:

A Footnote from *Ulysses*

"How can people point guns at each other? Sometimes they go off."
—BLOOM, IN *Ulysses*

"Love, says Bloom, I mean the opposite of hatred."

In the "Cyclops episode" of *Ulysses,* Bloom, a peaceful Odysseus, confronts the Irish revolutionary Cyclops, the violent "Citizen" who is a Sinn Feiner. This meeting takes place in a Dublin pub where the Citizen, accompanied by his ferocious dog, is drinking with others like himself. They are a typical group of toughs: aggressive, foul-mouthed, suspicious of anyone outside their own group, truculently xenophobic, united in a hatred of the English oppressor and in a desire to get rid of him by violence. Bloom, though uncircumcised, thrice baptized, and a loyal Dubliner, is not acceptable to them as "Irish." He is an outsider and a Jew. And he has "funny ideas." Furthermore, they suspect him of having slyly placed a hundred-to-five bet on the dark horse, the winner of the day's Gold Cup Race. They think he has gone to collect his bet, and that he is keeping quiet in order not to have to buy drinks all round.

Bloom tries to pacify them with conciliatory speeches about civilized life and love of neighbor, but the Citizen is not having any of that. When the party gets rough, Bloom is hurried out of the pub into a waiting vehicle. As a parting shot he taunts the Citizen with a reminder that Christ was a Jew. For this "blasphemy" the Citizen threatens to kill him and hurls a big tin biscuit box after the open jaunting car as it drives away. Parodying the style of Celtic epic and legend, Joyce brings to mind not only the heroes of Irish past but also Cyclops, blinded and enraged, hurling a huge stone after escaping Odysseus.

The Decline of Meaning

You may think me facetious for bringing this up, but the episode may be instructive as we consider Peace and Revolution! We are not used to considering moral and political issues in the light of contemporary literature, but perhaps we would be wise if we did so more often. Whatever we may think of Joyce's philosophy of life and of his art, there is no question that *Ulysses* is, among other things, an ironic moral cosmology, a literary commentary on the decay of Western civilization as exemplified by Dublin before World War I. The genius of James Joyce observes and describes the forces at work in that decaying society, looking back from the experience of World War I, which was in progress at the time when he wrote. Bloom is the central character of *Ulysses.* He is to a great extent an embodiment of the alienated, confused, money-minded, respectable middle-class Western man of the early twentieth century. He is a jumble of ineffective drives, confused ideas, mental clichés, frustrations, petty fears and more or less expedient strategies for meeting the problems and challenges of life. It is in this that Bloom re-lives, in his own very humble way, the adventures of the resourceful Odysseus. The mock-heroic style of Joyce's great comedy shows us, in Bloom, the decline of the classic, Greco-Roman and Christian civilization that first flowered in Homer. The nobility, the idealism, the chivalry, the humanity that we encounter in our cultural tradition have become, in Bloom, a pile of nondescript linguistic rubbish, sentimental jargon without any real force, based on no deep experience of life, but rather devised to justify alienation and evasion. And yet we note in passing that Bloom, when compared to the other characters in the book, not excluding Stephen, gives the impression of being more mature, more civilized, more experienced, even more humane, than they. Stephen of course is much more "cultured" than Bloom, but he is still somewhat callow and negative in his revolt against Dublin life. Bloom is the type who accepts modern life fully and adjusts to it willingly, because for him there is really no other. But his adjustment is seen to be equivocal and riddled with bad faith, in the full sense given to it by Sartre.

Now the importance of all this for our consideration of Peace and Revolution becomes clear when we note that some of the more important Joyce critics have given a positive and favorable reading of Bloom as *pacifist.* Yes, we learn that Bloom is really a reasonable man who sees the futility of force and conflict, and who lives by the conviction that "kindness overcomes power." And indeed all through the book we find Bloom accepting many hard knocks without protest. He is even a victim of real injustice, but he does not assert his rights. For instance, he knows that his wife is unfaithful to him that very afternoon and does nothing to stop it. He just ignores the whole thing. He pays no attention to implied or to explicit insults, and accepts the rather general contempt of others in good part. The climax of his "pacifism" is in his encounter with the Citizen and his expression of sentiments about civilization and love.

Now it must be said at once that these critics seem to underestimate the force of Joyce's irony. Joyce obviously does not accept Bloom's truisms about love at their face value—any more than the Citizen does. In fact Joyce inserts a famous and sardonic little aside about everybody loving somebody and God loving everybody: "Nurse loves the new chemist. Constable 14A loves Mary Kelly. Gerty McDowell loves the boy that has the bicycle. . . ." We have to consider the context. There has been an argument going on, the Citizen and his friends advocating that the English be thrown out of Ireland by force, Bloom protesting, defending the values of Western civilization and deploring the fact that violence merely perpetuates hatred among nations. "And what's *your* nation?" asks the Citizen with heavy sarcasm. All right, so Bloom will defend his *race,* too! A race that is "plundered, insulated and persecuted." He protests vehemently, and his protest meets with some sympathy, if not from the Citizen, at least from one of the others. "Right," says this other, but adds: "Stand up to it with force like men." As far as they are concerned, this is a challenge that Bloom simply cannot meet. His plea for love is nothing but a "collapse," "like a wet rag."

Poor Pacifism

Hatred and force, he says, are no use. They are "the opposite of what is really life." Joyce himself emphasizes the fact that Bloom's argument is all weakness, sentimentality, confusion. And Bloom runs out of the bar at once, only to return later and face real trouble.

Now it must be said first of all that whatever some Joyce critics may think of his intentions, Joyce has not portrayed, in Bloom, an authentic pacifist. Far from it. This "pacifism" is in line with everything else in Bloom. It is the expression of pathetic weakness, confusion, frustration and ambivalence. It is not the product of any serious moral conviction. It is not even one of his more significant velleities. It may indeed indicate a desire to be left in peace, a desire not to be rejected and injured. Surely that is not "pacifism" or "love of peace." Indeed Bloom himself later admits it. He wants to score as much as "they" do. He tells himself that with the jibe about Christ being a Jew he really did come out on top after all. "Got my own back there. What I said about his God made him wince!"

To say that Bloom is a pacifist and even to commend him for it certainly does no service whatever to pacifism or to the cause of peace. But the point I would like to make—and this I think fits in with Joyce's real intention—is that the Cyclops episode does in fact spell out the whole issue of Peace and Revolution in terms of popular contemporary cliché. Whatever may be the truth of the case, this is in fact the way the majority of people today continue to see the question of non-violence and force. This is the way all violent revolutionaries look at it, and it is also the way American public opinion and the established mass media of capitalism still generally regard it. If they are favorable, they see it more or less as the critics who "like" Bloom see it. There is a kind of heroism and nobility in *expressing these noble sentiments* and in *saying* that love is better than hatred. There is also something praiseworthy about refraining from violence in word or in act. This is an attitude which they feel to be nicer than its contrary. It appeals to them more than its contrary. They respond to it more than they do to its contrary. This reassures and pleases them—to hear a man affirm the priority of love! But to hear him affirm (with a few choice oaths) the prior efficacy of force, is disturbing and unpleasant. Very well. And yet they have no alternative to force. They prefer love as an idea, but when confronted with force, they have only two ways out: to run away or else to call the police. In the end they fall back on force to defend and to affirm love.

The Popular Image

As to those who, like the Citizen, have an open contempt for the civilization that Bloom does not want to see overthrown, they are in no doubt about what is really wrong with people who can't stand the idea of force. Such people are simply cowards, and they must be swept out of the way. They are slated for destruction with the structures they defend and justify with their humane inanities.

It is instructive to read the Cyclops episode again in a time that has become much more violent and much more revolutionary than the days before World War I. In fact, if we look back to Joyce's Dublin in 1904, we find an almost unbelievable era of peace, order and stability. The Citizen was of course a normal part of that culture: but there are many more like him today, whether in the Klan or in Black Power; in the CIA or in the Guerilla band; voting for Wallace or waving the Vietcong flag in demonstrations. It is therefore useful to spell out what Bloom's brand of "pacifism" means in the mind of the Citizen.

First of all, it is a lie. The pacifist, the nonviolent resister, in spite of subjective sincerity (even this is doubtful) is at once a crafty and ineffectual person. Ineffectual by definition, because his very ideas about love and peace mark him as cut off from reality. Ineffectual too, because he is doubtless masochistic, fear-ridden, passive, pathetic; he invites beatings. He exercises that sort of appeal on the sadism of the man of force. The Citizen is looking for an excuse, any excuse, to pick a fight with Bloom and mop up the floor with him. Bloom's defense of love is in fact a defense of himself, a pathetic appeal to be considered and accepted as a human being. But the Citizen does not want to waste any time considering a member of an out-group as a human being. In fact he simply wants to prove that Bloom's glorification of love is a mask of dishonesty and fear. Thus the man of force is intent above all on discrediting and unmasking the presumed bad faith of the pacifist, the nonviolent resister.

To do this, he assumes a secret dishonesty and a hook-up of some sort that presumably gives the pacifist a sinister undercover advantage, a quasi-superiority which, in spite of his surface innocuousness, makes him a real threat. So the Citizen assumes that Bloom is being both unjust and greedy in keeping his gains to himself. The modern man of force is convinced that the pacifist or the nonviolent resister is really allied with some hidden power group—generally the "Communists." In any case, it becomes not only possible but indeed honorable to unmask and destroy him.

The Language of Action

One of the main themes of *Ulysses* is the breakdown of language and of communication as part of the disruption of Western culture. The extraordinary linguistic richness of the book—which however comes out mostly in parody—only reminds us more forcefully how much further the breakdown has gone in the last fifty years. Pacifism and nonviolence are fully and consciously involved in this question of language. Nonviolence, as Gandhi conceived it, is in fact a kind of language. The real dynamic of nonviolence can be considered as a purification of language, a restoration of true communication on a human level, when language has been emptied of meaning by misuse and corruption. Nonviolence is meant to communicate love not in word but in act. Above all, nonviolence is meant to convey and to defend truth which has been obscured and defiled by political doubletalk.

The real lesson for us is this: we must clearly understand the function of nonviolence against the background of the collapse of language. It is no accident that Noam Chomsky, a leader in the Draft Resistance movement, is also an expert in the study of language. The special force of the Cyclops episode in *Ulysses* is that it shows how the language of pacifism and the language of force can both fit with equal readiness into a context of linguistic corruption. We have to be terribly aware of the fact that our pacifism and nonviolence can easily be nothing more than parodies of themselves. We must recognize the temptation to be quite content with this—to be content to express our weak convictions in weak and provisional terms, meanwhile waiting for an opportunity to abandon nonviolence altogether and go over to the side of force, on the ground that we have tried nonviolence and found it wanting.

He Shall Overcome

Has nonviolence been found wanting? Yes and no. It has been found wanting wherever it has been the nonviolence of the weak. It has not been found so when it has been the nonviolence of the strong. What is the difference? It is a difference of language. The language of spurious nonviolence is merely another, more equivocal form of the language of power. It is a different method of expressing one's will to power. It is used and conceived pragmatically, in reference to the seizure of power. But that is not what nonviolence is about, Nonviolence is not for power but for truth. It is not pragmatic but prophetic. It is not aimed at immediate political results, but at the manifestation of fundamental and crucially important truth. Nonviolence is not primarily the language of efficacy, but the language of *kairos*. It does not say "We shall overcome" so much as "This is the day of the Lord, and whatever may happen to us, *He* shall overcome."

And this, of course, is the dimension that is entirely absent from the Cyclops episode in *Ulysses*. Unhappily, it is too often absent from our world and our practice today. As a result people begin to imagine that to say "only force works" is to discredit nonviolence. This half-truth —that only force is efficacious—may turn out to be one of the most dangerous illusions of our time. It may do more than anything else to promote an irresponsible and meaningless use of force in a pseudo-revolution that will only consolidate the power of the police state. Never was it more necessary to understand the importance of genuine nonviolence as a power for real change because it is aimed not so much at revolution as at conversion. Unfortunately, mere words about peace, love and civilization have completely lost all power to change anything.

Breakthrough to Peace

The nineteenth century can be called an age of peace and comfort, though if we reflect a little we will remember the war in Crimea, the Indian Mutiny, the Opium War in China, the Franco-Prussian War and the bloody and utterly savage war between the northern and southern United States. In spite of these conflicts our grandfathers believed that war was gradually getting to be a thing of the past. They did not know that these were all preludes to the gigantic struggle which has continued to rend and batter the world of the twentieth century. But now in 1962 we are beginning to realize that our age has been practically nothing but one big fire of war dying down only to flame up in greater fury, growing in its appetite for violent destruction, and gradually threatening the very survival of civilized man.

The First World War, we are told, was not fully intended by anyone; but political and military strategists moved one step too far and could not turn back. The war was confidently and savagely fought with the expectation that it would end all wars and make the world finally and imperturbably safe for the free and comfortable life.

The very treaty which attempted to restore order to Europe and to guarantee that there would be no further conflict made another and greater war inevitable. And yet during the twenties and thirties, there was a succession of peace conferences, a procession of peace movements, not to mention the nonviolent revolution in India. Men studied, talked, agitated, prayed and suffered to bring about a permanent peace. Never had so much been said about peace, never had war been so thoroughly and universally execrated. Militarists remained, of course, but it cannot be denied that serious efforts at disarmament were made. So serious were these efforts that, when the Second World War broke out, the Western nations, particularly America, were not ready. Before Pearl Harbor the majority of Americans strenuously and articulately opposed entrance into the war. France, meanwhile, relied with blind faith on the Maginot Line, a complex and expensive system which proved completely useless against deadly new weapons of attack. The allies cannot be said to have "wanted" war. But they wanted a political and economic situation that made war inevitable.

In the unexampled and criminal frightfulness of World War II, massive attacks on defenseless civilian centers came to be accepted as perfectly normal in spite of protests of the Pope and other spokesmen for traditional ethics. It was believed that systematic terrorism was essential to beat down all resistance of the "Fascist war criminals" and bring them to an unconditional surrender that would definitely end all war. Finally the atomic bomb was dropped on Hiroshima and Nagasaki —the climax of this ruthless policy.

Yet at the very moment when the bomb fell, the cold war between America and Russia was already on. The threat of this bomb, which ended the hot war with Japan, was to be the chief weapon of the cold war. Instead of producing peace, the atom bomb started the most fantastic arms race in history.

Nuclear deterrence has proved to be an illusion, for the bomb deters no one. It did not prevent war in Korea, Indochina, Laos, the Congo. It did not prevent the Russian suppression of the Hungarian revolt. And now those who once relied on deterrence, on the threat of massive retaliation, are insensibly moving toward a policy that assumes a *first strike capacity*. This policy is dictated by the very weapons themselves. The missile armed with a nuclear warhead is the perfect weapon of offense, so perfect that no defense against it has yet been devised. An H-bomb is the cheapest of all mass engines of destruction. It costs only two hundred and fifty thousand dollars to make, and one can go all the way up the megaton scale without prohibitively increasing either the expense or the engineering difficulty. It has been said that the H-bomb "gives more destructive power for the dollar" than any other weapon in existence. Knowing man's love for a good bargain, this atrocious estimate should certainly give us food for thought.

There has been relatively little agitation for peace since World War II. One feels that public opinion has been embittered and disillusioned by the futility of the peace movements after the First World War. This disillusionment is of course compounded by the fact that the biggest "peace movement" in the world today is simply part of the Soviet propaganda front, and is another powerful psychological weapon in the cold war, cynically exploiting the deepest desires of modern man and his most pathetic need in what is frankly a war effort, leading inevitably to hot war or to revolution. In this grim situation, with the U.N. too weak and unsubstantial to offer any hope of a higher authority to restrain the lawless and truculent aspirations of national powers, we seem to be drifting helplessly toward another disaster which will make all previous wars look like rumbles in a back alley. As long as each nation remains the sole judge of its own case, and decides for itself what is right and wrong without further appeal except to the power of the bomb, it would seem that war must be inevitable. The question that now seems to preoccupy leaders and policy-makers is not whether war can be avoided, but whether war can be kept within "safe" limits.

In this situation, where the issues are too enormous for the mind of the average man to grasp, when the threat is too appalling for his political habits and instincts to instruct him adequately, the tendency is to take refuge in fanaticism or in passive desperation.

Fanatics yield to the pressures of inner resentment and frustration, and seek a show-down because they cannot bear the intolerable burden of waiting and uncertainty. The passive and the despairing accept the absurdity of life with a shrug and seek forgetfulness in an automatic, drugged existence which renounces all effort and all hope. In both cases people become more and more resigned to their destruction and to the destruction of the civilized world. Indeed, one gets the feeling that they are almost eager to see the whole thing blow up, and get it over with.

This precisely is the great danger. This is what the open mind, the humanist and Christian mind, the mind which desires the survival of reason and of life, must now confront most decisively. No one of us can say for sure what the future will bring, but we are not responsible for what is beyond our control. We are responsible for the present and for those present actions and attitudes of ours from which future events will develop. It is therefore supremely important that we get a grip on ourselves and determine that we will not relinquish either our reason or our humanity; that we will not despair of ourselves, or of man, or of our capacity to solve our problems; that we will make use of the faculties and resources we still have in abundance, and use them for positive and constructive action in so far as we can. We will resist the fatal inclination to passivity and despair as well as the fatuous temptation to false optimism and insouciance which condition us equally well to accept disaster. In a word we will behave as men, and, if Christians, then as members of Christ.

Our problem is a moral and spiritual problem. It is a problem of enormous and frightful complexity. We have no alternative but to face it, in all its ramifications, and do what we can about it. This is the duty which history itself has imposed on us, which our forefathers, in their mixture of wisdom and folly, have bequeathed to us. It will not do us any good to wish we were other than we actually are, or that we were in some other century, some other planet. We cannot escape present reality. We cannot all offer ourselves to be frozen up and comfortably hibernate through the critical years that are to come, in order to wake up painlessly in a new world.

But if we are to face the problem as it is, we must first of all admit its true nature. If it is a *moral* problem, then it implies the appropriate response of reason and of freedom. It implies choice, based on knowledge. It implies willingness to study, to reason, to communicate. It implies the capacity to judge. It implies not only that judgment which the individual makes in the secrecy of his conscience, but also political expression and action.

We must judge and decide not only as individuals, preserving for ourselves the luxury of a clean conscience, but also as members of society taking up a common burden and responsibility. It is all too easy to retire into the ivory tower of private spirituality and let the world blow itself to pieces. Such a decision would be immoral, an admission of defeat. It would imply a secret complicity with the overt destructive fury of fanatics.

Moral decisions have to be based on adequate knowledge. The scientist must tell us something reliable about the behavior of bombs and missiles. The political commentator must keep us in touch with the developments of strategy and with the plans that are being made for our defense or for our destruction. He must tell us what underlies the fair assurances we read in the mass media or hear in the speeches of the statesman and publicist. We must be informed of what goes on in the rest of the world, what is hoped and feared by our opposite numbers in the land of "the enemy." We must try to remember that the enemy is as human as we are, and not an animal or a devil.

Finally, we must be reminded of the way we ourselves tend to operate, the significance of the secret forces that rise up within us and dictate fatal decisions. We must learn to distinguish the free voice of conscience from the irrational compulsions of prejudice and hate. We must be reminded of objective moral standards, and of the wisdom which goes into every judgment, every choice, every political act that deserves to be called civilized. We cannot think this way unless we shake off our passive irresponsibility, renounce our fatalistic submission to economic and social forces, and give up the unquestioning belief in machines and processes which characterizes the mass mind. History is ours to make: now above all we must try to recover our freedom, our moral autonomy, our capacity to control the forces that make for life and death in our society.

It is necessary to discuss the fateful problems of our time, and independent minds have not hesitated to do so, even though the trend of the masses is toward an ever more submissive and inert acceptance of meaningless slogans. No such slogans will be found in this book. Nor do these writers offer easy solutions. Indeed, they do not pretend to an infallibility which can promise anything beyond the austerity of a task that may turn out to be fruitless. But they seek to offer sincere and unprejudiced judgments of our predicament and their analysis is not without very significant hopes, if only we can be faithful to the reason and wisdom which we have not yet irrevocably lost.

The fact remains that we may lose both, through our own fault, and forfeit our heritage of civilization and of humanity to enter a post-historic world of technological animals. There is no guarantee even now that reason can still prevail. But we must do what we can, relying on the grace of God for the rest.

The essays in this book attempt to break through thought barriers and open up rational perspectives. Hence each one of the writers assumes, in his own way, that the questions he raises are not already closed forever by prejudice or by the informal dictatorship of "thought control." If we assume that the basic questions have already been answered, our doom is sealed. On the contrary, if we recognize that we still have the obligation and, we hope, the time to reexamine certain fundamental assumptions, we may perhaps be able to open the way for developments in policy that will help future generations work out a fully constructive and peaceful solution.

The moral or political principles on which our most critical decisions are to be made may, in themselves, be relatively simple, but the assumptions on which they are based are immensely complicated. It is not difficult to appeal to traditional norms of justice and law, and apply them to our present situation in such a way as to come up with logical and plausible conclusions. But the very plausibility of the conclusions tends to be the most dangerous thing about them, if we forget that they may be based on premises which we take to be axiomatic and which, in fact, have been invalidated by recent developments of weapons technology. Indeed, the technological data on which we are basing our moral or political decision may be profoundly influenced by certain assumptions which have been fed into the computers in the first place. There is a very serious danger that our most crucial decisions may turn out to be no decisions at all, but only the end of a vicious circle of conjectures and gratuitous assumptions in which we unconsciously make the argument come out in favor of our own theory, our own favorite policy.

The written and spoken statements of nuclear "realists" seem to give grounds for very grave concern in this regard. It would be a disaster if ethical and political thought were to take too seriously the claims of men who dismiss the noxious effects of fallout as altogether negligible, and who minimize the destructive power of the bomb whenever they consider the possible destruction of our own cities. Yet on the basis of such conjectures as these, a moralist or a publicist, exercising a really decisive effect on a huge segment of public opinion, might issue a declaration in favor of nuclear war, and this judgment might itself be the deciding factor in swinging the whole policy of the United States in the direction of preemptive attack. Even more serious than this is the fact that the moral, or amoral preconceptions of the military mind, and particularly the oversimplified assessment of a political threat, implemented by a dogmatic and fanatical political creed, will certainly have grave influence upon military decisions at a high level.

It is therefore vitally important to create a general climate of rationality, and to preserve a broad, tolerant, watchful and humanist outlook on the whole of life, precisely in order that rash and absurd assumptions may not have too free a circulation in our society.

That is what these essays attempt to do. All of them, in their own way, approach the problems related to nuclear war with a freely questioning mind, in search of facts and principles which tend to upset the crude assumptions already too widely accepted by the majority, particularly in America. Hence these essays all share a common note of urgency and protest, and by that very fact alone they manifest their intention to continue fighting in defense of genuine democracy, freedom of thought, and freedom of political action.

One of the most absurd and dangerous of all prejudices is the popular assumption that anyone who doubts that the bomb is the only ultimate solution proves himself by that very fact to be subversive. For those who believe this, these essays will prove disturbing. The present writers prescribe austere remedies. They demand thought, patience, the willingness to face risks, in order to enter new and unexplored territory of the mind. They refuse to be satisfied with negativism and destruction, or with the despair that masks as heroism and prepares for the apocalyptic explosion in which all the humanized, social and spiritual values that we know will go up in radioactive smoke.

The perspectives in this book are, then, humanistic in the deepest and most spiritual sense of the word. They look beyond the interests of any restricted group toward the deepest and most critical needs of man himself. In so doing, they are, at least implicitly, faithful to the Judaeo-Christian tradition on which our civilization was built. There is no hope for us if we lose sight of these perspectives. There is no other human way out.

Christian Ethics and Nuclear War

When the preparations for the Second Vatican Council began to be discussed, a writer in *Réalités* produced an article which was not lacking in astute intuitions. It was called "The Last Chance Council." Doubtless this provoking title was dismissed by most of us Catholics as the flippancy of an irreligious mind. One feels nevertheless that the present cold war crisis has brought home, at least obscurely, to many Christians, whether Catholic or Protestant, a sense that the Church is now facing a test that may prove to be decisive and perhaps in some sense "final." Christianity may be on the point of being driven back into the catacombs and losing, in the process, millions of faithful.

Worse still, the possibility of the complete destruction of human society and even the extinction of life on the planet might, if Christians themselves were deeply involved in responsibility for it, be in some sense on their part a disastrous failure and betrayal. Though these fears have generated a climate of widespread uneasiness and even of implicit desperation, they are not without certain correlative hopes. We believe that the Church could not be brought face to face with any desperate situation which did not at the same time contain a challenge and a promise. For Christians to come "under judgment" in a historical crisis implies not more blind doom, but rather a difficult choice, a "temptation" if you like, and one in which the future of Christianity and of the whole world may hinge on the heroism and integrity of the faithful. In other words, we find ourselves confronting the possibility of nuclear war with more than the common and universal urgency, because we Christians are at least dimly aware that this is a matter of *choice* for us and that the future of Christianity on earth may depend on the moral quality of the decision we are making.

This is the climate in which all Christians are facing (or refusing to face) the most crucial moral and religious problem in twenty centuries of history.

It is doubtful whether for most Christians the real underlying religious issue is clearly visible. On the contrary, at least in America, the average priest and minister seems to react in much the same way as the average agnostic or atheist. The interests of the West, the NATO, and the Church are all confused with one another, and the possibility of defending the West with a nuclear first strike on Russia is accepted without too much hesitation as "necessary" and a "lesser evil." We assume without question that Western society equals Christendom and Communism equals Antichrist. And we are ready to declare without hesitation that "no price is too high" to pay for our religious liberty. The cliché sounds noble, perhaps, to those who are not shocked by its all too evident meaninglessness. The fact is that genocide *is* too high a price, and no one, not even Christians, not even for the highest ideals, has the right to take measures that may destroy millions of innocent noncombatants and even whole defenseless populations of neutral nations or unwilling allies. Note that some of these nations might be Christian, at least in principle. The bland assumption is always, of course, that nuclear warheads, ICBMs and Polaris submarines are dictated by "prudence," indeed by "Christian prudence." There seems to be very little awareness that this position is not only psychologically irresponsible, but plainly immoral according to all Christian standards and by that very fact supremely *imprudent*. Such thinking, or rather thoughtlessness, is due to the slow corruption of the Christian ethical sense by theorizing in a vacuum, juggling with moral clichés devoid of serious content, and the weakening of genuine human compassion. The scandalous consequence of this has been not only confusion, inertia, indecision and even culpable silence on the part of many Christian spokesmen, but worse still, some Christian leaders have actively joined in the cold war and call God Himself to justify the moral blindness and *hubris* of generals and industrialists, and to bless nuclear war as a holy and apocalyptic crusade. As C. Wright Mills has said, priests and ministers have fallen over one another to enlist in "the Swiss Guard of the power elite."

While this blindness and confusion are common to great numbers of Christians, nominal or otherwise, there are also strong and articulate movements against war. At this moment of crisis they are gaining in strength, in spite of the increasing pressure of suspicion and disapproval. For the unpleasant fact is that the Russians have succeeded in getting the cause of peace identified, in the popular mind, with the cause of the Soviet bloc. Hence anyone who dares to stand up for peace and disarmament in the West, by that very fact runs the risk of being called a fellow traveler. This is one of the most disturbing aspects of the thoughtless passivity, the crude opportunism and astonishing lack of discernment which have become characteristic of Western political thought in the cold war. But the fact that our politicians have let themselves be outmaneuvered by more subtle and better-organized adversaries does not dispense us from promoting reasonable and persistent peace negotiations, whether the position happens to be popular or not. It should be immediately clear to any objective observer that the Western defender of peace and of disarmament, even if he has no special ideology at all, is plainly concerned with the survival of Western freedom and democracy. This is especially true of Christian movements like the Fellowship of Reconciliation. In Europe the FOR unites Catholics and Protestants. In America it is exclusively Protestant, not by choice but due to unfortunate circumstances in this country. There has not hitherto been any Catholic peace movement in the United States if we except the *Catholic Worker* which, however, has lots of other irons in the fire. A *Pax* group, an offshoot of the English Pax movement, is now being formed to concentrate Catholic opposition to nuclear war in the United States and to articulate Christian policies for peace. Those who have joined fully expect to receive harsh criticism and opposition from their coreligionists, but they feel that the crisis is too serious for them to remain silent and inactive without incurring moral guilt. The members of *Pax* are not necessarily pure pacifists. They are opposed, however, to all nuclear war.

The popular image of the Catholic Church, particularly of American Catholicism, does not readily admit such a possibility as this. Catholics are regarded as a monolithic mass, directed passively from above, without thoughts or feelings of their own. The outspoken hostility with which right-wing Catholics have reacted to the encyclical *Mater et Magistra* as socialistic ought to warn the rest of men that the phenomenon of Catholic "passivity" is more complex than they realize.

Recent official statements of the American Catholic bishops deplore the irresponsibility and secularism which affect Catholics as much as everybody else. This would suggest that the American Catholic tends to be a passive unit in the affluent mass society of the U.S.A. and that he consecrates the values of this secular society with a few authoritative formulas he has heard in the pulpit.

This is especially true in the matter of war. It is commonly said, even by Catholics, that "the Church has never condemned nuclear war," which is completely false. Of course the Pope has never pronounced an *ex cathedra* definition which would formally outlaw nuclear war. Why should he? Does every *infima species* of mortal sin need to be defined and denounced by the extraordinary magisterium? Do we now need an *ex cathedra* fulmination against adultery before Catholics will believe themselves bound in conscience to keep the sixth commandment? There is no need for nuclear war to be solemnly outlawed by an extraordinary definition. It should not even need to be condemned by the ordinary papal teaching. In fact, however, it has been so condemned.

The Christmas messages of Pope Pius XII during and after World

War II became stronger and stronger in their denunciation of total war and all those policies by which the allies, with a "good conscience," forced the unconditional surrender of their enemies. Already in 1944, before Hiroshima, Pope Pius asserted that "the theory of war as an apt and proportionate means of solving international conflict is now out of date" and declared that the duty of banning all wars of aggression was binding on *all*. This duty "brooks no delay, no procrastination, no hesitation, no subterfuge." Few, it seems, were listening. The saturation bombing of open cities was purely and simply mass murder by Christian moral standards and it is sophistry to argue that because this was "tolerated" the H-bomb automatically becomes legitimate. Pope Pius XII denounced nuclear annihilation bombing very clearly and without any possibility of being mistaken. He declared that from the moment a weapon was so large and so destructive that it wiped out everything and everyone indiscriminately, it could not be tolerated by Christian morality. Here are his words:

> Should the evil consequences of adopting this method of warfare ever become so extensive as to pass utterly beyond the control of man, then indeed its use must be rejected as immoral. In that event it would no longer be a question of defense against injustice and necessary protection of legitimate possessions, but of the annihilation pure and simple of all human life within the affected area. That is not lawful on any title.
> (Address to the World Medical Association, September, 1954.)

We must note that this applies equally to offensive and defensive war. While it is obligatory to defend one's nation against unjust aggression, only legitimate means can be taken for this. And if the destructive effect of war is far greater than political injustice suffered, war is not legitimate. "If the damage caused by war is disproportionate to the injustice suffered, it may well be a matter of obligation to suffer the injustice," said Pope Pius XII to army doctors on October 19, 1953.

These are, of course, general statements of principle which are meant to be clarified by the bishops, theologians, and clergy. The Pope does not make individual moral decisions for all the members of the Church, but enunciates and defines the norms according to which they should make their personal decisions for themselves. Unfortunately, statements like this one on nuclear war, though dutifully reported in the press and respectfully noted by the faithful, are seldom really assimilated by them. That is why the serious moral implications of the measured Papal denunciations of nuclear war seem to have been overlooked.

The Popes have not merely been trying to say that nuclear war is not nice, but that it upsets traditional Catholic norms of the morality of war. In plain language this is an essentially new kind of war and one in which the old concept of the "just war" is irrelevant because the necessary conditions for such a war no longer exist. A war of total annihilation simply cannot be considered a "just war," no matter how good the cause for which it is undertaken.

Such is the view taken by no less authoritative a theologian than Cardinal Ottaviani, Secretary of the Holy Office. Writing before the development of the H-bomb, Cardinal (then Monsignor) Ottaviani says this without ambiguity:

> The war of their treatises is not the war of our experience. . . . Principles derive from the very nature of things: the difference between war as it was and war as we know it is *precisely one of nature*. . . . Modern wars can never fulfill the conditions which govern, theoretically, a just and lawful war. Moreover no conceivable cause could ever be sufficient justification for the evils, the slaughter, the moral and religious upheavals which war today entails.

Such is the thesis in an article entitled "War Is to Be Forbidden Entirely," published in Latin in his *Public Laws of the Church* (Rome, 1947). Unfortunately such opinions have not been widely disseminated, although Bishop Fulton J. Sheen has publically taken the same standpoint in this country. It must be said also that statements like this do not exclude the use of nuclear weapons in tactical warfare, assuming that such warfare can be "kept within limits," a possibility which hardly interests the military mind of 1962.

Perhaps the most cogent and articulate statements of Catholic opinion on nuclear war are now coming from Europe. A German Dominican, Fr. Franziskus Strattmann, has courageously broken through the conventional thought barriers to discover how, in the Middle Ages, the Gospel ethic was "supplemented—perhaps we must say stifled—by religiously neutral natural law," and from this developed the theory of just wars, whose elastic principles were to be stretched indefinitely by later casuistry until they have now reached the breaking point. He admits nevertheless that even the natural law clearly repudiates modern war. A recent collection of essays, *Nuclear Weapons and Christian Conscience* (London: Merlin Press, 1961), frankly takes the stand that the immoral hypotheses of "realists" who seek to justify nuclear war are "doing more from within to undermine Western civilization than the enemy can do from the outside." These Catholic writers protest with all their strength against the "habitual moral squalor" of the prevailing opportunism, and remind the Christian who may have forgotten the Cross that in a situation like ours we may be forced to choose "the ultimate weapon of meaningful suffering" or deny the Christian faith itself. It is absurd and immoral to pretend that Christendom can be defended by the H-bomb.

As Saint Augustine would say, the weapon with which we would attempt to destroy the enemy would pass through our own heart to reach him. We would be destroyed morally and no doubt physically as well. The H-bomb may possibly destroy Western society if it is used by Communists, but it will destroy Christendom spiritually if it is used as a weapon of aggression by Christians.

It must be noted that these Catholic writers are not formal pacifists. They admit the traditional theory of the "just war" but feel that this concept is no longer viable. At the same time they attack the extreme argument that Christianity must be by its very nature pacifistic. One of the writers blames this idealistic view for encouraging the opposite cynical extreme, "doublethink about double effect." The book questions the moral honesty of manufacturing and stockpiling nuclear weapons while "suspending the decision to use them." It questions the morality of using nuclear weapons even as a threat.

Another question: to what extent can the individual claim to remain uncommitted when his government pursues a policy that leads directly to nuclear war? One of the writers answers: "In modern warfare, responsibility for all that is not antecedently, clearly and publically ruled out must be accepted by anyone who in any way participates in waging the war." This means that if you go to work for Boeing with the impression that you will not have to build bombers, or for Chrysler missiles with a mental reservation that you won't manufacture anything with a warhead, you remain partly responsible for the nuclear war which you have helped to prepare, even though you may have had "good intentions" and desired nothing but to make an "honest living."

Problems facing the individual conscience are doubtless crucially important, but it would be of little use for individuals to fold their arms with a sweet smile and a pure heart and refuse to take part in political life. The moral and political problems are inextricable from one another, and it is only by sane political action that we can fully satisfy the moral requirements that face us today as Christians. The clarification of the basic moral issue of nuclear war is an all-important first step: but there is much to be done after that. What faces us all, Christians and non-Christians alike, is the titantic labor of trying to change the world from a camp of warring barbarians into a peaceful international community from which war has been perpetually banned. Chances of success in this task seem almost ludicrously impossible. Yet if we fail to face this responsibility we will certainly lose everything.

The immediate responsibility of Christians is to contribute whatever they can to an atmosphere of sanity and trust in which negotiation and disarmament may eventually become feasible. But if they continue in ignorance, suspicion, resentment and hatred of Communism, forgetting that the Communist, whatever his failings, is also a human being who might conceivably want peace, they may do more than anyone else to foment the blind, unchristian, murderous rage which makes war inevitable.

Christianity and Defense in the Nuclear Age

We have to recognize that the chief deficiency in theological evaluations of our present situation is that we have not at all caught up with the realities of our time. Our task at present cannot possibly be one of arriving at *clear and definite* solutions. It must first of all be a matter of estimating the work to be done, clearing ground, readjusting our views to the essentially new, tragically critical situation in which the entire human race finds itself. As Christians first of all, in a crisis where the very existence of man and the continuation of life itself are at stake, our duty to God the Creator becomes a duty to strive in every way to preserve and protect His creation. Our duty is to help save humanity for which Christ died. We cannot contemn man, or disregard his plight, and allege loyalty to abstract beliefs as an excuse, still less as a *reason* for policies based on hatred and destructiveness. To "kill Commies for Christ" is to admit that one has lost all sense of the meaning of the gospel of Christ.

It is in view of this task that we must first of all clearly state, not as a solution to problems, but as a prerequisite for considering the problem in its reality: that it is the unanimous judgment of *all* really serious religious, philosophical, social, psychological thought today that *total war* (whether nuclear or conventional) is both immoral and suicidal. This is so clear that it seems to require little discussion or proof. For a Catholic, there are the very clear statements of Pius XII and John XXIII. Even the theologians, whether Catholic or Protestant, who still insist that *war itself* can still be resorted to as a solution to international conflicts, and who therefore recommend strong military measures of defense, agree in practice that *total war* must be condemned not only as immoral but also as impractical and self-defeating. All who have a serious knowledge of the power of nuclear weapons and the extreme danger of the situation that has been created by the Cold War and the arms race realize that resort to a nuclear attack would unleash destruction which probably neither antagonist would survive.

This does not prevent politicians, and entire nations, from supporting a colossal war effort, on a scale never before dreamed of. It does not prevent the masses of "Christian" people from *taking it for granted* that nuclear war is not only a reasonable but even a Christian solution to the problem of Communism, at least in the sense that while no one "wants war," there is an inescapable necessity to act in a warlike and "tough" manner, to preserve our way of life and indeed our religion itself. It must be noticed that in doing this, Christians are actually aligning themselves with pragmatists for whom the moral issue is totally irrelevant. In taking this line of thought, Christians are working with the forces which are, in fact, most inimical to Christianity.

The problem, on the practical level, is urgent.

It is one in which Christians are and must be deeply involved. It is the problem of evaluating *the critical situation of humanity* in its totality, so that we may see the one problem of war in its whole context, and may also be able to work toward alternative solutions to international and national problems. It is a matter of primary urgency to see our way clear to other solutions than those presently being worked out by the military, by industry, and by the politicians who follow the suggestions and exhortations of the military-industrial complex.

The Christian has a duty, as a Christian, to contribute everything he can to help this great common work: *of finding nonmilitary and nonviolent ways of defending our rights, our interests, and our ideals.*

And yet in actual fact it seems that Christians, as much as anybody else, are contributing very much to the dangerous tensions and the irrational state of mind which is obsessed with the fear of disaster and is fixated on one hope: nuclear defense. It is Christians who are, as loudly as anyone else, clamoring for an unbeatable missile defense system—all of course in the name of "peace." And it is Christians who, as much as anybody else, are refusing even to consider possible alternatives to this line of action. It is Christians who most loudly and passionately support policies of overkill.

The following very schematic notes are an outline of a few approaches to the problem. They are more an evaluation of present modes of thought than a constructive program of change. We have to begin at the bottom, we are very poor in ideas and insights, we have barely started to wake up to our position.

One thing is very certain: inadequate and worn-out ideas must be discarded. Importance of our thinking and our information. Importance of a public opinion that is not fanatical and wild, but informed by reasonable as well as Christian principles and looking toward a worldwide cooperation in solving the critical problems of our time. We must recognize that fanatical nationalism and racism are prime causes of moral blindness—especially when they appeal most stridently to "moral principles."

1. *Imperfect Approaches:*
We rule out at the start all the extreme, fanatical, bellicose solutions. On the side of those who work for peace:

a. The conventional "pacifist" position is inadequate, if by this we mean a peace movement of individuals associated in a protest based on personal objections of conscience.

Not a question of individual conscience alone.

A problem for all men, a worldwide social question. Protest is not enough. Objection not enough. Personal withdrawal not enough.

b. A radical and sweeping policy of "unilateral disarmament." It is naïve, and would do more harm than good. Takes no account of important realities: the state of shock in which millions of people already are, and which would be magnified thousands of times over if the "only means of defense" were suddenly taken away. Might precipitate a war. On the other hand *unilateral initiatives* in *gradual* steps toward disarmament are imperative. These steps must be serious and courageous, and we must realize that they would add greatly to the prestige of the nation that could make them a sign of confidence, determination and strength. But such strength implies *alternatives* to military defense.

c. A purely "spiritual" witness. Is not enough. Simply to stand up and say that the world is wicked and is traveling toward an apocalyptic doom, and that the Christian is an individual witness, or the Church is a witness purely and simply calling man to repentance before it is too late. This is not enough. We must certainly bring the world to repentance, but we must engage with the rest of mankind in a collaborative work of social renewal, reconciliation, in a serious effort to bring about a peaceful world situation, in which men can work together to solve the enormous social problems posed by the technological and economic revolution of our time.

d. The "Just War"—"We must maintain peace, but we must also maintain justice." Characteristic of American theological thought, both Protestant and Catholic, is the idea that the *presence of nuclear weapons does nothing to alter the traditional just war theory*. I am not a "pacifist" in the sense that I would reject even the *theory* of the just war. I agree that even today a just war might *theoretically* be possible. But I also think we must take into account a totally new situation in which the danger of any war escalating to all-out proportions makes it imperative to find other ways of resolving international conflicts. In practice the just war theory has become irrelevant.

Niebuhr and Dunn: Let us examine their position. They

claim a "just war" is still possible and demand a strong defensive posture (military). Yet they make the following admissions:

i. The only form of just war they envisage is a *limited* war *of defense aimed at "preventing conquest and forcing an end of hostilities." No* war aiming to bring about the "unconditional surrender and punishment of aggression" can fit (they declare) this definition of a "just war." Presumably the action of Kennedy in the Cuba crisis fits the definition.

[*A Personal Opinion on the Cuba Crisis:* Conflict cannot be avoided. And at the present time the threat of violence in conflict is also to be expected. The fact that this is a "necessary" evil does not excuse us from trying our best to get into a situation where violence will NOT be so necessary and so imminent. Actually Kennedy's action was extremely risky. It nearly precipitated a nuclear war, and could have done so. But at the same time it can be said that it perhaps forestalled a nuclear war (the American military might have become exceedingly trigger-happy if a lot of missile bases were operative in Cuba). It is useless to expect all problems to be suddenly solved innocently without further ado. But are we going in the right direction at all? This was perhaps a "solution" of sorts, but it must not be regarded as *adequate* and taken as a pattern or precedent.]

ii. Niebuhr and Dunn then *exclude* a nuclear crusade against Communism and indeed the current war thinking does not clearly seem to fit their formula. Yet in effect they *are giving support* to the policies of Washington as they now are, in all their ambiguity. Hence their qualifications about limited war are practically irrelevant.

2. *A quick look at the military policies, and some of the contradictions involved for a Christian:*
   a. *Counterforce*—Theoretically this is a nuclear policy which can more easily be made to fit the moral theology books. It is a policy of preemptive attack on the enemy's missile bases (not on his cities). ACTUALLY IT IS THE MOST DANGEROUS POLICY. It is the one more and more favored in Washington, and the one which promises the most serious risk of preemptive first strike on the part of the enemy. And the inevitable consequences.
   b. *Deterrence*—The idea of threatening enemy cities from invulnerable missile sites. This might be harder to reconcile with the moral theology books, because the targets are frankly cities. But then the idea is that the missiles will "never be used." In practice, the missile sites invite preemptive first strike.
   c. In actual fact, both policies are in full swing (the "Mix").

   To support these policies is in effect to become a partner in extremely dangerous actions which, in the opinion of scientists like Leo Szilard, will lead to war within the next ten years. *Nuclear* war!

Note also the possibility of nuclear accidents, miscalculation, unintended acts of war.

Note some other ambiguities in our policy situation:

Our commitment to defend Berlin, which cannot possibly be defended with conventional weapons. Ergo: practical commitment to use of nuclear weapons even to "save face" if "necessary."

Note also: the theoretician who splits hairs about "just war" and makes nice distinctions in journals for experts is actually supporting the military mind and military policies, which imply no such fine distinctions at all.

We know that the military mind has one objective: to WIN at all costs. To completely subdue the adversary. This is common to extremists on both sides.

This is the thinking of the people who have the weapons on both sides.

The theologians may have nice thoughts about just war.

The military are above all concerned with *not being soft,* not showing fear, not being intimidated, not losing face.

This game of chicken by politicians and strategists is abetted and supported by Christians as a whole.

The state of affairs is this: men with nuclear weapons will use them when they think the situation is sufficiently critical. And they will not use them with any regard for restraints demanded by moral theologians.

To cooperate with them *now* is to share in their responsibility *then.*

3. *Summary of the Policy Situation:*

In theory our government rejects recourse to total nuclear war. We do not have a "policy of total war," the all-out destruction of Russia or China (though some extremists favor even that).

But the "mix" and the arms race add up, in fact, to a policy of total war. A policy of total war and unconditional victory is immoral and suicidal. What is essentially a power struggle is presented as an ideological and spiritual struggle, as a battle between light and darkness, and it is presented in such a way that CHRISTIANS ARE CONVINCED THERE IS NO OTHER WAY OF DEFENSE THAN MILITARY DEFENSE, that the surest defense is a fantastic arms build-up, and that the "strategists know best."

Hence it is taken for granted that any questioning of the present policies for defense is an implicit treason both to democracy and to Christianity. In actual fact, the first job we have is to open the way to clear thinking and investigation of *other methods of defense.*

It is definitely not a matter of renouncing defense, of giving in to Communism. It must be made quite clear that we intend to defend our ideals and our freedom. But that we also as Christians reject a form of defense which has now clearly become immoral and suicidal (we should have known this about war long ago, the First World War told us all we needed to know if earlier wars had not). And as Christians we want to take the lead in helping to discover the efficacy of *nonviolent methods of defense.*

4. *The Study of Alternatives:*
   a. Realize what we are up against. The military-industrial-political-academic complex, with the mass media at its disposal, is sold on military defense and the arms race and is obviously interested in ridiculing or discrediting all nonmilitary forms of defense—in fact all alternatives to the arms race.

      International negotiation for peace cannot be taken fully seriously in this climate, where it is assumed there is *no* alternative to nuclear armament on a colossal scale.
   b. Realize, however, that in the presence of formidable opposition and mistrust we must mobilize for the preservation of the human race, by a transformation of all the attitudes and methods that now govern our thought and action in politics.

      Christian thinking has to transform political attitudes!

      This means overcoming the "split" between the sacred and the profane, the spiritual and the political.
   c. We have got to get people to face the *moral evil* of nuclear war, and see the full moral and spiritual dimensions of the problem.
   d. We have got to support every kind of action that involves:
      —serious dialogue
      —genuine reciprocity
      —international understanding
      —social justice: removal of *causes* of war and unrest.
   e. We have got to see the spiritual and psychological evils in our own current social situation as a vitally important part of the problem:
      —boredom
      —tension
      —affluence
      —individualism and irresponsibility
   f. Study the positive meaning of nonviolent defense:
      —its *efficacy* as defense
      —its *clarity* in stating our will to resist
      —its *opportunities* for heroism and dedication.

Target Equals City[1]

There is one winner, only one winner, in war. The winner is war itself. Not truth, not justice, not liberty, not morality. These are the vanquished. War wins, reducing them to complete submission. He makes truth serve violence and falsehood. He causes justice to declare not what is just but what is expedient as well as cruel. He reduces the liberty of the victorious side to a servitude equal to that of the tyranny which they attacked, in defense of liberty. Though moralists may intend and endeavor to lay down rules for war, in the end war lays down rules for them. He does not find it hard to make them change their minds. If he could, he would change God's own mind. War has power to transmute evil into good and good into evil. Do not fear that he will not exercise this power. Now more than ever he is omnipotent. He is the great force, the evil mystery, the demonic mover of our century, with his globe of sun-fire, and his pillar of cloud. Worship him.

It took five years for war to turn the Christian ethic of the "just war" inside out. The years 1940 to 1945 completely revolutionized the moral thinking of the allies who were fighting totalitarianism with a *just cause* if ever there was one.

Certainly no cause can be absolutely just and pure. You can always find something wrong with it. But for those who accepted the traditional doctrine on war, there was not much doubt that Hitler was the aggressor, and that we were the defenders.

When the Japanese bombed Pearl Harbor, there was no question about the morality of America's entering the war to defend its rights.

1. The facts in this article are taken mostly from a recent detailed study of the events which shaped the decision to use the A-bomb at the end of World War II. *The Irreversible Decision, 1939–1950* by Robert C. Batchelder (Houghton Mifflin) is a clear and persuasive plea for a clear and definite ethical stand in regard to nuclear war, in place of the vague and unprincipled pragmatism which guides decisions today. Our meditation can serve as a review and a recommendation of this book.

Here was a very clear example of a "just cause" for war. Few doubted the fact. Those who did so were regarded as foolish because they were against all war on principle. They thought war was intrinsically evil. Twenty years later one is tempted to wonder if they were not more wise than men believed them to be.

At the end of World War II, many theologians openly began to discuss the question whether the old doctrine of the just war had any meaning. It seemed to them at that time that the obliteration bombing of cities on both sides, culminating in the total destruction of Hiroshima and Nagasaki by one plane with one bomb for each, had completely changed the nature of war. Traditional standards no longer applied because, for one thing, there was no longer any distinction made between civilian and combatant. Where this distinction was obliterated, or tended to be obliterated, war could not be considered just. Double effect could no longer be taken seriously when you "permitted" (without intending it) the slaughter of fifty thousand civilians in order to stop production in three or four factories. There was no proportion between the "permitted" evil and the "intended" good. (Investigation showed that even when there had been massive damage and countless deaths inflicted by obliteration bombing, the factories themselves were not always crippled for very long, and soon resumed production.)

Double effect was completely out of the question when the slaughter of civilians was explicitly *intended* as a means to "breaking enemy morale" and thus breaking his "will to resist." This was pure terrorism, and the traditional doctrine of war excluded such immoral methods. Traditional morality also excluded torture of prisoners, murder of hostages chosen at random, extermination of racial groups for no reason other than race, etc. These methods were practiced by the enemy, and after the war ended *they were bequeathed to the Western nations.* France in Algeria, for instance.

How did precision bombing, (allowed by traditional standards of justice) turn into obliteration bombing? How did ethical theory gradually come to defend obliteration bombing, and even mass destruction by atomic weapons? How did we gradually reach our present position where the traditional doctrine of the just war has been so profoundly modified that it is almost unrecognizable? How is it that we are now almost ready to permit any outrage, any excess, any horror, on the grounds that it is a "lesser evil" and "necessary" to save our nation?

The deliberate terroristic annihilation of defenseless civilians for military and political purposes, is perhaps not completely new. In all ages there has been calculated terrorism, the slaughter of innocents in war. It was never seriously considered as either very necessary or very useful in the actual process of winning a war. It was more or less of a "bonus." (You remember perhaps the report on the raid that annihilated Dresden? The city was full of refugees fleeing from the Russians in the east. The death of several thousand extra victims was announced with sober joy as a "bonus" by those who commanded the raid.)

Traditional Christian teaching, which deplored war itself even under the best of conditions, never hesitated to condemn terrorism in war as a very grave crime. Now terrorism is no longer taken so seriously. It has become "necessary," the "only effective defense," and of course defense is a "duty." Hence we are seriously told that it is the "duty" of our government to arm to the teeth with nuclear weapons capable of wiping out whole cities, whole nations. A conservative estimate declares that the United States probably now stocks the equivalent in explosive power of *ten tons of TNT for every human being on the face of the earth.* We are generously going beyond the limits of strict duty, just in case.

Terror from the air, as a deliberately planned policy, was characteristic of the Nazi and Fascist Axis. As a matter of fact the honor of having initiated it in Europe belongs to Catholic nations: Franco's Spain and Fascist Italy. The place? Guernica, a Christian city, in the Christian province of the Basques, in Christian Spain. Date: 1937. Also please remember Nanking, China. Same year. Not so many Christians. We protested.

Poland was the next victim. Reduced to nothing in a few days by the Luftwaffe. 1939. England came next.

It is to the everlasting credit of the British that although the civilians of England suffered one crushing blow after another, and saw whole sections of their cities reduced to rubble, the government declared that the RAF would abide by traditional methods, and would confine itself to the strategic bombing of military targets only. But since daylight raids were very costly, most of the attacks had to be carried out at night. This made precision bombing very difficult, and in the end civilians suffered more than industry. So "area bombing," the destruction of the whole neighborhood that included a military target, was already British policy by the time America came into the war. America determined to stick to the traditional ethical code. Roosevelt at first announced that the AAF would confine itself to strategic bombing.

By 1942, however, England abandoned its quixotic attachment to standards which were simply preventing the RAF raids from being fully effective. At least that was what the RAF thought. It was Air Marshal Sir Arthur Travers Harris who opened up with obliteration bombing against German cities in 1942. Not only was this aimed at the "sure" destruction of factories and military objectives that might otherwise be missed, but frankly and explicitly the intention was to "destroy enemy morale." "There are no lengths in violence to which we will not go" to achieve this end, declared Churchill. And another government spokesman, unidentified, said, "Our plans are to bomb, burn and ruthlessly destroy, in every way available to us, the people responsible for creating this war."

Here we have already one complete cycle. A country begins a defensive "just war." It starts by declaring its firm adherence to the ethical principles held by its Church, and by the majority of its civilian population. The nation accepts unjust suffering heroically. But then the military begins to grow impatient, seeing that its own methods of retaliation are not effective. It is *the military that changes the policy.* The new, more ruthless policy pays off. The civilian protest is silenced before it begins. Those who might otherwise have objected come to believe what they are told: "This will save lives. It is necessary to end the war sooner, and to punish the unjust aggressor."

The standards of justice are still in view—still *partially* in view. The injustice of the aggressor is very clearly seen. Justice in the use of means has been lost sight of, and what counts most is expediency.

We cannot lightly blame the courageous people who suffered so much and were so eager for the war to end. But . . . The allies had come around to adopting the same methods precisely, the same ruthless inhumanity which made the enemy unjust. Injustice was now common to both sides. Needless to say, both were now strenuously arguing and convincing themselves, in exactly the same terms, that their war effort was just, that their methods were just, and that it was necessary to do all that they did in order to win the victory, end the war quickly and "save lives."

Note also, on both sides there were sincere Catholics, encouraged by the clergy and by the Catholic press to accept and support these claims. There were therefore Catholics believing that each side was completely just. Catholics on both sides "served God" by killing each other. . . . What had become of the meaning of the doctrine of the "just war"? What had become of Christian ethics in this situation? Did anyone stop to reflect on the total absurdity of this self-contradiction on the part of Christians? Not the least appalling contradiction lay in the fact that German Christians heroically sacrificed themselves to defend a government that cruelly persecuted the Church. In defense of Hitler's neopaganism which advocated a totally immoral policy they fought their fellow Christians of France, England and America.

Just war? Just cause? Just methods? Double effect?

Now America was in the war. America was obviously going to follow the tactics England had been forced to take over from the Nazis by the very logic of the war. The USAF soon began obliteration bombing. A protest was published in *Fellowship,* the magazine of the Fellowship of Reconciliation, in 1944. Obliteration bombing was condemned by this magazine and by a group of Protestant ministers. The protest was taken seriously enough to get an official reply. Roosevelt said that these tactics were necessary to "shorten the war." There was a nationwide discussion of the issue. Americans were fifty to one against those who protested. They thought the moral scruples of these pacifists were ridiculous. To demand cessation of obliteration bombing was pure defeatism.

All distinction between precision bombing and obliteration bombing was forgotten in the general indignation. What mattered was to beat Hitler and right the wrong that had been done. Any methods that helped procure this end were justifiable.

One dissenting voice was that of a Catholic priest, Father John C. Ford, S.J., who argued that the obliteration bombing of cities was immoral and could not be defended by the principle of double effect.

Meanwhile the United States was working feverishly to develop the atomic bomb, believing that Hitler's scientists were on the point of perfecting this weapon that would multiply thousands of times the destructiveness of ordinary bombing.

However, before the atomic bomb was tested, the B29 bomber command in the Pacific had come to realize the failure of precision bombing of Japanese military targets. It was not possible to seriously slow down production by this means.

Early in 1945, General Curtis LeMay decided, on his own responsibility, to initiate a devastating new tactic of massive low-flying fire raids delivered at night.

On the night of March 9–10 the whole of Tokyo was set afire with napalm bombs. The blaze was so furious that it boiled the water of the canals. Fire storms consumed all the oxygen, and many who were not burned to death suffocated. So frightful were the effects of this raid that it claimed as many casualties as the Atom bombing of Hiroshima.

Some apologists for all-out war point to this fact, saying that since there is in reality no difference between total war carried on by conventional weapons and total war carried on by nuclear weapons, there is no new moral issue involved. On the contrary, this calls for a clarification of the real moral issue. The issue is precisely this: not that atomic and nuclear weapons are immoral while conventional weapons are just, but that *any resort to terrorism and total annihilation is unjust, whatever be the weapons it employs.*

The Tokyo raid, followed by similar raids on more than fifty other Japanese cities, was justified on the grounds that much of the Japanese war effort depended on the "phantom industry," the detailed piecework on small parts carried on by individuals in their homes. Hence residential areas came to be just as "legitimate" a target as factories themselves. This fact contributed to the loose generalization, now widely accepted, without further qualifications, that "in modern war everyone is to be considered a combatant." Hence even residential areas became "military targets." No more need for double effect!

Already in May and June of 1945 the American High Command was considering the choice of an appropriate target for the new bomb.

In discussing the choice of target, Truman and his advisers did not speak of this or that naval base, this or that fortress, this or that concentration of troops, this or that particular munitions plant. In Truman's own words: "Stimson's staff had *prepared a list of cities* in

Japan that might serve as targets. . . ." Later in the context Truman speaks of the entire city of Hiroshima as a "military target."

We must remember that in the list of cities originally considered was Kyoto, which is a religious and not a military center at all.

There were, of course, industries at Hiroshima, but its "military" importance was such that it had hardly been touched so far. It had even been neglected by LeMay's incendiaries.

In other words, the "targets" considered for the Atomic bomb were purely and simply cities. Any city at all, by the mere fact of being a city, was now a "military target." The fact that Kyoto was among them indicates that moral and psychological effect, in other words terrorism, was the dominant consideration in the minds of the high command.

Hiroshima was chosen in order that an "untouched" target might show the power of the bomb. The idea was to unleash the maximum destructive power on a civilian center, to obliterate that center and destroy all further will to resist in the Japanese nation. The word "target" and the word "city" had become completely identified.

Once again, moral thinking had gone through a full cycle in the short space of two or three years. The United States had entered the war with the conviction of the justice of its cause and with the firm intention to abide by just means.

However, it is possible that the notion of "just means" was much more nebulous in the American mind than it had been in the English. Moral thinking guided by pragmatic principles tends to be very vague, very fluid. Moral decisions were now a series of more or less opportunistic choices based on short-term guesses of possible consequences, rather than on definite moral principles.

It is quite certain that though the American public conscience was characterized by a certain undefined sense of decency and fittingness in these matters, a sense more or less attributable to the vestiges of Christian tradition, this "moral sense" easily yielded to the more practical dictates of the situation.

The moral decision to use the bomb, without warning, on a Japanese city was dictated by the urgent desire to end the war promptly, without having to sacrifice thousands of American combatants in the planned invasion of the Japanese archipelago. Once again, the idea was "to punish the unjust aggressor" and to "save American lives." Certainly few Americans, before the bomb was dropped, would have questioned the validity of these considerations. The war had to be ended, and this was the way to do it.

It was not generally known that Japan was trying to establish diplomatic contacts with the allies through Russia in order to work out a negotiated peace instead of the unconditional surrender relentlessly demanded by the allies. Neither invasion of Japan nor use of the bomb was absolutely necessary for peace. However, the war mentality of the time made it impossible for policy-makers to see this. They were convinced the bomb was necessary and their conviction overwhelmed all other considerations.

Nevertheless the use of the bomb on two open cities was a dire injustice and an atrocity.

Even after the war ended, a questionnaire conducted by *Fortune* revealed that half the respondents felt the decision to use the bomb on Hiroshima and Nagasaki had been right, while nearly a quarter of them *regretted that more atomic bombs* had not been used on other Japanese cities! Such was, and is, the general moral climate in the U.S.A.

At the same time, the terrible effects of the bomb produced a moral shock and profound revulsions in certain quarters in America. Religious groups and publications protested more or less vehemently. Catholic voices, notably those of the *Commonweal*, the *Catholic World* and, of course, the *Catholic Worker* were raised against the "sin" of the bomb. But it is to be noted that *America* already took a much more "realistic" and complacent view of the event.

In general, articulate protest against the bomb on moral grounds has been confined to a minority. The majority of Americans have "sincerely regretted" the necessity to use it, they have, in a word, "felt bad" about it. But that is all. These decent sentiments have very easily yielded to other, more "practical" considerations, and the foreign policy of our country since Hiroshima, while occasionally making perfunctory gestures of respect in the direction of the Deity, has been a policy of direct reliance on the threat of atomic and nuclear annihilation.

There have of course been repeated statements of unwillingness to carry out these threats, on the vague grounds that the consequences would be too awful. The American mind in general has, however, not questioned the fundamental propriety of using the bomb. This is practically taken for granted.

As the pressures of the cold war become more intense, the fallout shelter scare has had a direct and intimate connection with the policy of nuclear deterrence. It has been clearly and explicitly part of a campaign to "engineer consent" and make nuclear war thoroughly acceptable, at least as a reasonable possibility, in the American public mind. This, in turn, is intended to convince our enemies that we "believe in" the bomb, and that, though we still utter pious hopes that it will never be necessary, we thoroughly intend to use it if we feel ourselves to be sufficiently threatened.

Here, then, is the moral situation:

1. There has been a complete breakdown in the old notion of the "just war" as accepted for centuries by Christian ethics and international law. As far as policy-makers are concerned, this concept has now become completely irrelevant. It has been supplanted by the concept of "limited war," which has no ethical connotations, but is simply "tactical" and is designed to avoid the more disastrous effects of an

all-out war of annihilation. The "value" of a limited war, with or without tactical nuclear weapons, is that there is more of a chance that it may theoretically be "won" by one side or the other. At the same time, there seems to be every reason to believe that if one of the belligerents feels himself to be losing a limited war, he will resort to retaliation on the megatonic scale, and the war will become "total."

2. Moralists, while still clinging more or less resolutely to the idea that obliteration of civilian centers is evil (some show very little resolution in their attachment to this principle!) strive in general to patch up the traditional notion of just war and keep it functioning, by tying it up with the "limited" war of the tacticians. This ends by being a rather Pickwickian position, and in actual fact the moralists who still try to reconcile traditional notions with the new situation seek means of justifying massive nuclear retaliation as "self-defense."

Though no clear official pronouncement in this matter has been made by the Church, the repeated warnings of the Popes and their strong pleas for peace have insisted on the traditional principle that the rights of unarmed and noncombatant civilians must be respected and that failure to take these rights into account is a grave crime. Military policy, on the other hand, has completely discarded all consideration of these rights, except in perfunctory statements designed to assuage the scruples of the old-fashioned.

Theologians remain divided, but a strong and articulate group, especially in Europe, have taken their stand on the "relative pacifist" position which would outlaw all nuclear war and work for disarmament as the course of action most consistent with Christian morality.

It must be confessed that these issues are not as widely or as thoroughly discussed as they might be. The relative pacifist position does not get a very good hearing in the press, especially in the United States. The average Catholic is left with the impression that nuclear deterrence and the annihilation of Russian cities by H-bombs is *encouraged* by the Church, or at least left indifferently to the judgment of governments and military commands. The Church is by no means indifferent on this point. This fact is obscured because the moral thinking not only of the Christian laity but also of the clergy has been seriously confused by the mass media.

The Christian moral sense is being repeatedly eroded and worn down by the effect of the "cycles" we have described. A new policy is adopted on grounds that appear to be fully "just." Then, when the "ethical" means are found to be less expedient, more drastic measures are resorted to. Those violate justice, but the justification of them by publicists further weakens the moral sense of Christians. Occasional shocks momentarily reawaken this moral sense. There are protests and questions. Soothing answers are provided by policy-makers and religious spokesmen are ready to support them with new adjustments. A new cycle is prepared. Once again there is a "just cause." Few stop to think that what is now regarded complacently as "justice" was clearly a crime twenty years ago.

How long can Christian morality go on taking this kind of beating?

There is only one winner in war. That winner is not justice, not liberty, not Christian truth.

The winner is war itself.

The Machine Gun in the Fallout Shelter

The October issue of the *Catholic Worker* carried an article by me entitled "The Root of War" which is in reality an excerpt from a book to be published in December, *New Seeds of Contemplation.* This article did not intend to enter directly into the current controversy about the legitimacy of defending one's own safety in a fallout shelter by keeping others out at the point of a gun. However, discussion of the article has involved me in the controversy and therefore an explicit statement of my position has become necessary.

What precisely is the issue? Is it just a speculative question in moral philosophy? If so, the answer is simple. Speculatively, since every man retains a natural right to defend his life and protect his family, and indeed has an obligation to do so, especially where his family is concerned, there is no doubt that a man has a right to kill someone else if that is the only way he can protect his family and save his own life.

However this is more than a speculative question. This grave problem has to be seen in the light of very extraordinary circumstances. We are in the midst of what is perhaps the most crucial moral and spiritual crisis the human race has ever faced during its history. We are all deeply involved in this crisis, and consequently the way each individual faces the crisis has a definite bearing on the survival of the whole race. This does not mean that individual rights are to be sacrificed without further discussion. But it does mean that the *way* in which each individual protects his own rights is a matter of great importance. Therefore, while each individual certainly retains the right to defend his life and protect his own family, we run the risk of creating a very dangerous mentality and opening the way to moral chaos if we give the impression that from here on out it is just every man for himself, and the devil take the hindmost. This is not only fundamentally unchristian, but it is immoral on the purely natural level and is finally disastrous even to the political interests of our nation.

Here I would like to say in parentheses that I have not yet had an opportunity for studying the various statements that have been made by others on this question, and I am by no means accusing the writers who emphasize the right of self-defense of cynically opening the way to moral anarchy. I am just saying that if their position is not properly understood and qualified, many people may draw the wrong conclusions from it: for instance that the Church condones violence on the slightest pretext.

For that reason I think it is supremely important first of all to emphasize the *fully Christian view of the situation.* Certainly a man owes protection to his family and dependents. No one questions that. Let it be quite clear that even nonviolent resistance not only recognizes but emphasizes this fundamental duty. There is no such thing as legitimate nonviolent passivity in this case. It is not ethically permissible for a man to stand by and let his helpless dependents be killed or overrun. Nonviolent resistance is *active and positive.* It takes very definite steps to protect rights, but these steps are nonviolent in the sense that self-sacrifice for the sake of truth and rights takes precedence over everything else, and especially over the use of physical force against the aggressor. The nonviolent resister has the duty to lay down his life if necessary to protect the rights of his family. He is also ready to lay down his life in defense of the truth.

I admit that the practical question of how to resist nonviolently in the case we are discussing (the fallout shelter) presents very serious difficulties. Such a case would require a real mastery of the supremely difficult and heroic technique of nonviolent resistance. In practice, where nonviolent resistance is impossible, *then violent resistance must be used, rather than passive acquiescence.* I must emphasize this point very strongly, because it is generally unknown or misunderstood. Merely passive acquiescence in evil is in no sense to be dignified by the name of nonviolence. It is a travesty of Christian meekness. It is purely and simply the sin of cowardice. Those who imagine that this kind of apathy is nonviolent resistance are doing a great disservice to the cause of truth and confusing heroism with degenerate and apathetic passivity. Hence even the proponent of nonviolence will allow that in practice a man might use force to protect the safety of his family in a fallout shelter, assuming that he was not able to solve the problem in a legitimately nonviolent manner.

This does not alter the fact that it is both misleading and dangerous to place too much stress on the image of a man defending himself with a machine gun and to ignore other important Christian perspectives. There are other images we can keep in mind. Let us not forget that the supreme example of nonviolent resistance to evil is the Crucifixion of Our Lord Jesus Christ, in which the Incarnate Son of God destroyed sin by taking the sins of the world upon Himself and dying on the Cross, while forgiving the men who were putting Him to death. Far from being an act of mere helpless passivity, as Nietzsche and other moderns claim, this was a free and willing acceptation of suffering in the most positive and active manner. The activity in this case was hidden and spiritual. It was an exercise of the supremely dynamic spiritual force of divine Love. A Christian is committed to the belief that Love and Mercy are the most powerful forces on earth. Hence every Christian is bound by his baptismal vocation to seek, as far as he can, with God's grace to make those forces effective in his life, to the point where they dominate all his actions. Naturally, no one is bound to *attain* to the full perfection of charity. But a Christian who forgets that this is his goal ceases by that fact to live and act as a genuine Christian. We must strive, then, to imitate Christ and His sacrifice, in so far as we are able. We must keep in mind His teaching that supreme love consists in laying down one's life for one's friends. This means that a Christian will never purely and simply allow himself to develop a state of mind in which, forgetting his Christian ideal, he thinks in purely selfish and pragmatic terms. Our rights certainly remain, but they do not entitle us to develop a hard-boiled, callous, selfish outlook, a "me first" attitude. This is that rugged individualism which is so unchristian and which modern movements in Catholic spirituality have so justly deplored.

There is another and very grave aspect of the present problem. It is a purely practical and political aspect. What is going to happen to this country if it is suddenly attacked and all the citizens fly into a panic and start shooting each other up? Not only is this a very serious and actual danger, but it is undoubtedly *an important part in the well-calculated policy of Communism.* Why do you suppose Khrushchev has given worldwide publicity to his crescendo of nuclear tests? Do you suppose this has been totally unrelated to the near panic in some quarters in the United States? Let us consider for a moment a statement made some years ago by one of our own missile experts, Dr. James B. Edson. He says: "It is of course more artful and sophisticated and sometimes more economical to use one of the agents (nuclear, biological, or *psychological*) AS A CATALYST CAUSING THE TARGET TO DESTROY ITSELF BY ITS OWN ENERGY. THIS CAN BE DONE TO AMMUNITION DUMPS AND PEOPLE. IT CAN ALSO BE DONE TO ENEMIES AND NATIONS, CAUSING THEM TO MANEUVER ENDLESSLY IN RESPONSE TO THREATS THEY CANNOT FORESEE OR CANNOT FORESTALL."

In other words our moral theologians, in their innocence, do not take into account the almost infinitely subtle reasoning of the men of war. They do not reckon with the vast scope and probing calculations of power politicians and military technicians in the nuclear age. We are not just fighting with nuclear weapons. We are in a war that is total in the sense that it exploits every available resource, and one of the most explosive forces in this warfare is *the psychology of the helpless civilian.* Let us for the love of heaven wake up to the fact that our own minds are just as filled with dangerous power today as the nuclear bombs themselves. And let us be very careful how we unleash the pent-up forces in the minds of others. The hour is extremely grave. The guarded statements of moral theologians are a small matter compared to the constant deluge of irresponsible opinions, criminal half-truths and murderous images disseminated by the mass media. *This problem is going to be solved in our thoughts, in our spirit* or not at all. It is because the minds of men have become what they have become that the world is poised on the brink of total disaster. Those of us who can help in some feeble way to guide and educate consciences must take account of this fact, or also the consequences may be frightful. They may be frightful anyway, but at least we must take stock of our situation and strive as far as possible to reorientate ourselves in the light of conditions that often make theoretical solutions of moral cases pitifully inadequate.

Peace: A Religious Responsibility

Between 1918 and 1939 religious opposition to war was articulate and widespread, all over Europe and America. Peace movements of significant proportions were active in Germany, Britain, and the United States. Yet they were crushed without difficulty and almost without protest by totalitarian regimes on the one hand, and silenced by the outbreak of a clearly defensive war on the other. Since 1945 there has been nothing to compare with the earlier movements of protest. Instead we have witnessed the enormous and crudely contrived fiction of the Communist Peace Movement which has been accepted with disillusioned resignation on one side of the Iron Curtain while, on the other, it has managed to make almost all efforts of independent civilian or religious groups to oppose nuclear war seem dishonest or subversive.

Yet never was opposition to war more urgent and more necessary than now. Never was religious protest so badly needed. Silence, passivity, or outright belligerence seem to be characteristic official and unofficial Christian reactions to the H-bomb. True, there has been some theological and ethical debate. This debate has been marked above all by a seemingly inordinate hesitation to characterize the uninhibited use of nuclear weapons as immoral. Of course the bomb has been condemned without equivocation by the "peace Churches" (Quakers, Mennonites, etc.). But the general tendency of Protestant and Catholic theologians has been to consider how far nuclear war could be reconciled with the traditional "just war" theory. In other words the discussion has been not so much a protest against nuclear war, still less a positive search for peaceful solutions to the problem of nuclear deterrence and ever increasing cold-war obsessions, but rather an attempt to justify, under some limited form, a new type of war which is tacitly recognized as an imminent possibility. This theological thought has tended more and more to *accept* the evil of nuclear war, considering it a lesser evil than Communist domination, and looking for some practicable way to make use of the lesser evil in order to avoid the greater.

But it would seem that a genuinely religious perspective, especially a Christian perspective, should be totally different. Therefore the purpose of the present article is to stand back from the imminent risks of the cold-war crisis, seeking to judge the problem of nuclear war not in relation to what seem to be our own interests or even our own survival, but simply in the light of moral truth. A Christian ought to consider whether nuclear war is not in itself a moral evil so great that it *cannot* be justified even for the best of ends, even to defend the highest and most sacrosanct of values.

This does not imply a purely pacifist rejection of war as such. Assuming that a "just war" is at least a theoretical possibility and granting that in a just war Christians may be bound to defend their country, the question we want to examine here is whether or not the massive and unlimited use of nuclear weapons, or the use of them in a limited first strike which is foreseen as likely to set off a global cataclysm, can be considered under any circumstances just.

The great problem is in fact that both in the East and in the West nuclear weapons are taken for granted. Nuclear war is now assumed to be a rational option or at least nuclear deterrence is accepted as a reasonable and workable way of "preserving peace." The moral issue is generally set aside as irrelevant. But if in all these cases a use of nuclear weapons even to threaten total or quasi-total destruction of an enemy is immoral, then we are living in a completely noxious situation where most of our political, economic, and even religious thinking is inseparably bound up with assumptions that may ultimately prove criminal. And if this is so, we must be prepared to face terrible consequences. For moral truth is not a sentimental luxury. It is as much a necessity to man and his society as air, water, fire, food and shelter.

This essay takes the stand that the *massive and uninhibited use of nuclear weapons,* either in attack or in retaliation, is contrary to Christian morality. And the arguments will be drawn particularly from Catholic sources. Recent Popes have declared ABC warfare (that is, atomic, biological and chemical warfare) to be a "sin, an offense and an outrage" (Pius XII). It may be quite true that these Popes have also affirmed a nation's right to defend itself by *just means,* in a *just war.* It may also be true that a theological argument for the use of "tactical nuclear weapons" may be constructed on the basis of some of the Popes' statements. But when we remember that the twenty kiloton A-bomb that was dropped on Hiroshima is now regarded as "small" and a "tactical device" and when we keep in mind that there is every probability that a force that is being beaten with small nuclear weapons will resort to big ones, we can easily see how little moral value can be found in these theorizings.

"Tactical nuclear weapons" and "limited war" with conventional forces are of course proposed with the best intentions: as a "realistic" way to avoid the horror of total nuclear warfare. Since it is claimed that men cannot get along without some kind of war, the least we can do is to insure that they will only destroy one another in thousands instead of in millions. Yet curiously enough, the restraint that would be required to keep within these limits (a restraint that was unknown on either side after the early phases of World War II), would seem to demand as much heroism and as much control as disarmament itself. It would therefore appear more realistic as well as more Christian and more humane to strive to think of total peace rather than of partial war. Why can we not do this? If disarmament were taken seriously, instead of being used as a pawn in the game of power politics, we could arrive at a workable agreement. It might not be ideal, but it would certainly be at once safer, saner and more realistic than war, whether limited or total. But we make ourselves incapable of taking either disarmament or peace with total seriousness, because we are completely obsessed with the fury and the fantasies of the cold war. The task of the Christian is to make the thought of peace once again seriously possible. A step towards this would be the rejection of nuclear deterrence as a basis for international policy. Nuclear war is totally unacceptable. It is immoral, inhuman, and absurd. It can lead nowhere but to the suicide of nations and of cultures, indeed to the destruction of human society itself.

We must now face the fact that we are moving closer and closer to war, not only as a result of blind social forces but also as the result of our own decisions and our own choice. The brutal reality is that, when all is said and done, we seem to *prefer* war; not that we want war itself, but we are blindly and hopelessly attached to all that makes war inevitable.

I The Dance of Death

No one seriously doubts that it is now possible for man and his society to be completely destroyed in a nuclear war. This possibility must be soberly faced, even though it is so momentous in all its implications that we can hardly adjust ourselves to it in a fully rational manner. Indeed, this awful threat is the chief psychological weapon of the cold war. America and Russia are playing the paranoid game of nuclear deterrence, each one desperately hoping to preserve peace by threatening the other with bigger bombs and total annihilation.

Every step in this political dance of death brings us inexorably closer to hot war. The closer we get to hot war, the more the theoretical possibility of our total destruction turns into a real probability.

There is no control over the arbitrary and belligerent self-determination of the great nations ruled by managerial power elites concerned chiefly with their own self-interest. The UN is proving itself unable to fulfil the role of international arbiter and powerless to control the pugnacity of the nuclear club. Indeed, the big powers have been content to use the UN as a forum for political and propagandist wrestling matches and have not hesitated to take independent action that led to the discrediting of the UN whenever this has been profitable to them. Hence the danger that the uncontrolled power of nuclear weapons may break loose whenever one of the belligerents feels himself sufficiently strong and sufficiently provoked to risk an all-out war. Repeated threats to use the bomb have doubtless been mostly bluff, but one day somebody's bluff is going to be called, perhaps in a very drastic fashion.

Meanwhile the United States alone possesses a stockpile of nuclear weapons estimated at 60,000 megatons. This is enough to wipe out the present civilized world and to permanently affect all life on the planet earth. These nuclear bombs can be delivered by some 2,500 planes. It is no secret that such planes are constantly in the air, ready to strike. There are 200 missiles available to U.S. forces, mostly of intermediate range, and this does not suggest the immediate likelihood of a purely push-button war. But it is estimated that by 1963 there will be two thousand more of them, of which a large proportion will be intercontinental missiles based in "hard" installations. Attack on hard installations means ground bursts and therefore more fallout as well as more bombs. Hence even an attack concentrated on our missile bases is bound to have a destructive effect on many population centers.

An ICBM can carry an H-bomb warhead to a destination five thousand miles away, twenty times faster than the speed of sound. Intermediate-range missiles can be fired from submarines and deliver H-bombs which could reduce the eastern United States to a radioactive wasteland. H-bombs will soon be fitted to satellites and will be able to reach a target within a few minutes, without hope of interception.

It must be remembered that H-bombs are relatively cheap to produce, and it is not difficult to build and deliver big ones. Poison gas can also be delivered by long-range missiles. One such gas is manufactured in quantity by the U.S. Army Chemical Corps and it can exterminate whole populations of men as if they were insects. A similar nerve gas, originally developed by the Nazis, is manufactured in Soviet Russia. This gas is considered to be more effective against civilian populations than any nuclear agent. It leaves industry and property intact and there is no fallout! Shelters offer no protection against chemical agents.

In a word, the logic of deterrence has proved to be singularly illogical, because of the fact that nuclear war is almost exclusively offensive. So far there is no indication that there can be any really effective defense against guided missiles. All the advantage goes to the force that strikes first, without warning. Hence the multiplication of "hard" weapon sites, and of "deep shelters" becomes provocative and instead of convincing the enemy of our invulnerability, it only invites a heavier preemptive attack by bigger bombs and more of them. The cost of moving a significant portion of industry, business and the population underground is prohibitive and the whole idea is in itself nonsensical, at least as a guarantee of "peace."

Far from producing the promised "nuclear stalemate" and the "balance of terror" on which we are trying to construct an improbable peace, these policies simply generate tension, confusion, suspicion, and paranoid hate. This is the climate most suited to the growth of totalitarianism. Indeed, the cold war itself promises by itself to erode the last vestiges of true democratic freedom and responsibility even in the countries which claim to be defending these values. Those who think that they can preserve their independence, their civic and religious rights by ultimate recourse to the H-bomb do not seem to realize that the mere shadow of the bomb may end by reducing their religious and democratic beliefs to the level of mere words without meaning, veiling a state of rigid and totalitarian belligerency that will tolerate no opposition.

In a world where another Hitler and another Stalin are almost certain to appear on the scene, the existence of such destructive weapons and the moral paralysis of leaders and policy-makers combined with the passivity and confusion of mass societies which exist on both sides of the Iron Curtain, constitute the gravest problem in the whole history of man. Our times can be called apocalyptic, in the sense that we seem to have come to a point at which all the hidden, mysterious dynamism of the "history of salvation" revealed in the Bible has flowered into final and decisive crisis. The term "end of the world" may or may not be one that we are capable of understanding. But at any rate we seem to be assisting at the unwrapping of the mysteriously vivid symbols in the last book of the New Testament. In their nakedness they reveal to us our own selves as the men whose lot it is to live in a time of possibly ultimate decision. In a word, the end of our civilized society is quite literally up to us and to our immediate descendants, if any. It is for us to decide whether we are going to give in to hatred, terror and blind love of power for its own sake, and thus plunge our world into the abyss, or whether, restraining our savagery, we can patiently and humanely work together for interests which transcend the limits of any national or ideological community. We are challenged to prove we are rational, spiritual and humane enough to deserve survival, by acting according to the highest ethical and spiritual norms we know. As Christians, we believe that these norms have been given to us in the Gospel and in the traditional theology of the Church.

II The Christian as Peacemaker

We know that Christ came into this world as the Prince of Peace. We know that Christ Himself is our peace (Ephesians 2:14). We believe that God has chosen for Himself, in the Mystical Body of Christ, an elect people, regenerated by the Blood of the Savior, and committed by their baptismal promise to wage war upon the evil and hatred that are in man, and help to establish the Kingdom of God and of peace.

This means a recognition that human nature, identical in all men, was assumed by the Logos in the Incarnation, and that Christ died out of love for all men, in order to live in all men. Consequently we have the obligation to treat every other man as Christ Himself, respecting his life as if it were the life of Christ, his rights as if they were the rights of Christ. Even if the other shows himself to be unjust, wicked and odious to us, we cannot take upon ourselves a final and definitive judgment in his case. We still have an obligation to be patient, and to seek his highest spiritual interests. In other words, we are formally commanded to love our enemies, and this obligation cannot be met by a formula of words. It is not enough to press the button that will incinerate a city of five million people, saying in one's heart "this hurts me more than it hurts you," or declaring that it is all for love.

As Pope John XXIII pointed out in his first encyclical letter, *Ad Petri Cathedram*, Christians are obliged to strive for peace "with all the means at their disposal" and yet, as he continues, this peace cannot compromise with error or make concessions to it. Therefore it is by no means a matter of passive acquiescence in injustice, since this does not produce peace. However, the Christian struggle for peace depends first of all upon a free response of man to "God's call to the service of His Merciful designs" (Christmas message, 1958). Christ Our Lord did not come to bring peace to the world as a kind of spiritual tranquillizer. He brought to His disciples a vocation and a task, to struggle in the world of violence to establish His peace not only in their own hearts but in society itself. This was to be done not by wishing and fair words but by a total interior revolution in which we abandoned the human prudence that is subordinated to the quest for power, and followed the higher wisdom of love and of the Cross.

The Christian is and must be by his very adoption as a son of God, in Christ, a peacemaker (Matthew 5:9). He is bound to imitate the Savior who, instead of defending Himself with twelve legions of angels (Matthew 26:55), allowed Himself to be nailed to the Cross and died praying for His executioners. The Christian is one whose life has sprung from a particular spiritual seed: the blood of the martyrs who, without offering forcible resistance, laid down their lives rather than submit to the unjust laws that demanded an official religious cult of the emperor as God. That is to say, the Christian is bound, like the martyrs, to obey God rather than the state whenever the state tries to usurp powers that do not and cannot belong to it. We have repeatedly seen Christians in our time fulfilling this obligation in a heroic manner by their resistance to dictatorships that strove to interfere with the rights of their conscience and their religion.

Hence it must be stated quite clearly and without any compromise that the duty of the Christian as a peacemaker is not to be confused with a kind of quietistic inertia which is indifferent to injustice, accepts any kind of disorder, compromises with error and with evil, and gives in to every pressure in order to maintain "peace at any price." The Christian knows well, or should know well, that peace is not possible on such terms. Peace demands the most heroic labor and the most difficult sacrifice. It demands greater heroism than war. It demands greater fidelity to the truth and a much more perfect purity of conscience. The Christian fight for peace is not to be confused with defeatism. This has to be made clear because there is a certain complacent sophistry, given free currency by the theologians who want to justify war too easily, and who like to treat anyone who disagrees with them as if he were a practical apostate from the faith who had already surrendered implicitly to Communism by refusing to accept the morality of an all-out nuclear war. This, as any one can easily see, is simply begging the question. And one feels that those who yield to this temptation are perhaps a little too much influenced by the pragmatism and opportunism of our affluent society.

There is a lot of talk, among some of the clergy, about the relative danger of nuclear war and a "Communist takeover." It is assumed, quite gratuitously, that the Communist is at the gates, and is just about to take over the United States, close all the churches, and brainwash all the good Catholics. Once this spectral assessment of the situation is accepted, then one is urged to agree that there is only one solution: to let the Reds have it before they get our government and our universities thoroughly infiltrated. This means a preemptive strike, based not on the fact that we ourselves are actually under military attack, but that we are so "provoked" and so "threatened" that even the most drastic measures are justified.

If it is argued that there can be no proportion between the awful destruction wrought by nuclear war and the good achieved by exorcising this specter of Communist domination, the argument comes back: "better dead than Red." And this, in turn, is justified by the contention that the destruction of cities, nations, populations is "only a physical evil" while Communist domination would be a "moral evil."

It must be said at once that this has no basis in logic, ethics, politics or sound moral theology. Two quotations from Pope Pius XII will suffice to establish the true Catholic perspective on these points.

The destruction of cities and nations by nuclear war is "*only a physical evil*?" Pope Pius XII calls aggressive ABC warfare a "sin, an offense and an outrage against the majesty of God." And he adds: "It constitutes a crime worthy of the most severe national and international sanctions" (Address to the World Medical Congress, 1954). Fr. John Courtney Murray, S.J., whom no one can accuse of being a "pacifist" (he favors the licity of "limited nuclear war" and also believes that such a war would have practical value) has stated, "The extreme position of favoring a war . . . simply to kill off all Communists, cannot be a legitimate Catholic opinion."

The real issue here is not actually a moral principle so much as a state of mind. This state of mind is the one which we find in the American mass media. It is made up of a large number of very superficial assumptions about what is going on in the world and about what is likely to happen. We are in a sorry state, indeed, if our survival and indeed our Christian faith itself are left entirely at the mercy of such assumptions!

III Beyond East and West

We are no longer living in a Christian world. The ages which we are pleased to call the "ages of faith" were certainly not ages of earthly paradise. But at least our forefathers officially recognized and favored the Christian ethic of love. They fought some very bloody and unchristian wars, and in doing so, they also committed great crimes which remain in history as a permanent scandal. However, certain definite limits were recognized. Today a non-Christian world still retains a few vestiges of Christian morality, a few formulas and clichés, which serve on appropriate occasions to adorn indignant editorials and speeches. But otherwise we witness deliberate campaigns to oppose and eliminate all education in Christian truth and morality. Not only non-Christians but even Christians themselves tend to dismiss the Gospel ethic of nonviolence and love as "sentimental." As a matter of fact, the mere suggestion that Christ counselled nonviolent resistance to evil is enough to invite scathing ridicule.

It is therefore a serious error to imagine that because the West was once largely Christian, the cause of the Western nations is now to be identified, without further qualification, with the cause of God. The incentive to wipe out Bolshevism with H-bombs may well be one of the apocalyptic temptations of twentieth-century Christendom. It may indeed be the most effective way of destroying Christendom, even though man may survive. For who imagines that the Asians and Africans will respect Christianity and receive it after it has apparently triggered mass murder and destruction of cosmic proportions? It is pure madness to think that Christianity can defend itself by nuclear preemption. The mere fact that we now seem to accept nuclear war as reasonable and Christian is a universal scandal.

True, Christianity is not only opposed to Communism, but in a very real sense, at war with it. However this warfare is spiritual and ideological. "Devoid of material weapons," says Pope John, "the Church is the trustee of the highest spiritual power." If the Church has no military weapons of her own, it means that her wars are fought without violence, not that she intends to call upon the weapons of nations that were once Christian, in defense of the Gospel. Whatever we may think of the ethics of nuclear war, it is clear that the message of the H-bomb is neither salvation nor "good news."

But we believe, precisely, that an essential part of the "good news" is that spiritual weapons are stronger than material ones. Indeed, by spiritual arms, the early Church conquered the entire Roman world. Have we lost our faith in this "sword of the Spirit?" Have we perhaps lost all realization of its very existence?

Of course we must repudiate a tactic of inert passivity that purely and simply leaves man defenseless, without any recourse whatever to any means of protecting himself, his rights, or Christian truth. We repeat again and again that the right, and truth, are to be defended by the most efficacious possible means, and that the most efficacious of all are precisely the spiritual ones, which have always been the only ones that have effected a really lasting moral change in society and in man. The Church tolerates defensive use of weapons only in so far as men are unable to measure up to the stricter and more heroic demands of spiritual warfare. It is absolutely unchristian to adopt, in practice, a standard of judgment which practically rejects or ignores all recourse to the spiritual weapons, and relegates them entirely to the background as if they had no efficacy whatever, and as if material weapons (the bigger the better) were the ones that really counted.

It seems that a great deal of the moral discussion about nuclear war is based, in fact, on the assumption that spiritual weapons are quixotic and worthless and that material weapons alone are worthy of serious consideration. But this attitude is precisely what leads to a fundamental vitiation of the Church's traditionally accepted doctrine on the use of violence in war: it seeks in every possible way to evade the obligation to use war only as a last resort, purely in *defense*, and with the use of *just means only*.

Inevitably, as soon as the obsession with bigger and bigger weapons takes hold of us, we make it impossible for ourselves to consider the just rights of noncombatants. We twist and deform the truth in every possible way in order to convince ourselves that noncombatants are really combatants after all, and that our "attack" is in reality "defense," while the enemy's "defense" really constitutes an "attack." By such tactics we disqualify ourselves from receiving the guidance of light and grace which will enable us to judge as spiritual men and as members of Christ. Obviously, without this special gift of light, we remain utterly incapable of seeing or appreciating the superiority of spiritual weapons, prayer, sacrifice, negotiation, and nonviolent means in general.

This results in the unhappy situation that non-Christians with rather dubious doctrinal support in irreligious philosophies have been able to take over characteristically Christian spiritual methods, appropriating them to themselves and thus further discrediting them in the eyes of the orthodox believer who is already confused by the now instinctive justification of war and weapons as the "normal" Christian way of solving international problems.

We must remember that the Church does not belong to any political power bloc. Christianity exists on both sides of the Iron Curtain and we should feel ourselves united by very special bonds with those Christians who, living under Communism, often suffer heroically for their principles.

Is it a valid defense of Christianity for us to wipe out those heroic Christians along with their oppressors, for the sake of "religious freedom"?

Let us stop and consider where the policy of massive retaliation and worse still of preemptive strike may lead us. Are we to annihilate huge population centers, at the same time showering vast areas around them with lethal fallout? Do we believe it is necessary to do this in order to protect ourselves against the menace of world Communism?

In these countries which we may perhaps be ready to annihilate, the vast majority is not Communist. On the contrary, while the people have resigned themselves passively to Communist domination, and have become quite convinced that there is no hope to be looked for from us because we are their declared enemies, and intend to wipe them out, they are by no means Communists. They do not want war. They have, in many cases, lived through the horrors and sacrifices of total war and experienced things which we are barely able to imagine. They do not want to go through this again.

We, in the name of liberty, of justice, of humanity, are pursuing a policy which promises to crush them with even greater horror, except that it may be perhaps "merciful" that millions of them will simply be blown out of existence in the twinkling of an eye. Merciful? When many of them have a Christian background, many are faithful Christians?

What good will our belligerent policy do us in those countries? None at all. It will only serve to reinforce the fatalistic conviction of the necessity of armament and of war that has been dinned into these populations by the Communist minority which dominates them.

How do we justify our readiness to wage a war of this kind? Let us face the fact that we feel ourselves terribly menaced by Communism. Certainly we believe we have to defend ourselves. Why are we menaced? Because, as time goes on, the Communists have gained a greater and greater advantage over us in the cold war. Why have they been able to do this? This is a question of historic fact, which, however, is not absolutely clear, but anyone will admit that our very reliance on the massive power of the bomb has to a great extent crippled us and restricted our freedom to maneuver, and the Communists have been operating under the *protection* of this massive threat that is too enormous to let loose for any but the most serious causes. Hence, instead of the serious provocation, the massive attack, we are confronted with a multiplicity of little threats all over the world, little advances, little gains. They all add up, but even the total of all of them does not constitute a sufficient reason for nuclear war.

But we are getting mad, and we are beginning to be thoroughly impatient with the humiliation of constant defeat. The more humiliated we become, the worse we compromise our chances, the greater errors we make.

We used to have an unrivaled reputation among the backward peoples of the world. We were considered the true defenders of liberty, justice and peace, the hope of the future. Our anger, our ignorance and our frustration have made us forfeit this tremendous advantage.

IV *Moral Passivity and Demonic Activism*

One of the most disturbing things about the Western world of our time is that it is beginning to have much more in common with the Communist world than it has with the professedly Christian society of several centuries ago. On both sides of the Iron Curtain we find two pathological varieties of the same moral sickness: both of them rooted in the same basically materialistic view of life. Both are basically opportunistic and pragmatic in their own way. And both have the following characteristics in common. On the level of *morality* they are blindly passive in their submission to a determination which, in effect, leaves men completely irresponsible. Therefore moral obligations and decisions tend to become practically meaningless. At best they are only forms of words, rationalizations of pragmatic decisions that have already been dictated by the needs of the moment.

Naturally, since not everyone is an unprincipled materialist even in Russia, there is bound to be some moral sense at work, even if only as a guilt-feeling that produces uneasiness and hesitation, blocking the smooth efficiency of machinelike obedience to immoral commands. Yet the history of Nazi Germany shows us how appalling was the irresponsibility which would carry out even the most revolting of crimes under cover of "obedience" to "legitimately constituted authority" for the sake of a "good cause." This moral passivity is the most terrible danger of our time, as the American bishops have already pointed out in their joint letters of 1960 and 1961.

On the level of political, economic and military activity, this moral passivity is balanced, or overbalanced by a *demonic activism,* a frenzy of the most varied, versatile, complex and even utterly brilliant technological improvisations, following one upon the other with an ever more bewildering and uncontrollable proliferation. Politics pretends to use this force as its servant, to harness it for social purposes, for the "good of man." The intention is good. The technological development of power in our time is certainly a risk and challenge, but it is by no means intrinsically evil. On the contrary, it can and should be a very great good. In actual fact, however, the furious speed with which our technological world is plunging toward disaster is evidence that no one is any longer fully in control—least of all, perhaps, the political leaders.

A simple study of the steps which led to the dropping of the first A-bomb on Hiroshima is devastating evidence of the way well-meaning men, the scientists, generals and statesmen of a victorious nation, were guided step by step, without realizing it, by the inscrutable yet simple "logic of events" to fire the shot that was to make the cold war inevitable and prepare the way inexorably for World War III. This they did purely and simply because they thought in all sincerity that the bomb was the simplest and most merciful way of ending World War II and perhaps all wars, forever.

The tragedy of our time is then not so much the malice of the wicked as the helpless futility of the best intentions of "the good." There are warmakers, war criminals, indeed. They are present and active on *both sides*. But all of us, in our very best efforts for peace, find ourselves maneuvered unconsciously into positions where we too can act as war criminals. For there can be no doubt that Hiroshima and Nagasaki were, though not fully deliberate crimes, nevertheless crimes. And who was responsible? No one. Or "history." We cannot go on playing with nuclear fire and shrugging off the results as "history." We are the ones concerned.

In plain words, in order to save ourselves from destruction we have to try to regain control of a world that is speeding downhill without brakes because of the combination of factors I have just mentioned: almost total passivity and irresponsibility on the moral level, plus demonic activism in social, political and military life.

First of all we must seek some remedy in the technological sphere. We must try to achieve some control over the production and stockpiling of weapons. It is intolerable that such massive engines of destruction should be allowed to proliferate in all directions without any semblance of a long-range plan for anything, even for what is cynically called "defense." To allow governments to pour more and more billions into weapons that almost immediately become obsolete, thereby necessitating more billions for newer and bigger weapons, is one of the most colossal injustices in the long history of man. While we are doing this, two thirds of the world are starving, or living in conditions of subhuman destitution.

Far from demanding that the lunatic race for destruction be stepped up, it seems to me that Christian morality imposes on every single one of us the obligation to protest against it and to work for the creation of an international authority with power and sanctions that will be able to control technology, and divert our amazing virtuosity into the service of man instead of against him.

It is not enough to say that we ought to try to work for a negotiated disarmament, or that one power bloc or the other ought to take the lead and disarm unilaterally. Methods and policies can and should be fairly considered. But what matters most is the obligation to travel in every feasible way in the direction of peace, using all the traditional and legitimate methods, while at the same time seeking to improvise new and original measures to achieve our end.

Long ago, even before the A-bomb, Pope Pius XII declared it was our supreme obligation to make "war on war" (1944). At that time he stressed our moral obligation to ban all wars of aggression, stating this duty was binding on *all* and that it "brooks no delay, no procrastination, no hesitation, no subterfuge." And what have we seen since then? The A-bomb, the H-bomb, the ICBM, the development of chemical and bacteriological weapons, and every possible evasion and subterfuge to justify their use without limitation as soon as one or the other nation decides that it may be expedient!

Therefore a Christian who is not willing to envisage the creation of an effective international authority to control the destinies of man for peace is not acting and thinking as a mature member of the Church. He does not have fully Christian perspectives. Such perspectives must, by their very nature, be "catholic," that is to say worldwide. They must consider the needs of mankind and not the temporary expediency and shortsighted policy of a particular nation.

To reject a "worldwide" outlook, to refuse to consider the good of mankind, and to remain satisfied with the affluence that flows from our war economy, is hardly a Christian attitude. Nor will our attachment to the current payoff accruing to us from weapons make it any easier for us to see and understand the need to take the hard road of sacrifice which alone leads to peace!

Equally important, and perhaps even more difficult than technological control, is the restoration of some moral sense and the resumption of genuine responsibility. Without this it is illusory for us to speak of freedom and "control." Unfortunately, even where moral principles are still regarded with some degree of respect, morality has lost touch with the realities of our situation. Modern warfare is fought as much by machines as by men. Even a great deal of the planning depends on the work of mechanical computers.

Hence it becomes more and more difficult to estimate the morality of an act leading to war because it is more and more difficult to know precisely what is going on. Not only is war increasingly a matter for pure specialists operating with fantastically complex machinery, but above all there is the question of absolute secrecy regarding everything that seriously affects defense policy. We may amuse ourselves by reading the reports in mass media and imagine that these "facts" provide sufficient basis for moral judgments for and against war. But in reality, we are simply elaborating moral fantasies in a vacuum. Whatever we may decide, we remain completely at the mercy of the governmental power, or rather the anonymous power of managers and generals who stand behind the facade of government. We have no way of directly influencing the decisions and policies taken by these people. In practice, we must fall back on a blinder and blinder faith which more and more resigns itself to trusting the "legitimately constituted authority" without having the vaguest notion what that authority is liable to do next. This condition of irresponsibility and passivity is extremely dangerous. It is hardly conducive to genuine morality.

An entirely new dimension is opened up by the fantastic processes and techniques involved in modern war. An American President can speak of warfare in outer space and nobody bursts out laughing—he is perfectly serious. Science fiction and the comic strip have all suddenly come true. When a missile armed with an H-bomb warhead is fired by the pressing of a button and its target is a whole city, the number of its victims is estimated in "megacorpses"—*millions* of dead human beings. A thousand or ten thousand more here and there are not even matter for comment. To what extent can we assume that the soldiers who exercise this terrible power are worthy of our confidence and actually realize what they are doing? To what extent can we assume that in passively following their lead and concurring in their decision—at least by default—we are acting as Christians?

V *The Moral Problem*

In all-out nuclear war, there is no longer question of simply permitting an evil, the destruction of a few civilian dwellings, in order to attain a legitimate end: the destruction of a military target. It is well understood on both sides that all-out nuclear war is purely and simply massive and indiscriminate destruction of targets chosen not for their military significance alone, but for their importance in a calculated project of terror and annihilation. Often the selection of the target is determined by some quite secondary and accidental circumstance that has not the remotest reference to morality. Hiroshima was selected for atomic attack, among other reasons, because it had never undergone any notable air bombing and was suitable as an intact target to give a good idea of the effectiveness of the bomb.

It must be frankly admitted that some of the military commanders of both sides in World War II simply disregarded all the traditional standards that were still effective. The Germans threw those standards overboard with the bombs they unloaded on Warsaw, Rotterdam, Coventry and London. The Allies replied in kind with saturation bombing of Hamburg, Cologne, Dresden and Berlin. Spokesmen were not wanting on either side to justify these crimes against humanity. And today, while "experts" calmly discuss the possibility of the United States being able to survive a war if "*only fifty millions*" (!) of the population are killed, when the Chinese speak of being able to *spare* "three hundred million" and "still get along," it is obvious that we are no longer in the realm where moral truth is conceivable.

The only sane course that remains is to work frankly and without compromise for a supranational authority and for the total abolition of war. The pronouncements of the Holy See all seem to point to this as the best ultimate solution.

The moral duty of the Christian is by no means simple. It is far from being a neat matter of ethical principle, clear cut, well defined, and backed by a lucid authoritative decision of the Church. To make the issue seem too simple is actually to do a great disservice to truth, to morality and to man. And yet now more than ever we crave the simple and the clear solution. This very craving is dangerous, because the most tempting of all "simple" solutions are the ones which prescribe annihilation or submit to it without resistance. There is a grim joke underlying all this talk about "Red or dead." The inherent destructiveness of the frustrated mind is able to creep in here and distort the whole Christian view of life and of civilization by evading the difficult and complex way of negotiation and sacrifice, in order to resort, in frustrated desperation, to "magic" power and nuclear destruction. Let us not ignore this temptation, it is one of the deepest and most radical in man. It is the first of all temptations, and the root of all the others. "You shall be as gods. . . ." (Genesis 3:5).

On the contrary, our Christian obligation consists in being and remaining men, believing in the Word Who emptied Himself and became man for our sakes. We have to look at the problem of nuclear war from the viewpoint of humanity and of God made man, from the viewpoint of the Mystical Body of Christ, and not merely from the viewpoint of abstract formulas. Here above all we need a reasoning that is informed with compassion and takes some account of flesh and blood, not a legalistic juggling with principles and precedents.

In the light of these deep Christian truths we will better understand the danger of fallacious justifications of every recourse to violence, as well as the peril of indifference, inertia and passivity.

It is not a question of stating absolutely and infallibly that every Christian must renounce, under pain of mortal sin, any opinion that the use of the bomb might be legitimate. The H-bomb has not been formally and officially condemned, and doubtless it does not need to be condemned. There is no special point in condemning one weapon in order to give casuistical minds an opportunity to prove their skill in evasion by coming up with another, "licit" way of attaining the same destructive end. It is not just a matter of seeing how much destruction and murder we can justify without incurring the condemnation of the Church.

But I submit that at this time above all it is vitally important to avoid the "minimalist" approach. The issue of nuclear war is too grave and too general. It threatens everybody. It may affect the very survival of the human race. In such a case one is not allowed to take any but unavoidable risks. We are obliged to take the morally more secure alternative in guiding our choice. Let us remember too that while a doubt of the existence of an obligation leaves us with a certain freedom of choice, the doubt of an evil fact does not permit such freedom.

We may well dispute the legitimacy of nuclear war on principle: but when we face the *actual fact* that recourse to nuclear weapons may quite probably result in the quasi-total destruction of civilization, even possibly in the suicide of the entire human race, we *are absolutely obliged to take this fact into account and to avoid this terrible danger.*

It is certainly legitimate for a Catholic moralist to hold in theory that a limited nuclear war, in defense, is permitted by traditional Christian moral principles. He may even hold the opinion that the strategic use of nuclear, bacteriological and chemical weapons is theoretically permissible for defense, provided that there is a possibility that what we are defending will continue to exist after it has been "defended."

But when we come face to face with the terrible doubt of fact, *dubium facti,* the absolutely real and imminent probability of massive and uncontrolled destruction with the annihilation of civilization and of life, then there is no such latitude of choice. We are most gravely and seriously bound by all norms of Christian morality, however minimal, to choose the safer course and to try at all costs to avoid so general a disaster.

Let us remember that even if one were to admit the theoretical legitimacy of nuclear weapons for purposes of defense, that use would become gravely unjust, without a shadow of doubt, as soon as the effects of nuclear destruction overflowed upon neutral or friendly nations. Even though we may feel justified in risking the destruction of our own cities and those of the enemy, we have no right whatever to bring destruction upon helpless small nations which have no interest whatever in the war and ask only to survive in peace. It is not up to us to choose that *they* should be dead rather than Red.

Pope Pius XII said in 1954 (concerning ABC warfare, described above as a sin, an offense and an outrage against God): "Should the evil consequences of adopting this method of warfare *ever become so extensive as to pass entirely beyond the control of man, then indeed its use must be rejected as immoral.*" He adds that uncontrolled annihilation of life within a given area "IS NOT LAWFUL UNDER ANY TITLE."

Nor is it moral to overindulge in speculation on this dangerous point of "control." A lax interpretation of this principle would lead us to decide that a twenty megaton H-bomb dropped on Leningrad is "fully under control" because all its effects are susceptible to measurement, and we know that the blast will annihilate Leningrad while the fallout will probably wipe out the population of Helsinki and Riga, depending on the wind. Obviously what the Pope meant was much more strict than that. He meant that if there was uncontrolled annihilation of everybody in Leningrad, without any discrimination between combatants and noncombatants, enemies, friends, women, children, infants and old people, then the use of the bomb would be "not lawful under any title," especially in view of the "bonus" effects of fallout drifting over neutral territory, certainly without control. And I do not think "clean" bombs are going to get around this moral difficulty either.

Hence though nuclear warfare as such has not been entirely and formally condemned, the mind of the Church is obviously that every possible means should be taken to avoid it; and John XXIII made this abundantly clear in his Christmas Message of 1961 where he pleaded in most solemn terms with the rulers of all nations to "shun all thought of force" and remain at peace. The words of Pope John in this connection imply grave reservations even with regard to limited war which might possibly "escalate" and reach all-out proportions.

There can be no doubt whatever that the absence of formal condemnation cannot be twisted into a tacit official approval of all-out nuclear war. Yet it seems that this is what some of our theologians are trying to do.

On the contrary, out duty is to help emphasize with all the force at our disposal that the Church earnestly seeks the abolition of war; we must underscore declarations like those of Pope John XXIII pleading with world leaders to renounce force in the settlement of international disputes and confine themselves to negotiations.

Now let us suppose that the political leaders of the world, supported by the mass media in their various countries, and carried on by a tidal wave of greater and greater war preparations, see themselves swept inexorably into a war of cataclysmic proportions. Let us suppose that it becomes morally certain that these leaders are helpless to arrest the blind force of the process that has irresponsibly been set in motion. What then? Are the masses of the world, including you and me, to resign themselves to our fate and march to global suicide without resistance, simply bowing our heads and obeying our leaders as showing us the "will of God?" I think it should be evident to everyone that this can no longer, in the present situation, be accepted unequivocally as Christian obedience and civic duty.

It is true that Pope Pius XII in his Christmas Message of 1956 declared that a Catholic was bound in duty to help his country in a just war of defense. But to extend this to all-out nuclear war is begging the question because Papal pronouncements on nuclear war cast doubts upon its justice. No theologian, however broad, however lax, would insist that one was bound in conscience to participate in a war that was *evidently* leading to global suicide. Those who favor nuclear war can only do so by making all kinds of suppositions concerning the political and military facts: that it will be only a limited war or that the destructive effects of H-bombs are not as terrible as we have been told. However much they limit the scoresheet of megacorpses, it is difficult for us to admit the morality of all-out nuclear war.

This brings us face to face with the greatest and most agonizing moral issue of our time. This issue is not merely nuclear war, not merely the possible destruction of the human race by a sudden explosion of violence. It is something more subtle and more demonic.

If we continue to yield to theoretically irresistible determinism and to vague "historic forces" without striving to resist and control them, if we let these forces drive us to demonic activism in the realm of politics and technology, we face something more than the material evil of universal destruction. We face *moral responsibility for global suicide.* Much more than that, we are going to find ourselves gradually moving into a situation in which we are practically compelled by the "logic of circumstances" deliberately *to choose the course that leads to destruction.*

The great danger is then the savage and self-destructive commitment to a policy of nationalism and blind hate, and the refusal of all other policies more constructive and more in accordance with Christian ethical tradition. Let us realize that this is a matter of *choice,* not of pure blind determinism.

We all know the logic of temptation. We all know the confused, vague, hesitant irresponsibility which leads us into the situation where it is no longer possible to turn back, and how, arrived in that situation, we have a moment of clear-sighted desperation in which we freely commit ourselves to the course we recognize as evil. That may well be what is happening now to the whole world.

The free choice of global suicide, made in desperation by the world's leaders and ratified by the consent and cooperation of their citizens, would be a moral evil second only to the Crucifixion. The fact that such a choice might be made with the highest motives and the most urgent purpose would do nothing whatever to mitigate it. The fact that it might be made as a gamble, in the hope that some might escape, would never excuse it. After all, the purposes of Caiphas were, in his own eyes, perfectly noble. He thought it was necessary to let "one man die for the people."

The most urgent necessity of our time is therefore not merely to prevent the destruction of the human race by nuclear war. Even if it should happen to be no longer possible to prevent the disaster (which God forbid), there is still a greater evil than can and must be prevented. It must be possible for every free man to refuse his consent and deny his cooperation to this greatest of crimes.

VI The Christian Choice

In what does this effective and manifest refusal of consent consist? How does one "resist" the sin of genocide? Ideally speaking, in the imaginary case where all-out nuclear war seemed inevitable and the world's leaders were evidently incapable of preventing it, it would be legitimate and even obligatory for all sane and conscientious men everywhere in the world to lay down their weapons and their tools and starve and be shot rather than cooperate in the war effort. If such a mass movement should spontaneously arise in all parts of the world, in Russia and America, in China and France, in Africa and Germany, the human race could be saved from extinction. This is indeed an engaging hypothesis—but it is no more than that. It would be folly to suppose that men hitherto passive, inert, morally indifferent and irresponsible might suddenly recover their sense of obligation and their awareness of their own power when the world was on the very brink of war.

In any case, as has been said above, the ordinary man has no access to vital information. Indeed, even the politicians may know relatively little about what is really going on. How would it be possible to know when and how it was necessary to refuse cooperation? Can we draw a line clearly, and say precisely when nuclear war becomes so dangerous that it is suicidal? If a war of missiles breaks out, we will have at the most thirty minutes to come to our momentous conclusions —if we ever know what is happening at all. It seems to me that the time to form our conscience and to decide upon our course of action is *NOW*.

It is one thing to form one's conscience and another to adopt a specific policy or course of action. It is highly regrettable that this important distinction is overlooked and indeed deliberately obfuscated. To decide, in the forum of conscience, that one is obligated in every way, as a Christian, to avoid actions that would contribute to a world-wide disaster, does not mean that one is necessarily committed to absolute and unqualified pacifism. One may start from this moral principle, which is repeatedly set before us by the Popes and which cannot be seriously challenged, and one may then go on to seek various means to preserve peace. About these different means, there may be considerable debate.

Yet it seems clear to me that the enormous danger represented by nuclear weapons, and the near impossibility of controlling them and limiting them to a scale that would fit the traditional ethical theory of a just war, makes it both logical and licit for a Catholic to proceed, from motives of conscience, to at least a relative pacifism, and to a policy of nuclear disarmament.

In so doing, however, he has a strict obligation to see that he does not take a naïve and oversimplified position which would permit him to be ruthlessly exploited by the politicians of another nuclear power. The logic of all serious efforts to preserve peace demands that our very endeavors themselves do not help the war effort of the "enemy," and thus precipitate war. There is sometimes a danger that our pacifism may be somewhat shortsighted and immature. It may consequently be more an expression of rebellion against the status quo in our own country than an effective opposition to war itself.

In a word, there are three things to be considered: (1) Christian moral principles, which by their very nature favor peace, and according to which nuclear war remains, if not absolutely forbidden, at least of exceedingly dubious morality; (2) The facts about weapons systems and defense policies. Our moral decision, and the morality of our participation in the economic and political life of a society geared for nuclear war, demand imperatively that we realize the real nature of the military policies to which we contribute by taxation and perhaps also by our work in industry. So much in our national life is today centered on the most intense and most overwhelming arms race in the history of man. Everything points to the fact that these frightful weapons of destruction may soon be used, most probably on the highest and most expanded scale; (3) We must finally consider factors by which these military policies are dictated.

The Christian moral principles are relatively clear. While there is still intense debate over details, no Christian moralist worthy of the name can seriously defend outright a nuclear war of unqualified aggression.

The facts about ABC warfare are also clear enough. There is no question of the immense destructiveness of the weapons available to us. There is no question that the destruction of civilization and even global suicide are both possible. There is no question that the policies of the nuclear powers are geared for an all-out war of incredible savagery and destructive force.

What remains to be explored by the Christian is the area that is least considered, which also happens to be the area that most needs to be examined and is perhaps the one place where something can be done.

By what are our policies of hatred and destructiveness dictated? What seems to drive us inexorably on to the fate which we all dread and seek to avoid? This question is not hard to answer. What started the First World War? What started the Second World War? The answer is, simply, the rabid, shortsighted, irrational and stubborn forces which tend to come to a head in nationalism.

Christopher Dawson has said:

> The defeat of Hitlerism does not mean that we have seen the end of such movements. In our modern democratic world, irrational forces lie very near the surface, and *their sudden eruption under the impulse of nationalist or revolutionary ideologies is the greatest of all the dangers that threaten the modern world.* . . . It is at this point that the need for a reassertion of Christian principles becomes evident. In so far as nationalism denies the principle (of higher order and divine justice for all men) and sets up the nation and the national state as the final object of man's allegiance, *it represents the most retrograde movement the world has ever seen,* since it means a denial of the great central truth on which civilization

> was founded, and the return to the pagan idolatries of tribal barbarism.

Dawson then goes on to quote Pope Pius XII who distinguishes between "national life" and "nationalistic politics." National life is a combination of all the values which characterize a social group and enable it to contribute fruitfully to the whole policy of nations. Nationalistic politics on the other hand are divisive, destructive, and a perversion of genuine national values. They are "a principle of dissolution within the community of peoples."

This then is the conclusion: the Christian is bound to work for peace by working against global dissolution and anarchy. Due to nationalist and revolutionary ideologies (for Communism is in fact exploiting the intense nationalism of backward peoples), a world-wide spirit of confusion and disorder is breaking up the unity and the order of civilized society.

It is true that we live in an epoch of revolution, and that the breakup and re-formation of society is inevitable. But the Christian must see that his mission is not to contribute to the blind forces of annihilation which tend to destroy civilization and mankind together. He must seek to build rather than to destroy. He must orient his efforts towards world unity and not towards world division. Anyone who promotes policies of hatred and of war is working for the division and the destruction of civilized mankind.

We have to be convinced that there are certain things already clearly forbidden to all men, such as the use of torture, the killing of hostages, genocide (or the mass extermination of racial, national or other groups for no reason than that they belong to an "undesirable" category). The destruction of civilized centers by nuclear annihilation bombing is genocide.

We have to become aware of the poisonous effect of the mass media that keep violence, cruelty and sadism constantly present to the minds of unformed and irresponsible people. We have to recognize the danger to the whole world in the fact that today the economic life of the more highly-developed nations is in large part centered on the production of weapons, missiles and other engines of destruction.

We have to consider that the hate propaganda, and the consistent heckling of one government by another, has always inevitably led to violent conflict. We have to recognize the implications of voting for politicians who promote policies of hate. We must never forget that our most ordinary decisions may have terrible consequences.

It is no longer reasonable or right to leave all decisions to a largely anonymous power elite that is driving us all, in our passivity, towards ruin. We have to make ourselves heard.

Every individual Christian has a grave responsibility to protest clearly and forcibly against trends that lead inevitably to crimes which the Church deplores and condemns. Ambiguity, hesitation and compromise are no longer permissible. We must find some new and constructive way of settling international disputes. This may be extraordinarily difficult. Obviously war cannot be abolished by mere wishing. Severe sacrifices may be demanded and the results will hardly be visible in our day. We have still time to do something about it, but the time is rapidly running out.

Passivity and Abuse of Authority

The following very interesting texts are taken from the recently published diary of Father Ignace Lepp, *The Christian Failure* (Newman Press, 1962). They were written during the Nazi occupation of France, when many of the French clergy and the well-to-do laity collaborated with the puppet Vichy government anticipating the Nazi domination of Europe. They had no special love for the Nazis, but they passively accepted the totalitarian power of Hitler and preferred it to Communism. They were convinced that Europe had to be Nazi or Communist, and they chose Nazism as a "lesser evil" because they had hopes for the continued existence of the Church in France if they "played ball" with the conquerors.

Fr. Lepp attributed this mentality of the clergy in part to their seminary training which, he thought, made them unable to cope with the issue properly. They were not fully in touch with reality. They dealt only with abstract dilemmas, which could not really be resolved in practice, and which as a result left French Catholics more or less passive and submissive to an evil which they should have been able to resist.

One of the grave problems of religion in our time is posed by the almost total lack of protest on the part of religious people and clergy in the face of enormous social evils. It is not that these people are wicked or perverse (as the Communists would sometimes have us believe) but simply that they are no longer fully capable of *seeing and evaluating* certain evils as they truly are: as crimes against God and as betrayals of the Christian ethic of love. A case in point is the social injustice in the nominally "Catholic" countries of Latin America, against which the hierarchy has recently protested.

Another case is that of nuclear war, which the Popes have repeatedly denounced but which the majority of Catholics in America and other Western nations tend to accept passively and without question simply because it is "better than being a Communist." It is a "lesser evil." This, however, is not a serious moral judgment and is in no sense an answer. It represents nothing but a psychology of evasion, irresponsibility, and negativism, hiding behind such grandiose concepts as "defense of freedom and religion," "obedience to civil authority," "self-sacrifice" and so on.

It seems that a psychology of evasion and helplessness, glorified and encouraged by persons in authority who are able to take advantage of it, has gradually come to replace the true virtue of Christian obedience. This is a psychology of subservient opportunism which in reality has nothing Christian about it, but on the contrary gives ample scope for the irresponsibility of the mass mind and in the end threatens to destroy both Christian and democratic liberty.

True Christian obedience should liberate man from servitude to the "elements of this world" (cf. Galatians 4: 1–11) so that we may be able freely to obey civic authority when it is legal and just, and that in the presence of injustice and falsity we may "obey God rather than men" (cf. Acts 5: 17–32). But a pseudo-Christian obedience is nothing more than the mechanical and irrational submission of beings who have renounced freedom and responsibility in order to become cogs in an official machine. It is not the obedience of sons of God but the compliance of functionaries in a military bureaucracy. Here the supreme virtue is to agree with authority no matter whether it is right or wrong, to maintain one's position by flattery, compliance and mechanical efficiency. It is the obedience of an Eichmann who will commit any crime in order to retain his position in organized falsity and infamy.

The first text shows that typical members of the French clergy in 1942 thought Fr. Lepp was a rebel, a troublemaker and a madman because, instead of passively "obeying" an illegal government, he was aiding the publication of an underground Christian paper for the Resistance. For him to do this was, they felt, defying the manifest will of God by refusing to submit. For them, obedience was in reality opportunism and servility.

> Last night I had a heated discussion with a few fellow priests on the subject of the publication of the underground paper *Témoignage Chrétien.* They cannot understand why Catholics in public life and priests should edit this paper and it was no use my trying to point out that the Vichy government is not a divine institution. In the eyes of these well-meaning priests it is only communists, enemies both of God and of France, who are interested in sabotaging the efforts of the "national revolution" which this government claims as its own. At this moment when the allied landing in North Africa gives us more reason to doubt the final victory of the Nazis these good priests are still utterly convinced of it.
>
> It is not that they *want* German victory because not one of them upholds Nazi-ism but the training they received at the

> seminaries has formed their intellect on such exclusively abstract lines that they are unable to cope with practical life and they battle against dilemmas which exist only in their minds. Listening to them one would imagine that France and the world must choose either Hitler or Stalin—or, in other words, between a "New Europe" under Nazi leadership or the occupation of Europe by the "red hordes." Whatever the Nazi crimes, to these priests they seem less terrifying than the horrors for which the communists are responsible. It is quite impossible to convince them that there is a possibility of avoiding the domination of both Hitler and Stalin. And if one mentions the possible return of a French parliamentary democracy they repeat all the Vichy banalities about the corruption and decadence of the "people's republic" with a fervour worthy of a better cause.
>
> *The Christian Failure*, pp. 34–35

Note that a characteristic of this psychology is in fact a latent despair of freedom and of democratic government. The either/or complex, which resigns itself fatalistically to the supposed "choice" between Nazism and Communism is, in fact, flight from the difficulties and responsibilities without which democratic life and freedom are impossible.

But this evasion is really not a fully free and deliberate choice. It is rather a regressive and irresponsible capitulation to power: for since the Christian cannot, by definition, become an atheist Communist, he falls back on the other brand of totalitarianism which may still pretend to tolerate religion. In reality, this is a surrender of the Christian conscience to demonic forces at work for the destruction of society and of the Church.

The chief criterion of moral value comes to be "survival." Of course it is presented not just as the survival of the individual, but as "the freedom of religion," etc. Yet this also implies that the individual Catholic will retain his comfortable and privileged position . . . or so he thinks. For this, then, he will shut his eyes to monstrous evils, acquiesce in an unjust and tyrannical system, and prove himself obedient by never doing anything to rock the boat.

The next text shows the pitiful servility of this psychology, which goes to considerable trouble to invent good reasons, religious reasons, for its defection:

> It shocks me to think of all the Catholics who made no protest when some of their preachers had no scruples in flattering Pétain and acclaiming him as a sort of Joan of Arc. Even Péguy, the typical individualist, finds he is called upon to comply with the worst kind of pseudo-Christian principles. Pétain is known to be no more religious-minded than Paul

> Reynaud and yet all sorts of legends are invented to make him out a sort of saint. His entourage are shrewd enough to encourage these legends because they realise that numerically the Catholics are the only class on which the regime could stand. It seems as if the nostalgia for a theocratic regime is still prevalent among Catholics—how otherwise can one explain why the confusion between religious and political views is so welcome to them. Not only have the subsidies for denominational schools been welcomed with real gratitude but many people hope and trust that Pétain will restore the establishment of the Church in France.
>
> The authoritarian character of the Church has developed in many Catholics a tendency to evade all spiritual responsibility; they assert that the Church is the steward of eternal truth and then content themselves with repeating mechanically the liturgical and dogmatic formulas without making an intelligent effort to understand them and bring them to life. They seem to have lost the determination to obey moral laws; all they are concerned with is to be told by authority what to do and what not to do. I find it hard to believe that this is what Christ came for but, as far as the subconscious mind of many Catholics is concerned, a long time has elapsed since evangelical liberty was supplanted by pharisaical observance of the law. So it is not surprising that these Catholics also tend to evade the personal responsibilities in the sphere of temporal organizations. If a democracy is not to deteriorate into a mere demagogy each person must be prepared to look after his own affairs and to contribute to the affairs of the community. It is so much easier to leave it all trustingly to the leader—Franco in Spain, Pétain in France; even the atheists Mussolini and Hitler know how to make the most of this inertia. Our Lord had good reason to speak of "sheep" when he charged Peter to take care of his Church.
>
> Ibid. pp. 35–36

Fr. Lepp points out that this mentality may have in it something of a "nostalgia for the theocracy." Hence a wrong idea of obedience and false supernaturalism ought to be regarded as sources of dangerous confusion, when they destroy the distinction between the sacred and secular: in other words, when the authority of a secularist power is purely and simply identified with the divine authority and even usurps functions which rightly belong only to conscience.

Note that Fr. Lepp attributes this distortion of the right notion of Christian obedience to defects within the Church itself. Abuses of authority by ministers of the Church lead to a weakening of the moral sense of Christians, instead of strengthening it. The result of this is that in very grave social issues, where the conscience of the

Catholic layman should play a really positive and decisive part, the layman waits to be instructed by the priest who, in turn, being out of touch with the reality of the problem, hands down an abstract decision devoid of genuine moral seriousness. This results in an abdication of responsibility and passive submission to an evil that ought to be identified, denounced and resisted, not "obeyed." Thus by defection of the Christian conscience democracy degenerates into demagogy and Fascism—or Communism.

The last text shows to what extremes this psychology can lead. Emmanuel Mounier, protesting by a hunger strike against unjust imprisonment and being in danger of death, was refused absolution by a priest who could not conceive this resistance as anything other than rebellion against God. Yet in fact the resistance offered by Mounier was not only politically right, but was the answer demanded by Christian morality to injustice and untruth. It was Mounier who was obedient in all truth. The priest, misled by a defective formation, was betraying truth and justice. He was false to Christ.

Hence the ultimate danger of this thoroughly unchristian psychology is that it perverts the Christian conscience and punishes the Christian who, led by his moral sense and his Christian faith, seeks to offer heroic obedience to the will of God, and who therefore deserves all the support and comfort that the Church can give him.

> A friend of mine told me of the long hunger strike which Mounier has imposed on himself in prison. A few days ago he felt his strength fading and fearing to die almost at once he asked for a priest so that he could receive absolution and Holy Communion. But the priest (I shouldn't be surprised to hear that he was a "holy man") refused him absolution on the grounds that he had disobeyed legitimate authority and was not prepared to repent his disobedience. There seems no limit to the stupidity of men, even of priests. One sometimes needs great strength and pure faith not to be discouraged and to remain loyal to the Church almost, as it were, in spite of herself.
>
> Ibid., p. 34

In conclusion we must remark that this dangerous psychology is not always merely passive. It can become not only active but extremely aggressive and violent in support of a totalitarian myth. Once again, the ostensible motives may be "religious" but the fruits of cruelty, inhumanity, and fanaticism identify these motives as antichristian.

An Enemy of the State

On August 9, 1943, the Austrian peasant Franz Jägerstätter was beheaded by the German military authorities as an "enemy of the state" because he had repeatedly refused to take the military oath and serve in what he declared to be an "unjust war." His story has a very special importance at a time when the Catholic Church, in the Second Vatican Council, is confronting the moral problem of nuclear weaponry. This Austrian peasant was not only simultaneously a Catholic and a conscientious objector, but he was a fervent Catholic, so fervent that some who knew him believe him to have been a saint. His lucid and uncompromising refusal to fight for Germany in the Second World War was the direct outcome of his religious conversion. It was the political implementation of his desire to be a perfect Christian.

Franz Jägerstätter surrendered his life rather than take the lives of others in what he believed to be an "unjust war." He clung to this belief in the face of every possible objection not only on the part of the army and the state, but also from his fellow Catholics, the Catholic clergy and of course his own family. He had to meet practically every "Christian" argument that is advanced in favor of war. He was treated as a rebel, disobedient to lawful authority, a traitor to his country. He was accused of being selfish, self-willed, not considering his family, neglecting his duty to his children.

His Austrian Catholic friends understood that he was unwilling to fight for Hitler's Germany, but yet they argued that the war was justified because they hoped it would lead to the destruction of Bolshevism and therefore to the preservation of "European Christianity." He was therefore refusing to defend his faith. He was also told that he was not sufficiently informed to judge whether or not the war was just. That he had an obligation to submit to the "higher wisdom" of the state. The government and the Fuehrer know best. Thousands of Catholics, including many priests, were serving in the armies, and therefore he should not try to be "more Catholic than the Church."

He was even reminded that the bishops had not protested against this war, and in fact not only his pastor but even his bishop tried to persuade him to give up his resistance because it was "futile." One priest represented to him that he would have innumerable opportunities to practice Christian virtue and exercise an "apostolate of good example" in the armed forces. All these are very familiar arguments frequently met with in our present situation, and they are still assumed to be so conclusive that few Catholics dare to risk the disapproval they would incur by conscientious objection and dissent.

Jäggerstätter's fellow villagers thought his refusal was evidence of fanaticism due to his religious conversion at the time of his marriage in 1936, followed by an "excess of Bible reading." His conscientious objection is still not fully understood in his native village, though on the local war memorial his name has been added to those of the villagers who were killed in action.

The peasant refused to give in to any of these arguments, and replied to them with all simplicity:

> I cannot and may not take an oath in favor of a government that is fighting an unjust war. . . . I cannot turn the responsibility for my actions over to the Führer. . . . Does anyone really think that this massive blood-letting can save European Christianity or bring it to a new flowering? . . . Is it not more Christian to offer oneself as a victim right away rather than first have to murder others who certainly have a right to live and want to live—just to prolong one's own life a little while?

When reminded that most Catholics had gone to war for Hitler without any such qualms of conscience, he replied that they obviously "had not received the grace" to see things as they were. When told that the bishops themselves expressed no such objections he repeated that "they had not received the grace" either.

Jägerstätter's refusal to fight for Hitler was not based on a personal repugnance to fighting in any form. As a matter of fact Jägerstätter was, by temperament, something of a fighter. In his wilder youthful days he had participated rather prominently in the inter-village gang wars. He had also undergone preliminary military training without protest, though his experience at that time had convinced him that army life presented a danger to morals.

Shortly after Hitler took over Austria in 1938, Jägerstätter had a dream in which he saw a splendid and shining express train coming round a mountain, and thousands of people running to get aboard. "No one could prevent them from getting on the train." While he was looking at this he heard a voice saying: "This train is going to hell." When he woke up he spontaneously associated the "train" with Nazism. His objection to military service was, then, the fruit of a particular religious interpretation of contemporary political events. His refusal to fight was not only a private matter of conscience: it also expressed a deep intuition concerning the historical predicament of the Catholic Church in the twentieth century. This intuition was articulated in several long and very impressive meditations or "commentaries" in which he says:

> The situation in which we Christians of Germany find ourselves today is much more bewildering than that faced by the Christians of the early centuries at the time of their bloodiest persecution. . . . We are not dealing with a small matter, but the great (apocalyptic) life and death struggle has already begun. Yet in the midst of it there are many who still go on living their lives as though nothing had changed. . . . That we Catholics must make ourselves tools of the worst and most dangerous anti-Christian power that has ever existed is something that I cannot and never will believe. . . . Many actually believe quite simply that things have to be the way they are. If this should happen to mean that they are obliged to commit injustice, then they believe that others are responsible. . . . I am convinced that it is still best that I speak the truth even though it costs me my life. For you will not find it written in any of the commandments of God or of the Church that a man is obliged under pain of sin to take an oath committing him to obey whatever might be commanded him by his secular ruler. We need no rifles or pistols for our battle, but instead spiritual weapons—and the foremost of these is prayer.

The witness of this Austrian peasant is in striking contrast to the career of another man who lived and worked for a time in the nearby city of Linz: Adolf Eichmann.

The American sociologist Gordon Zahn, who is also a Catholic and a pacifist, has written an absorbing, objective, fully documented life of Jäggerstätter,[1] in which he studies with great care not only the motives and actions of the man himself, but the reactions and recollections of scores of people who knew him, from his family and neighbors to fellow prisoners and prison chaplains. One of the most striking things about the story is that repeated attempts were made to save the peasant-objector's life not only by his friends, by priests, by his attorney but even by his military judges (he was not in the hands of the SS).

Jäggerstätter could have escaped execution if he had accepted noncombatant service in the medical corps, but he felt that even this would be a compromise, because his objection was not only to killing other men but to the act of saving his own life by an implicit admission that the Nazis were a legitimate regime carrying on a just war. A few minutes before his execution Jägerstätter still calmly refused to sign a document that would have saved him. The chaplain who was present,

1. *In Solitary Witness* (New York: Holt, Rinehart & Winston, 1964).

and who had tried like everyone else to persuade the prisoner to save himself, declared that Jägerstätter "lived as a saint and died as a hero."

It is important to observe that though the Catholic villagers of his native St. Radegund still tend to regard Jägerstätter as an extremist and a fanatic, or even as slightly touched in the head, the priests who knew him and others who have studied him have begun to admit the seriousness and supernatural impact of his heroic self-sacrifice. There are some who do not hesitate to compare his decision with that of Thomas More.

One of the prison chaplains who knew him said: "Not for an instant did I ever entertain the notion that Jägerstätter was 'fanatic' or even possibly mentally deranged. He did not give the slightest impression of being so." And a French cellmate said of him that he was "one of the heroes of our time, a fighter to the death for faith, peace and justice."

Finally, it is interesting to read the very reserved judgment of the bishop who, when consulted by Jägerstätter about this moral problem, urged him to renounce his "scruples" and let himself be inducted into the army.

> I am aware of the "consistency" of his conclusions and respect them—especially in their intention. At that time I could see that the man thirsted after martyrdom and for the expiation of sin, and I told him that he was permitted to choose that path only if he knew he had been called to it through some special revelation originating from above and not in himself. He agreed with this. For this reason Jägerstätter represents a completely exceptional case, one more to be marveled at than copied.

The story of the Austrian peasant as told by Gordon Zahn is plainly that of a martyr, and of a Christian who followed a path of virtue with a dedication that cannot be fully accounted for by human motivation alone. In other words, it would seem that already in this biography one might find plausible evidence of what the Catholic Church regards as sanctity. But the Bishop of Linz, in hinting at the possibility of a special calling that might have made Jägerstätter an "exceptional case," does not mean even implicitly to approve the thesis that the man was a saint, still less a model to be imitated. In other words the bishop, while admitting the remote possibility of Catholic heroism in a conscientious objector, is not admitting that such heroism should be regarded as either normal or imitable.

The Second Vatican Council in its Constitution on the Church in the Modern World (n. 79) recognized, at least implicitly, the right of a Catholic to refuse on grounds of conscience to bear arms. It did not propose conscientious objection as a sweeping obligation. Nevertheless it clearly declared that no one could escape the obligation to *refuse obedience* to criminal orders issued by the state or the military command. The example of genocide was given. In view of the fact that total war tends more and more in fact to be genocidal, the Council's declaration obviously bears above all on war.

The Bishop of Linz, however, did not propose conscientious objection as a rational and Christian option. For him, the true heroes remain "those exemplary young Catholic men, seminarians, priests and heads of families who fought and died in heroic fulfillment of duty and in the firm conviction that they were fulfilling the will of God at their post. . . ."

It is still quite possible that even today after the Council and in an era of new war technology and new threats of global destruction, when the most urgent single problem facing modern man is the proliferation of atomic and nuclear weaponry, many Catholic bishops will continue to agree with this one. It is true, they admit that there is such a thing as an erroneous conscience which is to be followed provided it is "invincible." "All respect is due to the innocently erroneous conscience," says the Bishop of Linz, "it will have its reward from God."

Of whom is he speaking? Of the Catholic young men, the priests and the seminarians who died in Hitler's armies "in the firm conviction that they were fulfilling the will of God"? No. These, he says, were men (and the word is underlined) acting in the light of "a clear and correct conscience." Jägerstätter was "in error" but also "in good faith."

Certainly the bishop is entitled to his opinion: but the question of whose conscience was erroneous and whose was correct remains one that will ultimately be settled by God, not man. Meanwhile there is another question: the responsibility of those who help men to form their conscience—or fail to do so. And here, too, the possibility of firm convictions that are "innocently erroneous" gives food for some rather apocalyptic thought.

The real question raised by the Jägerstätter story is not merely that of the individual Catholic's right to conscientious objection (admitted in practice even by those who completely disagreed with Jägerstätter) but the question of the Church's own mission of protest and prophecy in the gravest spiritual crisis man has ever known.

A Martyr for Peace and Unity:

Father Max Josef Metzger (1887-1944)

Once again the civilized world sways on the brink of an abyss. This time the abyss seems to be bottomless. Once again the passions and confusions of social life have cruelly obscured the great problem of conscience that faces Christians in the twentieth century; that has, indeed, faced them for centuries. The problem of dissension, division and war. The Christian duty to fight for peace and unity.

Once again we confront the confusion between the obligation to respond without compromise to the Law of Christ, the Law of Peace, and the apparent duty to give first place to the warlike demands of the power politician. As Pope John XXIII has said in his Christmas Message of 1961: "All the teaching of Christ is an invitation to peace, for it proclaims the blessedness of peace. But (in politics) under the cloak of fair words, there is often a spirit opposed to peace." As we know, the great power blocs stand armed for mutual annihilation, each one claiming to be the only defender of "peace." Let us hope that the appeal of Pope John to "those responsible for forming public opinion" and to "the rulers of nations who hold in their hands the fate of mankind" may at last be heeded. He asks the propagandist in particular to "fear the severe judgment of God and to proceed with caution, governed by a sense of balance" instead of fomenting hatred among nations and races. Catholics at least are seriously bound in conscience to listen to this solemn warning of the Vicar of Christ, regarding hate propaganda and incitement to war, no matter how "good" the apparent cause may be.

When Hitler finally plunged the Western world into war by his attack on Poland, the German Catholics, and especially the German Catholic press, feeling that their duty was first of all to support

Reich und Volk, followed Hitler into battle without complaint. The Catholic who might perhaps have suffered from some pangs of conscience was officially reassured that this was a perfectly "just war." We who are far removed from the scene can judge the situation with critical and perhaps severe detachment. We can see, for instance, for what understandable reasons the German Catholic press at that time wanted to continue in existence and supported Hitler's war effort in order to avoid immediate suppression. We forget that here and there in the columns of Catholic papers and magazines were items which said much to those who knew how to read between the lines, and which could hardly be published without heroism on the part of those who knew how closely their proofs were scrutinized by the Gestapo.

And yet the lesson is inescapable in its tragic implications. In the modern godless world, where a heroic choice may be demanded, where peace and even the survival of mankind may conceivably depend on such a choice being made by Christians, we can blind our own conscience with a false conception of duty and of sacrifice which enables us quietly to participate in colossal injustices and barbarities, in order to preserve our institutional freedom of action. It is so easy to fear men more than God, so easy to feel that social ostracism is a greater danger than infidelity to conscience and to Christ. All our economic interests are there to persuade us that the side of God is the side on which our bread happens to be buttered. This does not imply that our moral obligations are always clear. But when such tremendous issues confront us, let us at least realize our moral risk. Let us at least consider that our obligation to Christ the King takes precedence over every other obligation. We must beware of seeing in our duties to Caesar a sweeping justification for cruelty, moral cowardice, infidelity, greed, and what Pope John has called the "callousness of the complacent man who pays no heed to the great cry of suffering which exists in the world."

The example of Max Josef Metzger, a Catholic priest executed by Hitler's Gestapo in the Brandenburg Prison, Berlin, on April 17, 1944, should make us realize that not everyone needs to be a passive utensil of the militarist. Father Metzger was a true patriot. He never failed his country, even though in Hitler's eyes he was a "traitor to the Reich and Führer." He died for Germany just as heroically and just as wholeheartedly as any soldier who fell on the battlefield. And he died for peace. It was indeed his attempts to work out a plan for peace in conjunction with bishops in other countries that was regarded by Hitler as "treason."

Father Metzger had been a chaplain in World War I. He had revolted against the senseless horrors of a war that achieved nothing, that only brought about moral and physical destruction and prepared the way for a still greater cataclysm.

Right after World War I he became a devoted worker in the

cause of peace. He was in contact with the International Fellowship of Reconciliation. He attended many peace conferences and congresses and founded a Secular Institute, the Society of Christ the King, devoted to the lay apostolate and works of mercy, particularly to work in the cause of international peace. He was also ardently devoted to the cause of Christian unity. He was, with Abbé Courturier in France, one of the most original and farsighted precursors of the present flourishing Catholic ecumenical movement. The best-known work of Father Metzger is the *Una Sancta* movement which began in 1939 with the retreat of a group of Catholic and Protestant clergymen, together, in search of a basis for agreement and fraternal union that would remotely prepare the way for Christian Unity. *Una Sancta* is today one of the most lively and flourishing of Catholic ecumenical endeavors.

Father Metzger was arrested three times before his last imprisonment which ended with his execution. He was jailed by the Gestapo in 1934, 1938, 1939 and finally in 1943. The first three prison terms involved sedulous examination of Father Metzger, in an effort to pin some kind of charge on him, and especially to implicate him in a conspiracy against the Führer. He was not engaged in any such conspiracy.

What finally emerged as "treason" sufficient to warrant a death sentence was his sincere, almost naïve effort to get a peace plan going which he thought would end the war. Through the intermediary of a Swedish woman, who was interested in *Una Sancta,* Father Metzger wanted to get letters out of Germany to bishops in various warring and neutral countries. He thought that the bishops would be able to influence their governments to seek a negotiated peace instead of the "unconditional surrender" that was to cost Germany so many burned and gutted cities, so many thousands of civilian dead. The Swedish lady was a Gestapo agent. The letters of Father Metzger, suggesting as they did that Germany needed to be "spared" and that the Reich would not come back to destroy all her enemies, was of course regarded as treason by Hitler.

Let us remember this formula: in the madness of modern war, when every crime is justified, the nation is always right, power is always right, the military is always right. To question those who wield power, to differ from them in any way, is to confess oneself subversive, rebellious, traitors. Father Metzger did not believe in power, in bombs. He believed in Christ, in unity, in peace. He died as a martyr for his belief.

Words of Father Metzger

1. I HAVE OPENED MY LIPS FOR THE PEACE OF THE WORLD AND THE UNITY OF CHRIST'S CHURCH. GOD HAS ACCEPTED IT AND I AM GLAD.

2. War owes its existence to the Father of lies. War is itself a lie. War is the kingdom of Satan, Peace is the Kingdom of God. The "just war" of which the moralists wrote in former days is now no longer possible. War today is a crime. We need to organize peace as men have organized war. Men of all peoples and nations, unite against the inhuman thing and declare that you will have no part in it, neither by taking up arms nor by transporting war materials nor in any other way.

3. IT IS HONORABLE TO DIE FOR ONE'S COUNTRY BUT STILL MORE HONORABLE TO DIE FOR RIGHTEOUSNESS AND PEACE.

4. Strive after love, strive unwearily after love, the selfless love that is ready for sacrifice.

5. God is love and those who live in Him cannot do anything else than bring forth the fruits of love.

6. THE NEED OF OUR DAY—AND THROUGH IT GOD IS SPEAKING TO US—IMPERATIVELY DEMANDS THE UTMOST EFFORT TO HEAL THE DISMEMBERMENT OF THE CHRISTIAN CHURCH, TO MAKE CHRIST'S KINGDOM OF PEACE EFFECTUAL THROUGHOUT THE WORLD.

7. Freedom is not a matter of space but of spirit.

8. The Apostle Paul speaks of being steadfast in the faith. That is certainly the special grace for which we all must pray, we who live in a world opposed to faith. I had never before understood as I do here how solitary are believing Christians in the world. (In prison, 1943.)

9. I am glad and carefree [in prison, 1943] since I have put myself and my fate entirely into God's hands. Why should I fear? I am never bored here, as I have so much work to occupy me; the day hardly seems long enough. My chief anxiety is for the future of our nation. I am ready to suffer for that, yet I hope I may be allowed to work for it also.

10. IT IS THE VERY EXPERIENCE OF THIS WRETCHED WAR THAT IT AROUSES IN COUNTLESS PEOPLE THE LONGING FOR A GREAT EFFORT TO SAVE THE HUMAN RACE, AN EFFORT TO OVERCOME THE APPARENT POWERLESSNESS OF CHRISTIANITY IN ITS INFLUENCE ON WORLD EVENTS. ONLY WHEN WAR HAS THROWN THE NATIONS INTO UNSPEAKABLE MISERY WILL THE WHOLE WORLD BEGIN TO LOOK FOR A GREAT WORD OF REDEMPTION. BUT WHAT IS NEEDED CAN BE ATTEMPTED ONLY BY FAITH. GLOOMY AND HALFHEARTED EFFORTS ARE BOUND TO FAIL.

11. The unity of Christendom was the last will and Testament of Jesus Christ. The disunion of Christendom today contradicts the purpose of Our Lord and is a stumbling block to the world. To overcome these divisions is the task of every disciple of Christ.

12. Anyone who is familiar with the inner development of the churches separated from us will admit the truth of the following statement, that dogmatic differences—however serious and important—are not today the main element which hinders reunion. Much more important is the spiritual attitude on both sides.

13. The president of the German Freethinkers' Union until a day or two ago occupied the bed next to mine. In spite of the gulf which in the eyes of the world divided us, we were nearer to one another than were others because of our mutual respect. I could see that he was a man of noble character, and one who was a good friend. I could imagine that in him there survived subconsciously something of the Christian education which had come down through centuries of German history. I would count such a man as among Christ's company more than many baptized persons whose soul has remained untouched by the Spirit of Christ.

14. A feeling of disdain came over me when I heard the death sentence. I knew there was no shame, only honor, in being declared dishonorable by such a court.

15. ONLY A GREAT VENTURE OF FAITH, HUMILITY AND LOVE CAN SOLVE THE PROBLEM OF THE FATE OF CHRISTENDOM.

The Answer of Minerva

Pacifism and Resistance in Simone Weil

Like Bernanos and Camus, Simone Weil is one of those brilliant and independent French thinkers who were able to articulate the deepest concerns of France and Europe in the first half of this century. More controversial and perhaps more of a genius than the others, harder to situate, she has been called all kinds of names, both good and bad and often contradictory: Gnostic and Catholic, Jew and Albigensian, medievalist and modernist, Platonist and anarchist, rebel and saint, rationalist and mystic. De Gaulle said he thought she was out of her mind. The doctor in the sanatorium at Ashford, Kent, where she died (August 24, 1943) said, "She had a curious religious outlook and (probably) no religion at all." In any case, whatever is said about her, she can always be treated as "an enigma." Which is simply to say that she is somewhat more difficult to categorize than most people, since in her passion for integrity she absolutely refused to take up any position she had not first thought out in the light of what she believed to be a personal vocation to "absolute intellectual honesty." When she began to examine any accepted position, she easily detected its weaknesses and inconsistencies.

None of the books of Simone Weil (seventeen in French, eight in English) were written as books. They are all collections of notes, essays, articles, journals and letters. Though she has conquered a certain number of fans by the force of her personality, most readers remember her as the author of some fragment or other that they have found in some way both impressive and disconcerting. One cannot help admiring her lucid genius, and yet one can very easily disagree with her most fundamental and characteristic ideas. But this is usually because one does not see her thought as a whole. The new biography by Jacques Cabaud [1] not only tells of her active and tormented life,

1. Jacques Cabaud, *Simone Weil* (Harvill Press, 1964, 392 pp, ill.).

but studies in detail a large number of writings (of which a complete bibliography is given), together with the testimony of those who knew her. Cabaud has also avoided treating Simone Weil either as a problem or as a saint. He accepts her as she evidently was. Such a book is obviously indispensable, for without such a comprehensive and detached study it would be impossible to judge her reasonably. In fact, no one who reads this book carefully and dispassionately can treat Simone Weil merely as an enigma or a phenomenon, still less as deluded or irrelevant. Few writers have more significant thoughts on the history of our time and a better understanding of our calamities. On the other hand, probably not even Mr. Cabaud would claim that this book says the last word on Simone Weil or that it fully explains, for instance, her "Christian mysticism" that prompted her of deliberate purpose to remain outside the Church and refuse baptism even on the point of death because she felt that her natural element was with "the immense and unfortunate multitude of unbelievers." This "unbeliever," we note, was one who had been "seized" by Christ in a mystical experience the marks of which are to all appearances quite authentic, though the Catholic theologian has trouble keeping them clearly in a familiar and traditional focus. (Obviously, one of her charisms was that of living and dying as a sign of contradiction for Catholics, and one feels that the climate of Catholic thought in France at the time of Vatican II has been to some extent affected by at least a vague awareness of her experiences at Solesmes and Marseilles.)

Though her spirit was at times explicitly intended to be that of the medieval Cathars and though her description of her mystical life is strongly Gnostic and intellectual, she has had things to say of her experience of suffering and of her understanding of the suffering of Christ which are not only deeply Christian but also speak directly to the anguish and perplexity of modern man. This intuition of the nature and meaning of suffering provides, in Simone Weil, the core of a metaphysic, not to say a theology, of nonviolence. A metaphysic of nonviolence is something that the peace movement needs.

Looking back at Simone Weil's participation in the peace movement of the thirties, Cabaud speaks rather sweepingly of a collapse of pacifism in her thought and political action. It is quite true that the pacifism of the thirties was as naïve as it was popular, and that for many people at that time pacifism amounted to nothing more than the disposition to ignore unpleasant realities and to compromise with the threat of force as did Chamberlain at Munich. It is also true that Simone Weil herself underestimated the ruthlessness of Hitler at the time of the Munich crisis though her principles did not allow her to agree with the Munich pact. Cabaud quotes a statement of Simone Weil accusing herself of a "criminal error committed before 1939 with regard to pacifist groups and their actions." Her tolerance of a passive and inert pacifism was regarded by her as a kind of cooperation with "their disposition towards treason" which, she said, she did not see because she was disabled by illness (Cabaud, p. 197). This reflects her disgust with Vichy and with former pacifists who now submitted to Hitler without protest. But we cannot interpret this statement to mean that after Munich and then the fall of France Simone Weil abandoned all her former principles in order to take up an essentially new position in regard to war and peace. This would mean equating her "pacifism" with the quietism of the uncomprehending and the inert. It would also mean failure to understand that she became deeply committed to nonviolent resistance. Before Munich the emphasis was, however, on nonviolence, and after the fall of France the emphasis was on *resistance,* including the acceptance of resistance by force where nonviolence was ineffective.

It is unfortunate that Cabaud's book does not sufficiently avoid the usual cliché identification of pacifism as such with quietist passivity, and nonresistance. Simone Weil's love of peace was never sentimental and never quietistic; and though her judgment sometimes erred in assessing concrete situations, it was seldom unrealistic. An important article she wrote in 1937 remains one of the classic treatments of the problem of war and peace in our time. Its original title was: "Let us not start the Trojan War all over again." It appears in her *Selected Essays* as "The Power of Words." Cabaud analyzes it in his book (pp. 155–160) where he says that it marks a dividing line in her life. It belongs, in fact, to the same crucial period as her first mystical experiences.

There is nothing mystical about this essay. It develops a theme familiar to Montaigne and Charron—the most terrible thing about war is that, if it is examined closely, it is discovered to have no rationally definable objective. The supposed objectives of war are actually myths and fictions which are all the more capable of enlisting the full force of devotion to duty and hatred of the enemy when they are completely empty of content. Let us briefly resume this article, since it contains the substance of Simone Weil's ideas on peace and is (apart from some of her topical examples) just as relevant to our own time as it was to the late thirties.

The article begins with a statement which is passed over by Cabaud, and which is very important for us. Simone Weil remarks that while our technology has given us weapons of immense destructive power, the weapons do not go off by themselves (we hope). Hence it is a primordial mistake to think and act as if the weapons were what constituted our danger, rather than the people who are disposed to fire them off. But more precisely still: the danger lies not so much in this or that group or class but in the climate of thought in which all participate (not excluding pacifists). This is what Simone Weil set herself to understand. The theme of the article is, then, that war must be regarded as a problem to be solved by rational analysis and action, not as a fatality to which we must submit with bravery or desperation. We see immediately that she is anything but passively resigned to the evil of war. The acceptance of war as an unavoidable fatality she clearly saw to be the root of the power politician's ruthless and obsessed commitment to violence.

This, she believed, was the "key to our history."

If in fact conflicting statesmen faced one another only with clearly defined objectives that were fully rational, there would be a certain measure and limit which would permit of discussion and negotiation. But where the objectives are actually nothing more than capital-letter slogans without any intelligible content whatever, there is no common measure, therefore no possibility of communication, and hence no possibility of avoiding war except by ambiguous compromises, or by agreements that are not intended to be kept. Such agreements do not really avoid war. And of course they solve no problems.

The typology of the Trojan war, "known to every educated man," illustrates this. The only one, Greek or Trojan, who had any interest in Helen, was Paris. No one, Greek or Trojan, was fighting for Helen, but for the "real issue" which Helen symbolized. Unfortunately, there was no real issue at all for her to symbolize. Both armies, in this war, which is the type of all wars, were fighting in a moral void, motivated by symbols without content, which in the case of the Homeric heroes took the form of gods and myths. Simone Weil considered that this was relatively fortunate for them since their myths were thus kept within a well-defined area. For us, on the other hand (since we imagine that we have no myths at all), myth actually is without limitation and can easily penetrate the whole realm of political, social and ethical thought. Thus, instead of going to war because the gods have been arguing among themselves, we go because of "secret plots" and sinister combinations, because of political slogans elevated to the dignity of metaphysical absolutes: "Our political universe is peopled with myths and monsters—we know nothing there but absolutes." We shed blood for high-sounding words spelled out in capital letters. We seek to impart content to them by destroying other men who believe in enemy-words, also in capital letters.

But how can men really be brought to kill each other for what is objectively void? The nothingness of national, class or racial myth must receive an apparent substance, not from intelligible content but from the *will to destroy and be destroyed*. (We may observe here that the substance of idolatry is the willingness to give reality to metaphysical nothingness by sacrificing to it. The more totally one destroys present realities and alienates oneself to an object which is really void, the more total is the idolatry, i.e., the commitment to the falsehood that the non-entity is an objective absolute. Note here that in this context the God of the mystics is not "an object" and cannot be described properly as "an entity" among other entities. Hence one of the marks of authentic mysticism is that God as experienced by the mystic can in no way be the object of an idolatrous cult.)

The will to kill and be killed grows out of sacrifices and acts of destruction already performed. As soon as the war has begun, the first dead are there to demand further sacrifice from their companions since they have demonstrated by their example that the objective of the war is such that no price is too high to pay for its attainment. This is the "sledgehammer argument," the argument of Minerva in Homer: "You must fight on, for if you now make peace with the enemy, you will offend the dead."

These are cogent intuitions, but so far they do not add anything beyond their own vivacity to the ideas that prevailed in the thirties. In effect, everyone who remembered the First World War was capable of meditating on the futility of war in 1938. Everyone was still able to take sarcastic advantage of slogans about "making the world safe for democracy." But merely to say that war was totally absurd and totally meaningless, in its very nature, was to run the risk of missing the real point. Mere words without content do not suffice, of themselves, to start a war. Behind the empty symbols and the objectiveless motivation of force, there is a real force, the grimmest of all the social realities of our time: collective power, which Simone Weil, in her more Catharist mood, regarded as the "Great Beast." ("How will the soul be saved," she asked her philosophy students in the Lycée, "after the Great Beast has acquired an opinion about everything?")

The void underlying the symbols and the myths of nationalism, of capitalism, Communism, Fascism, racism, totalism, is in fact filled entirely by the presence of the Beast. We might say, developing her image, that the void thus becomes an insatiable demand for power, which sucks all life and all being into itself. Power is thus generated by the plunge of real and human values into nothingness, allowing themselves to be destroyed in order that the collectivity may attain to a theoretical and hopeless ideal of perfect and unassailable supremacy: "What is called national security is a chimerical state of things in which one would keep for oneself alone the power to make war while all other countries would be unable to do so. . . . War is therefore made *in order to keep or to increase the means of making war.* All international politics revolve in this vicious circle." "But," she adds, "why must one be able to make war? This no one knows any more than the Trojans knew why they had to keep Helen."

Nevertheless, when Germany overran France she herself found a reason for joining the resistance: the affirmation of human liberty against the abuse of power. "All over the world there are human beings *serving as means to the power of others without having consented to it.*" This was a basic evil that had to be resisted. The revision of Simone Weil's opinion on pacifism and nonviolence after Munich does not therefore resolve itself, as Cabaud seems to indicate, with a practical repudiation of both. Munich led her to clarify the distinction between ineffective and effective nonviolence. The former is what Gandhi called the nonviolence of the weak, and it merely submits to evil without resistance. Effective nonviolence ("the nonviolence of the strong") is that which opposes evil with serious and positive resistance, in order to overcome it with good. Simone Weil would apparently have added that if this nonviolence had no hope of success, then evil could be resisted by force. But she hoped for a state of affairs in which human conflict could be resolved nonviolently rather than by force. However, her notion of nonviolent resistance was never fully developed. If she had survived (she would be fifty-six now) she might possibly have written some exciting things on the subject.

Once this is understood, then we can also understand Simone Weil's revulsion at the collapse of that superficial and popular pacifism of Munich, which, since it was passive and also without clear objective, was only another moment in the objectiveless dialectic of brute power. And we can also understand the passion with which she sought to join the French resistance. But she did not change her principles. She did not commit herself to violent action, but she did seek to expose herself to the greatest danger and sacrifice, nonviolently. Though her desire to form a "front line nursing corps" (regarded by De Gaulle as lunacy) were never fulfilled, she nevertheless worked—indeed overworked—until the time of her death, trying to clarify the principles on which a new France could be built. She never gave up the hope that one might "substitute more and more in the world effective nonviolence for violence."

Auschwitz: A Family Camp

On December 20, 1963, twenty-two former SS men who had played important parts in the "final solution of the Jewish question" at Auschwitz went on trial at Frankfort. The trial lasted twenty months. Scores of survivors of the camp, together with many other witnesses, testified to the massive torture and butchery accomplished twenty years before, in that curious place "far away, somewhere in Poland." The testimony does not make pleasant reading. It fills a book [1] in large format running to nearly 450 pages: and this is only a summary of the most important points. The defendants were convicted and sentenced to prison terms, which they have all appealed. The most curious thing about the trial is that the defendants confidently and consistently denied almost everything. Finally the judge remarked in astonishment that he had "yet to meet anyone who had done anything at Auschwitz"! There was, in other words, a marked contrast between the unanimity of the witnesses saying black and the unanimity of the defendants saying white. Still more curiously, these same defendants had previously admitted much more of the dark side of the picture themselves. But now this has been "forgotten." They have somehow changed their minds. Hannah Arendt, in an important introduction, interprets this to mean that the German public has tacitly come to terms with the grim past. It has now apparently accepted these men, and many others like them.

In spite of the general tone of outrage still noticeable on the level of the court and of the better newspapers, the defendants themselves remained contemptuous and at ease, certain of ultimate freedom and confident that they had the tacit approval of their peers. Keeping this in mind, we now turn to the book. We reflect on the workings of a death factory where some three or four million people were barbarously

1. *Auschwitz*, by Bernd Naumann, translated by Jean Steinberg, with an introduction by Hannah Arendt (London: Pall Mall Press, 1966), 433 pp.

destroyed. Yet to judge by the testimony of these men who have been sentenced to prison for literally thousands of murders each, the camp was an innocent establishment, a place for "protective custody." It doubtless knew its moments of austerity, but on the whole, it was simply a camp where people went to be "reeducated." At times, it almost sounds like fairyland. . . .

Fairyland in Poland

Chief among the defendants was Robert Mulka. In July, 1942, Mulka became deputy of the camp commandant, Hoss. Though second in command for about a year, he claimed to know nothing about the fact that many prisoners seemed to be dying and of course issued no orders that had any connection with these unfortunate occurrences. When questioned about his duties he said he had worried a lot about whether or not the camp could afford some entertainers he wished to bring there. He sometimes encountered death close at hand when he paraded at the honor funeral of one of the SS guards. Gas chambers? Yes, he had heard something about them over the camp grapevine. "Word," he said, "got out in the course of time." Crematory furnaces? He admitted having seen a red glow in the sky and wondered what it was: rumor had supplied details. When pressed to explain why he had not tried to discover the facts himself, he said there was "no one to ask." Not even Commandant Hoss? No, the commandant was an "opaque man." Were there no orders about the "special treatment" of "asocial elements" and the "disinfection" of undesirables? He admitted that "there were probably some general instructions" which of course bypassed his own department, for he was after all only second in command. Confronted with orders signed by himself he offered no explanation. At the end of the trial, when the prosecution was asking that Mulka be given life imprisonment for more than 36,500 murders, Mulka himself simply asked the court to consider "all the circumstances which at the time brought me into my conflict situation."

The other defendants all said the same. Even those who were accused of selecting the prisoners for extermination, of driving them into the gas chambers, naked, with dogs turned loose and tearing their flesh. Of beating them to death on the "Boger swing" in "rigorous interrogations." Of injecting phenol into their hearts and killing them. Of wiping them out in shootings that lasted two or three hours. All these people were strangely unaware that Auschwitz had been an extermination camp and that they had been the exterminators. They admitted there were gas chambers "somewhere near the barracks." (And where were the barracks? "Somewhere near the gas chambers!") Yes, sometimes one drove a truck up "near the barracks" and one became aware that "people were busy doing something." It was even observed that "some prisoners were lying around." Resting perhaps? Since resting was not the usual thing at Auschwitz, were they perhaps dead? Altogether hard to say. One had failed to notice.

What about "cap shooting," making the prisoners throw their caps away, ordering them to run over to pick up the caps, and then shooting them for "trying to escape"? What about genuine escape attempts (some of which even succeeded)? One of the former SS guards assured the court that there were no attempted escapes. Who would want to escape? Auschwitz, he said, was after all, "a family camp." Another of the defendants, when obligingly describing the camp layout, asked the court if it would like him to point out on the map the place where he had made "a children's playground with sandboxes for the little ones."

Yes, there were even little ones in Auschwitz. They were marked out for play.

"The children were playing ball," says a former prisoner, "and waiting unsuspectingly. . . . A woman guard came, and clapped her hands, and called out: 'All right now, let's stop. Now we take showers.' And then they ran down the steps into the room in which they undressed. And the guard took a little girl on her arm and carried her down. And the child pointed to the eagle emblem on the cap of the SS woman and asked: 'What kind of birdie is that?' And that was the last I saw and heard of the child."

The Installations

No need to describe Auschwitz, the two huge death camps about three miles apart, the guard towers, the high barbwire fences charged with thousands of volts, the barracks, the gas chambers, the furnaces burning day and night. The evil-smelling smoke. The glare in the night sky visible for miles. The ramp where the long freight trains arrived, the "transports" jammed with prisoners, men, women, children, from all parts of Europe. On the ramp, those selected for immediate gassing were told by a gesture to go to the right. Selection depended to some extent on the caprice or mood of the one in charge. But one could be "selected" in the camp itself. If a prisoner became seriously ill or too weak to work. If the barracks were getting too crowded. If conditions became inconvenient, efficiency might demand a housecleaning.

Delousings were not working properly in the woman's camp. And a new doctor came along and solved the problem in a businesslike manner. "He simply had an entire block gassed." Having thus disposed of seven hundred and fifty women prisoners, he cleaned out the block, disinfected it, thoroughly deloused another batch of prisoners and moved them in. "He was the first to rid the entire women's camp of lice."

If Auschwitz was one of the main centers for the "final solution of the Jewish question" we must also remember it dealt with other problems too. Polish intellectuals and members of the Polish resistance were sent here for torture and liquidation. Thousands of Russian prisoners of war were exterminated at Auschwitz. According to the written testimony of one of the defendants (a deposition handed to the British at the end of the war) twelve thousand Russian prisoners of war reached Auschwitz early in 1942. In six months, there were only one hundred and fifty of them still alive. "Thousands of prisoners of war were shot in a copse near Birkenau" (wrote the defendant Perry Broad). They were "buried in mass graves . . . the fisheries began to complain that the fish in the ponds in the vicinity of Birkenau were dying. Experts said this was due to the pollution of the ground water through cadaveric poison. . . . The summer sun was beating down on Birkenau, the bodies . . . started to swell up and a dark red mass started to seep through the cracks of the earth. . . ." This called for a quick and efficient solution, since the camp authorities did not like bad publicity. Twenty or thirty "very reliable SS men" were picked for the job. They had to sign a statement that if they violated their oath of secrecy or even hinted at the nature of their job they would be punished by death. This special detail then rounded up prisoners to do the digging. The prisoners chosen were Jews. The bodies of the Russians were exhumed and burned. "For weeks, thick white smoke continued to rise from that isolated tract of land." There were rumors. Prisoners who refused to do this job were shot. The others did not survive to tell about it. The SS men on this unpleasant detail were rewarded with "special rations from the SS kitchen: 1 quart of milk, sausages, cigarettes and of course liquor." This, it turned out, was standard practice and applied also to those who had the tiresome job of beating prisoners to death, or shooting them at the Black Wall, or pushing them into the gas. When things were very busy the SS men were seen to be pretty drunk. On one such occasion an SS man, trying to show off his marksmanship, unfortunately shot a colleague. He was, of course, punished. One of the SS men, Klehr, was a male nurse—a "medical orderly." He specialized in injecting his patients in the heart with phenol and thus solving all their problems at once. He was also a notorious drunk, and was sometimes so intoxicated that he could no longer carry on the selections of appropriate candidates for the gas chamber. "Such selections had to be interrupted."

Klehr also had other hobbies. He was in charge of some rabbits: perhaps they were used for scientific experiments like the prisoners. At any rate he was so interested in the rabbits that he often "injected the prisoners two at a time because he wanted to get back to his rabbits." Such was the testimony of a former prisoner who had to hold the patients whom Klehr was injecting. One day the prisoner looked up and recognized the next patient in line. It was his father. Klehr was in a hurry and did not stop to ask why the prisoner was crying. He did so the next day, however. "Why," said Klehr in a burst of arbitrary generosity, "you should have told me. I would have let him live!"

Favors were sometimes done at Auschwitz! The prisoner, however, had feared to speak, convinced that if he did so he would have got a shot of phenol in the heart himself.

The Children of Zamosc

Klehr took care of one hundred and twenty Polish children from a village called Zamosc. They were killed in two batches: eighty the first day, the rest on the day after. Their parents were dead and no one quite knew what to do with them. They played in the courtyard of the hospital. "A ball had somehow turned up." Maybe that was when there were sandboxes. Another witness mentioned a balloon. But eventually the children were lined up and filed into the "examination room." Klehr was waiting for them with the syringe and the saucer of phenolic acid. The first ones screamed. After that it was somehow quieter. In the silence of the barrack, one heard the bodies falling off the chair and thumping onto the wooden floor. But Klehr did not do it all. Maybe he got bored and went to his rabbits, handing over the syringe. Scherpe, who took over, broke down under the strain and ran out of the room, refusing to kill any more children. A third SS man had to supply and finish the work begun. Reason for the death of the little boys from Zamosc? As a precaution against "immorality" in the camp. Auschwitz had to be very, very clean!

Other scenes with children: Outside the gas chambers and crematories where mothers with children were sent immediately upon arrival. The mothers sometimes tried to hide the children under the piles of clothing. "Sometimes the voice of a little child who had been forgotten would emerge from beneath a pile of clothing. . . . They would put a bullet through its head."

Sometimes, children were not sent at once for "special treatment." They might be kept handy for medical experiments. In the interests of science! Or they might even be assigned to useful work. One witness who entered Auschwitz at fourteen and survived testified that he was on the cart detail that removed ashes from the crematory. "We got ashes from Crematory III and scattered them on the icy roads. When there were no people in the gas chambers, the capo let us warm ourselves there." Another less bucolic scene: an SS man who threw living children into the flames and boiling human fat of the open cremation pyres. And finally this, from a witness: "Early in the morning I saw a little girl standing all by herself in the yard . . . wearing a claret-colored dress and [she had] a little pigtail. She held her hands at her side like a soldier. Once she looked down, wiped the dust off her shoes and again stood very still. Then I saw Boger come into the yard. He took the child by her hand—she went along very obediently—and stood her with her face to the Black Wall. Once she turned around. Boger again turned her head to the wall, walked back, and shot. . . ."

Exceptionally gentle for Boger, one of the most brutal professional butchers in the camp. He was sometimes seen to pick up little children by the heels and smash their heads against a brick wall. . . . But that was during a moment of stress in the mass liquidation of the Gypsy compound.

The Language of Auschwitz

Language itself has fallen victim to total war, genocide and systematic tyranny in our time. In destroying human beings, and human values, on a mass scale, the Gestapo also subjected the German language to violence and crude perversion.

In Auschwitz secrecy was emphasized. "If you talk about what you can see from here," one prisoner was told, "you'll go through the chimney." Written records were kept cryptic, evasive. Great care was taken to destroy as much paperwork as possible before the Russians arrived. Even mention of corporal punishment was taboo. Any open reference to the realities of life and death in the camp was regarded as treason. Any guard, doctor, prison administrator who let out the truth could be severely punished for "defeatist talk."

This circumlocution was itself highly significant. It admitted the sinister and ironic fact that even knowledge of the truth about Auschwitz could furnish a formidable propaganda weapon to the enemies of the Reich. The very irony of the fact should have raised some urgent questions about the principle behind the camp. But the function of doubletalk and doublethink is to say everything without raising inconvenient questions. Officialese has a talent for discussing reality while denying it and calling truth itself into question. Yet the truth remains. This doubletalk is by its very nature invested with a curious metaphysical leer. The language of Auschwitz is one of the vulnerable spots through which we get a clear view of the demonic.

Gestapo doubletalk encircles reality as a doughnut encircles its hole. "Special treatment," "special housing." We need no more than one lesson, and we gain the intuition which identifies the hole, the void of death, in the heart of the expression. When the circumlocution becomes a little more insistent ("recovery camps for the tired") it brings with it suggestions of awful lassitude, infinite hopelessness, as if meaning had now been abolished forever and we were definitively at the mercy of the absurd.

"Disinfectants," "materials for resettlement of Jews," "ovaltine substitute from Swiss Red Cross"—all references to Zyklon B! When a deadly poison gas is referred to as a soothing, restorative, a quasi-medicine to put babies to sleep, one senses behind the phrase a deep hatred of life itself. The key to Auschwitz language is its pathological joy in death. This turns out to be the key to all officialese. All of it is the celebration of boredom, of routine, of deadness, of organized futility. Auschwitz just carried the whole thing to its logical extreme, with a kind of heavy lilt in its mockery, its oafish love of death.

"Work makes free"—the sign over the gate of Auschwitz—tells, with grim satisfaction, the awful literal truth: "Here we work people to death." And behind it the dreadful metaphysical admission: "For us there is only one freedom, death."

"To the Bath," said the sign pointing to the gas chambers. (You will be purified of that dirty thing, your life!) And as a matter of fact the gas chambers and crematories were kept spotlessly clean. "Nothing was left of them [the victims] not even a speck of dust on the armatures."

"Assigned to harvest duty"—this, in the record of an SS man, meant he had been posted to Auschwitz. The double meaning of "harvest" was doubtless not random. It has an apocalyptic ring.

Yet the Gestapo people had an acute sense of the importance of words. One of them became quite excited in court, over the distinction between "transferred" and "assigned."

Those who tortured escapees or resistors (and resistance could be expressed even by an expressionless face) praised the "Boger Swing" as their most effective language machine. The victim was hung from a horizontal pole, upside down, by wrists and ankles. He was whipped so vigorously that he often spun clean round on the pole. "You'll learn to talk, we have language for you," said the Gestapo men. "My talking machine will make you talk," said Boger, who was proud of his invention. In fact he has earned himself a place in history on account of it. Not an enviable place.

One of the results of the Frankfort trial is that it makes an end of the pure Auschwitz myth: the myth of demented monsters who were twice our size, with six eyes and four rows of teeth, not of the same world as ourselves. The demonic sickness of Auschwitz emanated from ordinary people, stimulated by an extraordinary regime. The trial brought out their variety, their ordinariness, their shades of character, and even their capacity of change. In strict justice to Klehr, it must be said that he was profoundly affected by a visit from his wife in 1944, "a good kind woman . . . her two children were decent and well brought up." She did not suspect that her husband was involved in murder, but she knew that everything was not well at the camp. A witness overheard her saying to him, "I heard that terrible things happen here. I hope you're not involved." Klehr replied that he "cured people." But after his wife's visit, he began to treat prisoners more decently and to react against the camp methods. He even volunteered for frontline duty, and when his request was refused, he denounced a brutal camp officer and had him transferred, thus improving conditions.

It is nevertheless eerie to read the testimony of a witness who had been a neighbor of the defendant Dr. Capesius in Bucharest, and met him on the ramp where he sent her sisters, brothers and father to the gas chamber. "I still knew Dr. Capesius from Bucharest. . . . We lived in the same building. He was a representative of Bayer. Sometimes I spoke to him and his wife. . . ." The witness had even had coffee with Capesius and his wife in a park. That was the last time she saw him until 1944, at Auschwitz. "I recognized him right away. . . . I was happy to see him. When I stood in front of him all he said was, 'How old are you?' and sent me to the right." However, it may be noted that in sending her to the right he had saved her life. Not even Boger can be regarded without qualification as a pure monster. Auschwitz becomes a little more horrible when we have to admit that Boger too is a human being.

Boger and his colleagues were all more or less the products of a society at least as respectable and as civilized as that of New York or London. They had all received an education, some of them higher education. They had been brought up, it is said, in "Christian homes," or at least in middle-class homes—not quite the same, but Christianity has been willing to overlook the possible difference. Before Hitler, they lived and moved among "respectable people" and since Hitler they have done the same. How is it that for twelve years in between they could beat and bash and torment and shoot and whip and murder thousands of their fellow human beings, *including even their former neighbors and friends,* and think nothing of it?

In the first place it would be wrong to say that they all thought nothing of it. One among the defendants who comes close to being tragic is Dr. Lucas. We sense in him a complex, lonely, tormented character who knew he was involved in a wrong that he could not entirely escape. Perhaps he might have escaped it. No one will ever be able to say with finality. But in any event he elected to go along with the system, to participate in the "selections," while at the same time practicing the ambivalent quasi-unconscious resistance technique of the "good soldier Schweik." Witness after witness spoke out in favor of Dr. Lucas. He was different from the others. Yes, he sent people to their death, but many witnesses recognized that he had saved their lives. Still he remained identified with the machinery of organized murder, and recognized that in so doing he had ruined his own life. Another who admitted that Auschwitz had been a doubtful quality in his life was Stark. He had gone to the camp as an SS guard when still in his teens. He had not yet finished school. Shooting, beating and killing were, for him, normal facts of life. He accepted them without question. He had practically grown up under Hitler and did not learn the difference until later. "I regret the mistakes of my past," he said, "but I cannot undo them."

What about Boger? Though he consistently denied everything said by witnesses, in the end his defense was content to ask for leniency rather than life imprisonment, on the grounds that Boger had merely done his duty as a good policeman.

This seems to sum up Boger's rather aggrieved view of his own case. Boger defended his "swing" right to the end. How could one refuse a conscientious police official the right to use "rigorous methods of interrogation"? Boger bluntly addressed the court on the virtues and necessity of these methods. They were highly practical. His defense lawyer expostulated with the Jury: "The swing was not intended as torture: it was the only effective means of physical suasion."

The shocking thing about the views of both Boger and his lawyer is that they are evidently quite sincere. Not only that, they are views with which, it is assumed, other people will sympathize without difficulty.

In his final statement to the court, Boger made a distinction between the genocidal extermination of the Jews, which he admitted was perhaps a bit rough, and what he himself thought most important at the time: "*the fight against the Polish resistance movement and Bolshevism.*"

Boger's case has now become an open appeal to the "good Germans" who, he assumes, agree with him; they will easily approve the rigors of his interrogation methods since they were justified by anti-Communism.

At this point, there swims into view a picture taken at another investigation, (hardly a trial) in the state of Mississippi. We see the smiling, contemptuous, brutal faces of the police deputies and their colleagues who are allegedly the murderers of three civil rights workers in the summer of 1964. Whatever may have been the facts in the case, one feels that in Mississippi and Auschwitz the basic assumptions are not very different. Instead of seeing the Bogers and Klehrs of Auschwitz as fabulous, myth-sized and inhuman monsters, we come to recognize that people like them are in fact all around us. All they need is the right kind of crisis, and they will blossom out.

Salutary Reflections

Such is the first conclusion. We have learned to associate the incredible brutality and inhumanity of Auschwitz with ordinary respectable people, in an extraordinary situation.

Second: Auschwitz worked because these people wanted it to work. Instead of resisting it, rebelling against it, they put the best of their energies into making genocide a success. This was true not only of one or two psychopaths but of an entire bureaucratic officialdom, including not only the secret police and Nazi party members but also managers and employees of the industries which knowingly made use of the slave labor provided in such abundance by the camp.

Third: although it was usual to argue that "they had no choice" and that they were "forced" to comply with orders, the trial showed a more complex and less excusable picture of the defendants. Almost all of them committed gratuitous acts of arbitrary cruelty and violence which were forbidden even by the Gestapo's own rules. Some were even punished by the SS for these violations. Was there no choice? There are on record refusals of men who simply would not take part in murder and got themselves transferred. Why was not this done more often? Let us clearly spell out two of the circumstances. Auschwitz was safe. One was not at the front, and there was practically no danger from bombing planes. And there were privileges: the work was no doubt disagreeable to some, but there were extra rations, smokes, drinks. Finally, there can be little doubt that many of these men tortured and killed because they thoroughly enjoyed it.

Fourth: what does all this add up to? Given the right situation and another Hitler, places like Auschwitz can be set up, put into action, kept running smoothly, with thousands of people systematically starved, beaten, gassed, and whole crematories going full blast. Such camps can be set up tomorrow anywhere and made to work with the greatest efficiency, because there is no dearth of people who would be glad to do the job, provided it is sanctioned by authority. They will be glad because they will instinctively welcome and submit to an ideology which enables them to be violent and destructive without guilt. They are happy with a belief which turns them loose against their fellow man to destroy him cruelly and without compunction, as long as he belongs to a different race, or believes in a different set of semi-meaningless political slogans.

It is enough to affirm one basic principle: ANYONE BELONGING TO CLASS X OR NATION Y OR RACE Z IS TO BE REGARDED AS SUBHUMAN AND WORTHLESS, AND CONSEQUENTLY HAS NO RIGHT TO EXIST. All the rest will follow without difficulty.

As long as this principle is easily available, as long as it is taken for granted, as long as it can be spread out on the front pages at a moment's notice and accepted by all, we have no need of monsters: ordinary policemen and good citizens will take care of everything.

A Devout Meditation in Memory of Adolf Eichmann

One of the most disturbing facts that came out in the Eichmann trial was that a psychiatrist examined him and pronounced him *perfectly sane*. I do not doubt it at all, and that is precisely why I find it disturbing.

If all the Nazis had been psychotics, as some of their leaders probably were, their appalling cruelty would have been in some sense easier to understand. It is much worse to consider this calm, "well-balanced," unperturbed official conscientiously going about his desk work, his administrative job which happened to be the supervision of mass murder. He was thoughtful, orderly, unimaginative. He had a profound respect for system, for law and order. He was obedient, loyal, a faithful officer of a great state. He served his government very well.

He was not bothered much by guilt. I have not heard that he developed any psychosomatic illnesses. Apparently he slept well. He had a good appetite, or so it seems. True, when he visited Auschwitz, the Camp Commandant, Hoss, in a spirit of sly deviltry, tried to tease the big boss and scare him with some of the sights. Eichmann was disturbed, yes. He was disturbed. Even Himmler had been disturbed, and had gone weak at the knees. Perhaps, in the same way, the general manager of a big steel mill might be disturbed if an accident took place while he happened to be somewhere in the plant. But of course what happened at Auschwitz was not an accident: just the routine unpleasantness of the daily task. One must shoulder the burden of daily monotonous work for the Fatherland. Yes, one must suffer discomfort and even nausea from unpleasant sights and sounds. It all comes under the heading of duty, self-sacrifice, and obedience. Eichmann was devoted to duty, and proud of his job.

The sanity of Eichmann is disturbing. We equate sanity with a sense of justice, with humaneness, with prudence, with the capacity to love and understand other people. We rely on the sane people of the world to preserve it from barbarism, madness, destruction. And now it begins to dawn on us that it is precisely the *sane* ones who are the most dangerous.

It is the sane ones, the well-adapted ones, who can without qualms and without nausea aim the missiles and press the buttons that will initiate the great festival of destruction that they, *the sane ones,* have prepared. What makes us so sure, after all, that the danger comes from a psychotic getting into a position to fire the first shot in a nuclear war? Psychotics will be suspect. The sane ones will keep them far from the button. No one suspects the sane, and the sane ones will have *perfectly good reasons,* logical, well-adjusted reasons, for firing the shot. They will be obeying sane orders that have come sanely down the chain of command. And because of their sanity they will have no qualms at all. When the missiles take off, then, *it will be no mistake.*

We can no longer assume that because a man is "sane" he is therefore in his "right mind." The whole concept of sanity in a society where spiritual values have lost their meaning is itself meaningless. A man can be "sane" in the limited sense that he is not impeded by his disordered emotions from acting in a cool, orderly manner, according to the needs and dictates of the social situation in which he finds himself. He can be perfectly "adjusted." God knows, perhaps such people can be perfectly adjusted even in hell itself.

And so I ask myself: what is the meaning of a concept of sanity that excludes love, considers it irrelevant, and destroys our capacity to love other human beings, to respond to their needs and their sufferings, to recognize them also as persons, to apprehend their pain as one's own? Evidently this is not necessary for "sanity" at all. It is a religious notion, a spiritual notion, a Christian notion. What business have we to equate "sanity" with "Christianity"? None at all, obviously. The worst error is to imagine that a Christian must try to be "sane" like everybody else, that we *belong* in our kind of *society.* That we must be "realistic" about it. We must develop a *sane* Christianity: and there have been plenty of sane Christians in the past. Torture is nothing new, is it? We ought to be able to rationalize a little brainwashing, and genocide, and find a place for nuclear war, or at least for napalm bombs, in our moral theology. Certainly some of us are doing our best along those lines already. There are hopes! Even Christians can shake off their sentimental prejudices about charity, and become sane like Eichmann. They can even cling to a certain set of Christian formulas, and fit them into a Totalist Ideology. Let them talk about justice, charity, love, and the rest. These words have not stopped some sane men from acting very sanely and cleverly in the past. . . .

No, Eichmann was sane. The generals and fighters on both sides, in World War II, the ones who carried out the total destruction of entire cities, these were the sane ones. Those who have invented and developed atomic bombs, thermonuclear bombs, missiles; who have planned the strategy of the next war; who have evaluated the various possibilities of using bacterial and chemical agents: these are not the crazy people, they are the *sane* people. The ones who coolly estimate how many millions of victims can be considered expendable in a nuclear war, I presume they do all right with the Rorschach ink blots too. On the other hand, you will probably find that the pacifists and the ban-the-bomb people are, quite seriously, just as we read in *Time,* a little crazy.

I am beginning to realize that "sanity" is no longer a value or an end in itself. The "sanity" of modern man is about as useful to him as the huge bulk and muscles of the dinosaur. If he were a little less sane, a little more doubtful, a little more aware of his absurdities and contradictions, perhaps there might be a possibility of his survival. But if he is sane, too sane . . . perhaps we must say that in a society like ours the worst insanity is to be totally without anxiety, totally "sane."

II

THE NONVIOLENT ALTERNATIVE

Danish Nonviolent Resistance to Hitler

One of the rare glimmers of humanity and reason in the detailed history of Eichmann's patient labors to exterminate the Jews, as recorded by Hannah Arendt's recent series of articles in *The New Yorker,* was the nonviolent resistance offered by the entire nation of Denmark against Nazi power mobilized for genocide.

Denmark was not the only European nation that *disagreed* with Hitler on this point. But it was one of the only nations which offered explicit, formal and successful nonviolent resistance to Nazi power. The adjectives are important. The resistance was successful because it was explicit and formal, and because it was practically speaking unanimous. The entire Danish nation simply refused to cooperate with the Nazis, and resisted every move of the Nazis against the Jews with nonviolent protest of the highest and most effective caliber, yet without any need for organization, training, or specialized activism: *simply by unanimously and effectively expressing in word and action the force of their deeply held moral convictions.* These moral convictions were nothing heroic or sublime. They were merely *ordinary.*

There had of course been subtle and covert refusals on the part of other nations. Italians in particular, while outwardly complying with Hitler's policy, often arranged to help the Jews evade capture or escape from unlocked freight cars. The Danish nation, from the King on down, formally and publically rejected the policy and opposed it with an open, calm, convinced resistance which shook the morale of the German troops and SS men occupying the country and changed their whole outlook on the Jewish question.

When the Germans first approached the Danes about the segregation of Jews, proposing the introduction of the yellow badge, the government officials replied that the King of Denmark would be the first to wear the badge, and that the introduction of any anti-Jewish measures would lead immediately to their own resignation.

At the same time, the Danes refused to make any distinction between Danish and non-Danish Jews. That is to say, they took the German Jewish refugees under their protection and refused to deport them back to Germany—an act which considerably disrupted the efficiency of Eichmann's organization and delayed anti-Jewish operations in Denmark until 1943 when Hitler personally ordered that the "final solution" go into effect without further postponement.

The Danes replied by strikes, by refusals to repair German ships in their shipyards, and by demonstrations of protest. The Germans then imposed martial law. But now it was realized that the German officials in Denmark were changed men. They could "no longer be trusted." They refused to cooperate in the liquidation of the Jews, not of course by open protest, but by delays, evasions, covert refusals and the raising of bureaucratic obstacles. Hence Eichmann was forced to send a "specialist" to Denmark, at the same time making a concession of monumental proportions: all the Jews from Denmark would go only to Theresienstadt, a "soft" camp for privileged Jews. Finally, the special police sent direct from Germany to round up the Jews were warned by the SS officers in Denmark that Danish police would probably forcibly resist attempts to take the Jews away by force, and that there was to be no fighting between Germans and Danes. Meanwhile the Jews themselves had been warned and most of them had gone into hiding, helped, of course, by friendly Danes: then wealthy Danes put up money to pay for transportation of nearly six thousand Jews to Sweden, which offered them asylum, protection and the right to work. Hundreds of Danes cooperated in ferrying Jews to Sweden in small boats. Half the Danish Jews remained safely in hiding in Denmark, during the rest of the war. About five hundred Jews who were actually arrested in Denmark went to Theresienstadt and lived under comparatively good conditions: only forty-eight of them died, mostly of natural causes.

Denmark was certainly not the only European nation that *disapproved* more or less of the "solution" which Hitler had devised for the *Judenfrage.* But it was the only nation which, as a whole, expressed a forthright moral objection to this policy. Other nations kept their disapproval to themselves. They felt it was enough to offer the Jews "heartfelt sympathy," and, in many individual cases, tangible aid. But let us not forget that generally speaking the practice was to help the Jew at considerable profit to oneself. How many Jews in France, Holland, Hungary, etc., paid fortunes for official permits, bribes, transportation, protection, and still did not escape!

The whole Eichmann story, as told by Hannah Arendt (indeed as told by anybody) acquires a quality of hallucinatory awfulness from the way in which we see how people in many ways exactly like ourselves, claiming as we do to be Christians or at least to live by humanistic standards which approximate, in theory, to the Christian ethic, were able to rationalize a conscious, uninterrupted and complete cooperation in activities which we now see to have been not only criminal but diabolical. Most of the rationalizing probably boiled down to the usual half-truths: "What can you do? There is no other way out, it is a necessary evil. True, we recognize this kind of action to be in many ways 'unpleasant.' We hate to have to take measures like these: but then those at the top know best. It is for the common good. The individual conscience has to be overruled when the common good is at stake. Our duty is to obey. The responsibility for these measures rests on others . . . and so on."

Curiously, the Danish exception, while relieving the otherwise unmitigated horror of the story, actually adds to the nightmarish and hallucinated effect of incredulousness one gets while reading it. After all, the Danes were not even running a special kind of nonviolent movement. They were simply acting according to ordinary beliefs which everybody in Europe theoretically possessed, but which, for some reason, nobody acted on. Quite the contrary! Why did a course of action which worked so simply and so well in Denmark not occur to all the other so-called Christian nations of the West just as simply and just as spontaneously?

Obviously there is no simple answer. It does not even necessarily follow that the Danes are men of greater faith or deeper piety than other western Europeans. But perhaps it is true that these people had been less perverted and secularized by the emptiness and cynicism, the thoughtlessness, the crude egoism and the rank amorality which have become characteristic of our world, even where we still see an apparent surface of Christianity. It is not so much that the Danes were Christians, as that they were *human.* How many others were even that?

The Danes were able to do what they did because they were able to make decisions that were based on clear convictions about which they all agreed and which were in accord with the inner truth of man's own rational nature, as well as in accordance with the fundamental law of God in the Old Testament as well as in the Gospel: thou shalt love thy neighbor as thyself. The Danes were able to resist the cruel stupidity of Nazi anti-Semitism because this fundamental truth was *important* to them. And because they were willing, in unanimous and concerted action, to stake their lives on this truth. In a word, *such action becomes possible where fundamental truths are taken seriously.*

Man Is a Gorilla with a Gun

Reflections on a Best Seller

"Extrapolation," say the dictionaries, "is the method of finding by calculation, based on the known terms of a series, other terms, whether preceding or following." The method belongs to mathematics and works efficiently when dealing with number and quantity. When it is transferred to the realm of quality and of organic life, more still to that of history and of culture, it tends to lose its precisely exact scientific quality and becomes a venture in creativity, or, at any rate, a work of fantasy. "Imagination" now takes the place of "calculation" and there can be no doubt that the scientist who seeks to learn the origin of man from a fossilized remnant of a skull that might have belonged to a man or to a baboon must be blessed with a creative imagination as well as with a scientifically exact intelligence. I suppose that when Robert Ardrey, a playwright rather than a professional scientist, subtitles his book [1] "A *personal* investigation into the animal origins and nature of man" he is serving notice that he intends to extrapolate with unrestrained imaginative abandon. At any rate, this is what he does!

There is of course a good basis of scientific evidence in *African Genesis*. The most recent discoveries of paleontology made in Africa, especially the most notable, those of Leakey at Olduvai in Tanganyika, give very convincing indications that the origin of man was in Africa, not in Asia. But the most significant element in the new discoveries is the apparent use of tools and weapons by anthropoid apes. It is not true, as Ardrey seems to think, that these discoveries were totally unknown to everyone before his book appeared to dispel the shrouds of obscurantism with which jealous and less inspired scientists attempted to conceal them. But no matter. The cloak and dagger atmosphere is apparently an essential part of this "personal" extrapolation, which is nothing if not melodramatic. As a matter of fact, one could be grateful

1. Robert Ardrey, *African Genesis* (New York: Atheneum Publishers, 1961).

to Mr. Ardrey for giving us some precise information about these new discoveries, if the information was not buried in autobiographical reminiscence, pungent anecdote and pages of philosophical improvisation.

On the basis of the possibility that there were, in Africa, perhaps a million years ago, tool-and-weapon-using anthropoids, Mr. Ardrey delivers a very aggressive homily on atheistic evolutionism. He attacks not only the traditional Christian world view but also, much more radically, the world views of Marx, Freud, Darwin and practically everyone else you can think of. One theory of man after another is tossed out the window with glorious enthusiasm: and all because some ape picked up the leg bone of an antelope and used it to crack the skull of one of his fellows. This is all we need in order to entirely reconstruct all social philosophy, all history, all anthropology, all psychology, all economics. For Mr. Ardrey, this one monumental act of violence explains everything.

Homo sapiens (including modern man) is the direct "legitimate" descendent of a transitional, carnivorous, erect-walking and weapon-using anthropoid. Because this ape was no ordinary mild-mannered vegetarian ape, but a ruthless "killer ape," man emerged. Man is, according to Ardrey, the child not only of the ape but of the weapon. It was "the weapon that fathered man." The consequence follows immediately. Man is by his very nature an inventor and user of weapons. The essence of human nature is therefore not so much rationality as trigger-happiness, or at least club-happiness. Even sex is set aside as a secondary, relatively meaningless urge compared with man's essential drive to beat up anything and anyone that threatens to invade his "territory." Yes, "territory" is very important here, crucially important. Man is not really interested in woman, in love, in the warmth of satisfied yearning (as Freud may have thought). Man is not so deeply engaged in making a living that his very existence is shaped and dominated by the system of production (according to Marxian dogma). Man is an ape that goes berserk when he thinks he is running out of *lebensraum,* and I must admit that Mr. Ardrey's description of two rival teams of howling monkeys trying to jam each other's broadcasts is very suggestive of modern political life.

The chief contention of Robert Ardrey's high-powered social message is that any philosophy, religious or otherwise, which takes an optimistic view of man, regards him as basically rational and progressive, and postulates that he can better himself by improving his social system, is basically a "romantic illusion." It is absurd, says Mr. Ardrey, to hope that man can some day reach the point where he will settle his difference over "territory" by means of arbitration rather than by bombs. It is fortunate that some members of the human race are still capable of thinking otherwise (for instance Pope John XXIII in his encyclical *Pacem in Terris*).

Quite apart from religious faith and Christian hope, it seems to me that Mr. Ardrey's thesis negates any real value there may be in evolutionism. After all, the theory of natural selection postulates that a species is able to survive by progressive adaptation to new and more difficult conditions. We armed gorillas have now reached a rather crucial point in our evolutionary development in which it would seem that if we cannot get beyond the stage where we were a million years ago, in other words, if we cannot settle our problems by reason instead of with clubs, we are soon going to be as extinct as any dinosaur. The amusing thing about all this is that we are a species that has been given the *choice* of survival or non-survival. We have very large skulls and, presuming there is still something inside of them, it is up to us to make use of them for something besides inventing ways to blow ourselves up.

And that is what one regrets about a book like this. The author has a great deal of imagination and yet not quite enough. He is totally and slavishly committed to a philosophy of ironbound determinism which is dominated by one inexorable obsession: that ape with the club. *Because* man descended in a direct line from an ape with a club, then he is predetermined to be a killer, he is before all else a killer, and it is folly to even consider him being anything else. Mr. Ardrey confesses himself to be firmly convinced of "man's pristine depravity." Thus he is committed to a world view in which violence, barbarism, murder, and every form of depravity are bound to prevail. As a priest, I am prompted to reflect that this is where you end up when you lose your grasp on the real import of the higher religions. No man can really exist completely without religion. If he gets rid of a good one, he will unconsciously exchange it for a bad one. If he is impatient of "myth" in higher religion then he will end up fabricating a myth of his own, and organizing his own crude fantasies into another homemade "system" which pleases him better—perhaps with unfortunate consequences.

Now Mr. Ardrey's exploits in myth-making are not hard to observe. They are evident on every page of his book. To take just one example: on page twenty-one, he wants to give a brief description of Lake Victoria, as the spot near which man came into existence. There are innumerable ways in which one could describe Lake Victoria. Out of several hundred possible qualifiers Mr. Ardrey, characteristically, selects the following: "A hundred miles to the east spreads *sprawling* and *enormous* the *cynically smiling* face of Lake Victoria, *poisonous with disease, crawling with crocodiles,* the probable focus of our earliest human experience." I submit that people who read books like this need a little elementary training in semantics, in the interests of their basic mental and spiritual hygiene. Such a sentence (and there are hundreds like it in the book), has one function above all others: it bludgeons the reader into emotional submission, and subjects him to a crude impression of violence and evil, so that his intelligence raises no objections to the author's thesis. The author pressures the reader into an emotional acceptance of man's pristine depravity by suggesting that the very place where man came into being was itself sinister and depraved.

This kind of thinking is all too common in the twentieth century. It abounded in the Europe of Mussolini, of Hitler, of Goebbels. The Second World War was the direct consequence of this kind of high-powered emotional conditioning. The Nazi dogma of race, blood and land developed an ideology of war and conquest out of just this kind of emotionally loaded anthropology. Everyone is aware that Hitler's thought was, in part, simply a crudely misunderstood mishmash of popular evolutionism.

Nothing can better dispose us for a third world war than the conviction that we are doomed to fight anyway, that our enemies are all well-armed gorillas too, and the only smart thing to do is to let them have it before they ambush us. In the chaotic atmosphere of a nation torn by race riots, deafened by the stridency of hate groups and of fanatics, it is understandable that readers may derive a kind of comfort from this mythology—made to order for readers of Ayn Rand. They will do so all the more readily because there is an unquestionably important basis of scientific data mixed in with the theatrical rhetoric and sermonizing of *African Genesis*. One can only repeat, by way of conclusion, that this is an age in which every man owes it to himself to get at least a nodding acquaintance with that technique of interpretation called semantics. One of the best and most readable authors in this field at the moment is S. I. Hayakawa. You should get to know him.

Saint Maximus the Confessor on Nonviolence

Many Christians are so disturbed by the hostility of enemies of Christianity that they have become convinced that hatred of these enemies is a proof of love for Christ, and that the will to destroy them is a pledge of their own salvation. At such a time it is necessary to go back to the sources and try to recover the true Christian meaning of the first and all-embracing commandment to love all men including our enemies. Failure to understand and observe this commandment brings down the wrath of God on our civilization and means damnation for those Christians who are willfully blind to the clearly expressed teaching of Christ and of the Church from the Apostolic times down to John XXIII and Paul VI. This obligation is not a merely theoretical matter, or something that calls for a rectification of one's inner intentions, without any effect on one's outward conduct. It is on the contrary one of the crucial ways in which we give proof in practice that we are truly disciples of Christ.

Therefore it may be useful to present here a few excerpts from one of the great theologians of the Greek Church, Saint Maximus the Confessor (seventh century) on the love of enemies. These quotations are taken from his book on the ascetic life, which is to say that they are part of a context in which he deals with the essentials of Christian holiness.

The theme of the book is our response to the call of Christ who came into the world offering us the gift of salvation, which we will receive if we obey His commandments and become followers of His example. In this book, which is a dialogue between the master and his disciple, the master at one point reminds the disciple of the Christian's obligation to renounce his selfish desires, because "no man can serve two masters" (Matthew 6:24) and if one follows his own desires he will not take seriously the commandments of Christ, but will seek to evade them. The disciple protests that after all the love of food, comfort, money, possessions, praise, etc., are all good natural desires. If they are good, and if they come from God, why should we renounce them?

It is in replying to this objection that the master brings up the subject of our relations with our enemies: in fact, it is because we love money, possessions, comfort, etc., more than other men that we enter into conflict with our fellow man, in order to take for ourselves what we do not wish to share with him, even if in order to fulfill our desires we must destroy our enemies.

The master continues:

> It is true that we can please God by making a good use of the things He has given to us. Nevertheless we are weak, and our spirit is weighed down by matter, so that now we prefer profane and material things to the commandment of love. Because we are attached to these things we fight against other men, whereas we ought to prefer love for our fellow man to every visible thing and even to love for our own body. Such preference as this would be the sign of our authentic love of God, as the Lord said Himself in the Gospel: "He who loves me, keeps my commandments" (John 14:15). And what is this commandment which proves our love for Him? Let us hear Him tell us Himself: "This is my commandment: that you love one another" (John 15:12).
>
> Do you now see that this love for one another is the proof of our love for God, and this is the way to fulfil all the other commandments? It is for this reason that He commands anyone who would like to become His disciple in truth, to renounce all his possessions rather than to become attached to these things.

At this point the disciple protests again: how can he love another man who hates him? This is the usual justification of all emnities: we always claim it is the enemy who hates us. We assert that nothing we can do will make him treat us fairly or kindly. He is indeed confirmed in evil, since he is a kind of diabolical being: how could he otherwise be our enemy? He envies us, he insults us, he is always trying to deceive us. This is, of course, characteristic of enemies! They are always trying to deceive. We do not reflect that perhaps our enemy sees in us the mirror image of what we see in him. Has he perhaps reason to think that we hate him and wish to destroy him? That we would gladly trick him? That our claim to be ready to come to an agreement with him is itself a trick, because our invitation to negotiate is always offered in terms that we know he cannot possibly accept? Is that why he treats us accordingly?

The master replies to this allegation that love of enemies is simply impossible. It is, after all, important to show that it is *not* impossible, for if the love of enemies is impossible Christ could not have commanded it, and in fact those who today say that we are not seriously obliged to love our enemies are contending that Christ could not have meant what He said when He told us to do this. The master's reply:

> Of course it is impossible for snakes and wild beasts, dominated by their instincts, to keep from resisting with all their power anyone who causes them to suffer. But for us, created in the image of God, guided by reason, to whom it has been given to know God, who have received our law from Him, it is indeed possible not to have an aversion for those who cause us pain. It is possible for us to love those who hate us. And so when the Lord says "Love your enemies and do good to those who hate you" (Matthew 5:44) and all that follows, He is not commanding the impossible, but obviously what is possible. Otherwise, He would not punish those who disobey this command.

That it is possible to love our enemies and not retaliate by meeting hatred with hatred is shown by the example not only of the Lord Himself, but also of His disciples, the saints, the martyrs, and thousands of heroic Christians who have taken His commandment seriously. What was possible for them can, with God's grace, become possible for us. Meanwhile, if it does happen to be impossible for some of us to love our enemies, there must be a reason for it. The reason is that we love money and possessions more than we love our fellow man, and so when he seems to threaten our material interests, we are compelled to hate him.

The master continues:

> We are held by the love of material things and the attraction of pleasure, and since we prefer these things to the commandment of the Lord, we become incapable of loving those who hate us. Rather we find that because of these very things we are often in conflict with those who love us. In this we show that we are even worse than wild animals or snakes. For this reason we are incapable of following the footsteps of the God-man and also incapable of even understanding the aim He has in view. But knowledge of this aim would give us strength.

Here the master puts his finger on the center of the trouble. When we are dominated by a selfish and materialistic scale of values, we are not only unable to love our enemies, we even hate our friends when they come between us and our love for possessions and pleasures. And since this is the case, we are completely unable to see any point in the idea of loving our enemies. We cannot really believe it is commanded us because we are not even able to grasp what it is all about in the first place.

The disciple naïvely objects that he has left the world and abandoned all possessions in order to become a monk, and even then he is not able to love a brother, another monk, if the latter hates him. Why is this? he inquires. Is there some way in which he can learn to love his brother from his heart?

At this the master returns to the question of *understanding what the Lord has in view when he commands us to love our enemies:*

> Even one who thinks he has renounced everything in the world still remains unable to love those who make him suffer, as long as he has not yet truly understood the Lord's aim in giving us this commandment. But if the grace of God once gives him the capacity to see this aim, and if, having seen it, he conforms his life to it with fervor, then he will become able to love even those who hate and torment him. The Apostles did this, once they had received knowledge of the Lord's aim. . . .

Here the master returns to the theme which is central to the whole treatise on the ascetic life: the Word became Flesh in order to save man. To be precise, Jesus made Himself subject to the Law in order to carry out the injunctions of the Law as Man and thus accomplish in Himself what Man had been unable to do since Adam. All the Law and the Prophets are contained in the twofold commandment of Love. "You shall love the Lord your God with your whole heart and your neighbor as yourself" (Matthew 22:37–40).

The demon, says the master, seeing Jesus keeping the Law, wished to make Him break the Law. Therefore he tempted Him in the desert with those things which men ordinarily, in their weakness, prefer to the Law: food, money and honors. But having failed in this, the demon then sought to tempt Him with hatred by raising up enemies to plot against Him. But instead of hating His enemies, the Lord continued to love them and even laid down His life for them.

> Out of love for His enemies, the Lord fought against the evil instigator of their hatred. . . . He was not weary of doing good to those who were stirred up to hate Him, even though they might have refused the temptations of the evil one. He endured blasphemies; He accepted suffering with patience and showed them every kind of love. In this way He fought against the evil one who was the instigator of their actions. He fought by kindness for those who were burning with hatred towards Him. A strange, new kind of warfare! In exchange for hate, He returns only love! By his kindness, He casts out the father of evil. It was for this reason that He endured so much evil from them; or rather to speak more accurately, it was for their sakes that He, as man, fought even to death in order to obey the com-

> mandment of Love. . . . Hence the Apostle tells us that we "should have in ourselves that same mind which was that of Christ" (Philippians 2:5).
>
> This then was the Lord's aim: to obey His Father, as man, even to the point of dying, and to fight against the demon by submitting to those sufferings which the demon inflicted on Him through those whom he incited to hatred. It is thus, in allowing Himself freely to be overcome, that He overcame the evil one who planned to win and who had already wrested the world out of the Lord's grasp.
>
> Thus the Lord was crucified in weakness (2 Corinthians 13:4) and by means of this "weakness" He destroyed death . . . and in the same way Paul "gloried in his infirmities in order that the power of Christ might rest on him" (2 Corinthians 12:9).

After this the master goes on to quote many New Testament texts on the courageous acceptance of suffering, on the love of enemies, on inflexible patience under persecution. The most important thing is to *understand* how important all these things are in the Christian life, and to see how they are essential for anyone who wants to attain his aim as a Christian, namely, salvation in imitation of Christ, in participation in the sufferings of Christ, in order to vanquish the enemy of Christ by the power of Christ's love.

Hence the disciple must learn that the love of enemies is not simply a pious luxury, something that he can indulge in if he wants to feel himself to be exceptionally virtuous. It is of the very essence of the Christian life, a proof of one's Christian faith, a sign that one is a follower and an obedient disciple of Christ.

The point the master is making is this: that a superficial and even illusory Christianity is one which professes faith in Christ by verbal formulas and external observance, but which in fact denies Christ by refusing to obey His commandment to love. Since no man can serve two masters, and since the Christian life is a bitter struggle to keep the commandments of Christ in spite of everything in order to hold fast to our faith in Him and not deny Him, the enemy of Christ seeks in every way to make us deny the Lord in our lives and in our actions, even though we may remain apparently faithful to Him in our words and in our worship. He does this by leading us to hate others on account of our attachment to money and pleasure or, when we have apparently renounced these, to hate others when they attack us in our own person or in the society to which we belong. But in all these cases we must see that the evil that is done to us, apparently, by others, is a summons to greater faith and to heroic obedience to the word of the Gospel.

The significant thing for us, in this remarkable passage from the Greek saint, is that he portrays nonviolent resistance under suffering and persecution as the normal way of the Christian, and shows that the Christian who has recourse to force and hatred in order to protect himself is, in fact, by that very action, denying Christ and showing that he has no real understanding of the Gospel.

Very often people object that nonviolence seems to imply passive acceptance of injustice and evil and therefore that it is a kind of co-operation with evil. Not at all. The genuine concept of nonviolence implies not only active and effective resistance to evil but in fact a *more effective* resistance. Saint Maximus takes pains to make very clear the absolutely uncompromising obligation to resist evil.

But the resistance which is taught in the Gospel is aimed *not at the evildoer but at evil in its source.* It combats evil as such by doing good to the evildoer, and thus overcoming evil with good (Romans 12:21), which is the way our Lord Himself resisted evil.

On the other hand, merely to resist evil with evil, by hating those who hate us and seeking to destroy them, is actually no resistance at all. It is active and purposeful collaboration in evil. It brings the Christian into direct and intimate contact with the same source of evil and hatred which inspires the acts of his enemy. It leads in practice to a denial of Christ and to the service of hatred rather than love.

How do we learn to love our enemy? By seeing him as a brother who is tempted as we are, and attacked by the same real enemy which is the spirit of hatred and of "Antichrist." This same enemy seeks to destroy us both by arming us against one another.

The master continues:

> If you meditate without ceasing on these truths you will be able to see through all the deceptions of the evil one in this regard, provided that you also understand that your brother is moved by an evil power to hate, just in the same way that you too are tempted. If you understand this you will pardon your brother. If you refuse to fall into the trap, you will be resisting the Tempter who wishes to make you hate your brother who is tempted. . . . Resist the devil, and he will fly from you (James 4:1). Meditating on these things you will understand the aim which the Lord and the Apostles had in view, to love men, to have compassion for those who fall into sin, and thus by love to hold in check the malice of the demon.
>
> *But if we are negligent, lazy, and blinded in spirit by carnal desires, then we do not make war on the demons but on ourselves and our brothers. Indeed by such things we place ourselves in the service of the demons and in their name we fight against our fellow man.*

The Gospel does, indeed, teach us to make war—but only on our real enemies, lest we serve our enemies and the enemies of Christ by making war on our brothers.

A Tribute to Gandhi

In 1931 Gandhi, who had been released from prison a few months before, came to London for a conference. The campaign of civil disobedience which had begun with the Salt March had recently ended. Now there were to be negotiations. He walked through the autumn fogs of London in clothes that were good for the tropics, not for England. He lived in the slums of London, coming from there to more noble buildings in which he conferred with statesmen. The English smiled at his bald head, his naked brown legs, the thin underpinnings of an old man who ate very little, who prayed. This was Asia, wise, disconcerting, in many ways unlovely, but determined upon some inscrutable project and probably very holy. Yet was it practical for statesmen to have conferences with a man reputed to be holy? What was the meaning of the fact that one could be holy, and fast, and pray, and be in jail, and be opposed to England all at the same time?

Gandhi thus confronted the England of the depression as a small, disquieting question mark. Everybody knew him, and many jokes were made about him. He was also respected. But respect implied neither agreement nor comprehension. It indicated nothing except that the man had gained public attention, and this was regarded as an achievement. Then, as now, no one particularly bothered to ask if the achievement signified something.

Yet I remember arguing about Gandhi in my school dormitory: chiefly against the football captain, then head prefect, who had come to turn out the flickering gaslight, and who stood with one hand in his pocket and a frown on his face that was not illuminated with understanding. I insisted that Gandhi was right, that India was, with perfect justice, demanding that the British withdraw peacefully and go home; that the millions of people who lived in India had a perfect right to run their own country. Such sentiments were of course beyond comprehension. How could Gandhi be right when he was *odd*? And how could I be right if I was on the side of someone who had the wrong kind of skin, and left altogether too much of it exposed?

A counter argument was offered but it was not an argument. It was a basic and sweeping assumption that the people of India were political and moral infants, incapable of taking care of themselves, backward people, primitive, uncivilized, benighted, pagan, who could not survive without the English to do their thinking and planning for them. The British Raj was, in fact, a purely benevolent, civilizing enterprise for which the Indians were not suitably grateful. . . .

Infuriated at the complacent idiocy of this argument, I tried to sleep and failed.

Certain events have taken place since that time. Within a dozen years after Gandhi's visit to London there were more hideous barbarities perpetuated in Europe, with greater violence and more unmitigated fury than all that had ever been attributed by the wildest imaginations to the despots of Asia. The British Empire collapsed. India attained self-rule. It did so peacefully and with dignity. Gandhi paid with his life for the ideas in which he believed.

As one looks back over this period of confusion and decline in the West, the cold war, and the chaos and struggle of the world that was once colonial, there is one political figure who stands out from all the rest as an extraordinary leader of men. He is radically different from the others. Not that the others did not on occasion bear witness to the tradition of which they were proud because it was Christian. They were often respectable, sometimes virtuous men, and many of them were sincerely devout. Others were at least genteel. Others, of course, were criminals. Judging by their speeches, their programs, their expressed motives were usually civilized. Yet the best that could be said of them may be that they sometimes combined genuine capability and subjective honesty. But apart from that they seemed to be the powerless victims of a social dynamic that they were able neither to control nor to understand. They never seemed to dominate events, only to rush breathlessly after the parade of cataclysms, explaining why these had happened, and not aware of how they themselves had helped precipitate the worst of disasters. Thus with all their good intentions, they were able at best to rescue themselves after plunging blindly in directions quite other than those in which they claimed to be going. In the name of peace, they wrought enormous violence and destruction. In the name of liberty they exploited and enslaved. In the name of man they engaged in genocide or tolerated it. In the name of truth they systematically falsified and perverted truth.

Gandhi on the other hand was dedicated to peace, and though he was engaged in a bitter struggle for national liberation, he achieved this by peaceful means. He believed in serving the truth by nonviolence, and his nonviolence was effective in so far as it began first within himself.

It is certainly true that Gandhi was not above all criticism; no man is. But it is evident that he was unlike all the other world leaders of his time in that his life was marked by a wholeness and a wisdom, an integrity and a spiritual consistency that the others lacked, or manifested only in reverse, in consistent fidelity to a dynamism of evil and destruction. There may be limitations in Gandhi's thought, and his work has not borne all the fruit he himself would have hoped. These are factors which he himself sagely took into account, and having reckoned with them all, he continued to pursue the course he had chosen simply because he believed it to be true. His way was no secret: it was simply to follow conscience without regard for the consequences to himself, in the belief that this was demanded of him by God and that the results would be the work of God. Perhaps indeed for a long time these results would remain hidden as God's secret. But in the end the truth would manifest itself.

What has Gandhi to do with Christianity? Everyone knows that the Orient has venerated Christ and distrusted Christians since the first colonizers and missionaries came from the West.

Western Christians often assume without much examination that this oriental respect for Christ is simply a vague, syncretistic and perhaps romantic evasion of the challenge of the Gospel: an attempt to absorb the Christian message into the confusion and inertia which are thought to be characteristic of Asia. The point does not need to be argued here. Gandhi certainly spoke often of Jesus, whom he had learned to know through Tolstoy. And Gandhi knew the New Testament thoroughly. Whether or not Gandhi "believed in" Jesus in the sense that he had genuine Christian faith in the Gospel would be very difficult to demonstrate, and it is not my business to prove it or disprove it. I think that the effort to do so would be irrelevant in any case. What is certainly true is that Gandhi not only understood the ethic of the Gospel as well, if not in some ways better, than many Christians, but he is one of the very few men of our time who applied Gospel principles to the problems of a political and social existence in such a way that his approach to these problems was *inseparably* religious and political at the same time.

He did this not because he thought that these principles were novel and interesting, or because they seemed expedient, or because of a compulsive need to feel spiritually secure. The religious basis of Gandhi's political action was not simply a program, in which politics were marshalled into the service of faith, and brought to bear on the charitable objectives of a religious institution. For Gandhi, strange as it may seem to us, political action had to be by its very nature "religious" in the sense that it had to be informed by principles of religious and philosophical wisdom. To separate religion and politics was in Gandhi's eyes "madness" because his politics rested on a thoroughly religious interpretation of reality, of life, and of man's place in the world. Gandhi's whole concept of man's relation to his own inner being and to the world of objects around him was informed by the contemplative heritage of Hinduism, together with the principles of Karma Yoga which blended, in his thought, with the ethic of the Synoptic Gospels and the Sermon on the Mount. In such a view, politics had to be understood in the context of service and worship in the ancient sense of *leitourgia* (liturgy, public work). Man's intervention in the active life of society was at the same time by its very nature *svadharma,* his own personal service (of God and man) and worship, *yajna.* Political action therefore was not a means to acquire security and strength for one's self and one's party, but a means of witnessing to the truth and the reality of the cosmic structure by making one's own proper contribution to the order willed by God. One could thus preserve one's integrity and peace, being detached from results (which are in the hands of God) and being free from the inner violence that comes from division and untruth, the usurpation of someone else's *dharma* in place of one's own *svadharma.* These perspectives lent Gandhi's politics their extraordinary spiritual force and religious realism.

The success with which Gandhi applied this spiritual force to political action makes him uniquely important in our age. More than that, it gives him a very special importance for Christians. Our attitude to politics tends to be abstract, divisive and often highly ambiguous. Political action is by definition secular and unspiritual. It has no really religious significance. Yet it is important to the Church as an institution in the world. It has therefore an *official* significance. We look to the Church to clarify principle and offer guidance, and in addition to that we are grateful if a Christian party of some sort comes to implement the program that has thus been outlined for us. This is all well and good. But Gandhi emphasized the importance of the individual person entering political action with a fully awakened and operative spiritual power in himself, the power of *Satyagraha,* nonviolent dedication to truth, a religious and spiritual force, a wisdom born of fasting and prayer. This is the charismatic and personal force of the saints, and we must admit that we have tended to regard it with mistrust and unbelief, as though it were mere "enthusiasm" and "fanaticism." This is a lamentable mistake, because for one thing it tends to short-circuit the power and light of grace, and it suggests that spiritual dedication is and must remain something entirely divorced from political action: something for the prie-dieu, the sacristy or the study, but not for the marketplace. This in turn has estranged from the Church those whose idealism and generosity might have inspired a dedicated and creative intervention in political life. These have found refuge in groups dominated by a confused pseudo-spirituality, or by totalitarian messianism. Gandhi remains in our time as a sign of genuine union of spiritual fervor and social action in the midst of a hundred pseudo-spiritual crypto-fascist, or Communist movements in which the capacity for creative and spontaneous dedication is captured, debased and exploited by false prophets.

In a time where the unprincipled fabrication of lies and systematic violation of agreements has become a matter of course in power politics, Gandhi made this unconditional devotion to truth the mainspring of his social action. Once again, the radical difference between him and other leaders, even the most sincere and honest of them, becomes evident by the fact that Gandhi is chiefly concerned with truth and with service, *svadharma,* rather than with the possible success of his tactics upon other people, and paradoxically it was his religious conviction that made Gandhi a great politician rather than a mere tactician or operator. Note that *satyagraha* is matter for a vow, therefore of worship, adoration of the God of truth, so that his whole political structure is built on this and his other vows (*Ahimsa,* etc.) and becomes an entirely religious system. The vow of *satyagraha* is the vow to die rather than say what one does not mean.

The profound significance of *satyagraha* becomes apparent when one reflects that "truth" here implies much more than simply conforming one's words to one's inner thought. It is not by words only that we speak. Our aims, our plans of action, our outlook, our attitudes, our habitual response to the problems and challenges of life "speak" of our inner being and reveal our fidelity or infidelity to ourselves. Our very existence, our life itself contains an implicit pretention to meaning, since all our free acts are implicit commitments, selections of "meanings" which we seem to find confronting us. Our very existence is "speech" interpreting reality. But the crisis of truth in the modern world comes from the bewildering complexity of the almost infinite contradictory propositions and claims to meaning uttered by millions of acts, movements, changes, decisions, attitudes, gestures, events, going on all around us. Most of all a crisis of truth is precipitated when men realize that almost all these claims are in fact without significance when they are not in great part entirely fraudulent.

Satyagraha for Gandhi meant first of all refusing to say "nonviolence" and "peace" when one meant "violence" and "destruction." However, his wisdom differed from ours in this: he knew that in order to speak truth he must rectify more than his inner *intention.* It was not enough to say "love" and *intend* love thereafter proving the sincerity of one's own intentions by demonstrating the insincerity of one's adversary. "Meaning" is not a mental and subjective adjustment. For Gandhi, a whole lifetime of sacrifice was barely enough to demonstrate the sincerity with which he made a few simple claims: that he was not lying, that he did not intend to use violence or deceit against the English, that he did not think that peace and justice could be attained through violent or selfish means, that he did genuinely believe they could be assured by nonviolence and self-sacrifice.

Gandhi's religio-political action was based on an ancient metaphysic of man, a philosophical wisdom which is common to Hinduism, Buddhism, Islam, Judaism, and Christianity: that "truth is the inner law of our being." Not that man is merely an abstract essence, and that our action must be based on logical fidelity to a certain definition of man. Gandhi's religious action is based on a religious intuition of *being* in man and in the world, and his vow of truth is a vow of fidelity to being in all its accessible dimensions. His wisdom is based on experience more than on logic. Hence the way of peace is the way of truth, of fidelity to wholeness and being, which implies a basic respect for life not as a concept, not as a sentimental figment of the imagination, but in its deepest, most secret and most fontal reality. The first and fundamental truth is to be sought in respect for our own inmost being, and this in turn implies the recollectedness and the awareness which attune us to that silence in which alone Being speaks to us in all its simplicity.

Therefore Gandhi recognized, as no other world leader of our time has done, the necessity to be free from the pressures, the exorbitant and tyrannical demands of a society that is violent because it is essentially greedy, lustful and cruel. Therefore he fasted, observed days of silence, lived frequently in retreat, knew the value of solitude, as well as of the totally generous expenditure of his time and energy in listening to others and communicating with them. He recognized the impossibility of being a peaceful and nonviolent man if one submits passively to the insatiable requirements of a society maddened by overstimulation and obsessed with the demons of noise, voyeurism and speed.

"Jesus died in vain," said Gandhi, "if he did not teach us to regulate the whole life by the eternal law of love." Strange that he should use this expression. It seems to imply at once concern and accusation. As Asians sometimes do, Gandhi did not hesitate to confront Christendom with the principles of Christ. Not that he judged Christianity, but he suggested that the professedly Christian civilization of the West was in fact judging itself by its own acts and its own fruits. There are certain Christian and humanitarian elements in democracy, and if they are absent, democracy finds itself on trial, weighed in the balance, and no amount of verbal protestations can prevent it from being found wanting. Events themselves will proceed inexorably to their conclusion. *Pacem in Terris* has suggested the same themes to the meditation of modern Europe, America and Russia. "Civilization" must learn to prove its claims by a capacity for the peaceful and honest settlement of disputes, by genuine concern for justice toward people who have been shamelessly exploited and races that have been systematically oppressed, or the historical preeminence of the existing powers will be snatched from them by violence, perhaps in a disaster of cosmic proportions.

Gandhi believed that the central problem of our time was the acceptance or the rejection of a basic law of love and truth which had been made known to the world in traditional religions and most clearly by Jesus Christ. Gandhi himself expressly and very clearly declared himself an adherent of this one law. His whole life, his political action, finally even his death, were nothing but a witness to his commitment. "IF LOVE IS NOT THE LAW OF OUR BEING THE WHOLE OF MY ARGUMENT FALLS TO PIECES."

What remains to be said? It is true that Gandhi expressly disassociated himself from Christianity in any of its visible and institutional forms. But it is also true that he built his whole life and all his activity upon what he conceived to be the law of Christ. In fact, he died for this law which was at the heart of his belief. Gandhi was indisputably sincere and right in his moral commitment to the law of love and truth. A Christian can do nothing greater than follow his own conscience with a fidelity comparable to that which Gandhi obeyed what he believed to be the voice of God. Gandhi is, it seems to me, a model of integrity whom we cannot afford to ignore, and the one basic duty we all owe to the world of our time is to imitate him in "disassociating ourselves from evil in total disregard of the consequences."

Faith and Violence

By Way of Preface

The Hassidic rabbi Ball-shem-tov once told the following story. Two men were traveling through a forest. One was drunk, the other was sober. As they went, they were beset by robbers, beaten, robbed of all they had, even their clothing. When they emerged, people asked them if they got through the wood without trouble. The drunken man said: "Everything was fine: nothing went wrong: we had no trouble at all!"

They said: "How does it happen that you are naked and covered with blood?"

He did not have an answer.

The sober man said: "Do not believe him: he is drunk. It was a disaster. Robbers beat us without mercy and took everything we had. Be warned by what happened to us, and look out for yourselves."

For some "faithful"—and for unbelievers too—"faith" seems to be a kind of drunkenness, an anaesthetic, that keeps you from realizing and believing that anything can ever go wrong. Such faith can be immersed in a world of violence and make no objection: the violence is perfectly all right. It is quite normal—unless of course it happens to be exercised by Negroes. Then it must be put down instantly by superior force. The drunkenness of this kind of faith—whether in a religious message or merely in a political ideology—enables us to go through life without seeing that our own violence is a disaster and that the overwhelming force by which we seek to assert ourselves and our own self-interest may well be our ruin.

Is faith a narcotic dream in a world of heavily-armed robbers, or is it an awakening?

Is faith a convenient nightmare in which we are attacked and obliged to destroy our attackers?

What if we awaken to discover that *we* are the robbers, and our destruction comes from the root of hate in ourselves?

Abbey of Gethsemani
ADVENT, 1967

Part One: Toward a Theology of Resistance

Theology today needs to focus carefully upon the crucial problem of violence. The commandment "Thou shalt not kill" is more than a mere matter of academic or sentimental interest in an age when man not only is more frustrated, more crowded, more subject to psychotic and hostile delusion than ever, but also has at his disposition an arsenal of weapons that make global suicide an easy possibility. But the so-called nuclear umbrella has not simplified matters in the least: it may have (at least temporarily) caused the nuclear powers to reconsider their impulses to reduce one another to radioactive dust. But meanwhile "small" wars go on with unabated cruelty, and already more bombs have been exploded on Vietnam than were dropped in the whole of World War II. The population of the affluent world is nourished on a steady diet of brutal mythology and hallucination, kept at a constant pitch of high tension by a life that is intrinsically violent in that it forces a large part of the population to submit to an existence which is humanly intolerable. Hence murder, mugging, rape, crime, corruption. But it must be remembered that the crime that breaks out of the ghetto is only the fruit of a greater and more pervasive violence: the injustice which forces people to live in the ghetto in the first place. The problem of violence, then, is not the problem of a few rioters and rebels, but the problem of a whole social structure which is outwardly ordered and respectable, and inwardly ridden by psychopathic obsessions and delusions.

It is perfectly true that violence must at times be restrained by force: but a convenient mythology which simply legalizes the use of force by big criminals against little criminals—whose small-scale criminality is largely *caused* by the large-scale injustice under which they live—only perpetuates the disorder.

Pope John XXIII in *Pacem in Terris* quoted, with approval, a famous saying of Saint Augustine: "What are kingdoms without justice but large bands of robbers?" The problem of violence today must be traced to its root: not the small-time murderers but the massively organized bands of murderers whose operations are global.

This book is concerned with the defense of the dignity and rights of man against the encroachments and brutality of massive power structures which threaten either to enslave him or to destroy him, while exploiting him in their conflicts with one another.

The Catholic moral theology of war has, especially since the Renaissance, concerned itself chiefly with casuistical discussion of how far the monarch or the sovereign state can justly make use of force. The historic context of this discussion was the struggle for a European balance of power, waged for absolute monarchs by small professional armies. In a new context we find not only a new struggle on a global scale between mammoth nuclear powers provided with arsenals capable of wiping out the human race, but also the emergence of scores of small nations in an undeveloped world that was until recently colonial. In this Third World we find not huge armed establishments but petty dictatorships (representing a rich minority) opposed by small, volunteer guerrilla bands fighting for "the poor." The Great Powers tend to intervene in these struggles, not so much by the threat and use of nuclear weapons (with which, however, they continue to threaten one another) but with armies of draftees and with new experimental weapons which are sometimes incredibly savage and cruel and which are used mostly against helpless non-combatants. Although many churchmen, moved apparently by force of habit, continue to issue mechanical blessings upon these draftees and upon the versatile applications of science to the art of killing, it is evident that this use of force does not become moral just because the government and the mass media have declared the cause to be patriotic. The cliché "my country right or wrong" does not provide a satisfactory theological answer to the moral problems raised by the intervention of American power in all parts of the Third World. And in fact the Second Vatican Council, following the encyclical of John XXIII *Pacem in Terris*, has had some pertinent things to say about war in the nuclear era.

To assert that conflict resolution is one of the crucial areas of theological investigation in our time is not to issue an *a priori* demand for a theology of pure pacifism. To declare that *all* use of force in any way whatever is by the very fact immoral is to plunge into confusion and unreality from the very start, because, as John XXIII admitted, "unfortunately the law of fear still reigns among peoples" and there are situations in which the only way to effectively protect human life and rights is by forcible resistance against unjust encroachment. Murder is not to be passively permitted, but resisted and prevented—and all the more so when it becomes mass murder. The problem arises not when theology admits that force can be necessary, but when it does so in a way that implicitly favors the claims of the powerful and self-seeking establishment against the common good of mankind or against the rights of the oppressed.

The real moral issue of violence in the twentieth century is obscured by archaic and mythical presuppositions. We tend to judge violence in terms of the individual, the messy, the physically disturbing, the personally frightening. The violence we want to see restrained is the violence of the hood waiting for us in the subway or the elevator. That is reasonable, but it tends to influence us too much. It makes us think that the problem of violence is limited to this very small scale, and it makes us unable to appreciate the far greater problem of the more abstract, more global, more organized presence of violence on a massive and corporate pattern. Violence today is *white-collar violence, the systematically organized bureaucratic and technological destruction of man.*

The theology of violence must not lose sight of the real problem, which is not the individual with a revolver but *death and even genocide as big business.* But this big business of death is all the more innocent and effective because it involves a long chain of individuals, each of whom can feel himself absolved from responsibility, and each of whom can perhaps salve his conscience by contributing with a more *meticulous efficiency* to his part in the massive operation.

We know, for instance, that Adolph Eichmann and others like him felt no guilt for their share in the extermination of the Jews. This feeling of justification was due partly to their absolute obedience to higher authority and partly to the care and efficiency which went into the details of their work. This was done almost entirely on paper. Since they dealt with numbers, not with people, and since their job was one of abstract bureaucratic organization, apparently they could easily forget the reality of what they were doing. The same is true to an even greater extent in modern warfare in which the real moral problems are not to be located in rare instances of hand-to-hand combat, but in the remote planning and organization of technological destruction. The real crimes of modern war are committed not at the front (if any) but in war offices and ministries of defense in which no one ever has to see any blood unless his secretary gets a nosebleed. Modern technological mass murder is not directly visible, like individual murder. It is abstract, corporate, businesslike, cool, free of guilt feelings and therefore a thousand times more deadly and effective than the eruption of violence out of individual hate. It is this polite, massively organized white-collar murder machine that threatens the world with destruction, not the violence of a few desperate teen-agers in a slum. But our antiquated theology, myopically focused on *individual* violence alone, fails to see this. It shudders at the fantasm of muggings and killings where a mess is made on our own doorstep, but blesses and canonizes the antiseptic violence of corporately organized murder because it is respectable, clean, and above all profitable.

In another place I have contrasted, in some detail, the mentality of John XXIII on this point with the mentality of Machiavelli (see *Seeds of Destruction,* Part III). Machiavelli said: "There are two methods of fighting, one by law and the other by force. The first method is that of men, the second of beasts; but as the first method is often insufficient, one must have recourse to the second." I submit that a theology which merely seeks to justify the "method of beasts" and to help it disguise itself as law—since it is after all a kind of "prolongation of law"—is not adequate for the problems of a time of violence.

On the other hand we also have to recognize that when oppressive power is thoroughly well established, it does not always need to resort openly to the "method of beasts" because its laws are already powerful—perhaps also bestial—enough. In other words, when a system can, without resort to overt force, *compel* people to live in conditions of abjection, helplessness, wretchedness that keep them on the level of beasts rather than of men, it is plainly violent. To make men live on a subhuman level against their will, to constrain them in such a way that they have no hope of escaping their condition, is an unjust exercise of force. Those who in some way or other concur in the oppression—and perhaps profit by it—are exercising violence even though they may be preaching pacifism. And their supposedly peaceful laws, which maintain this spurious kind of order, are in fact instruments of violence and oppression. If the oppressed try to resist by force—which is their right—theology has no business preaching nonviolence to them. Mere blind destruction is, of course, futile and immoral: but who are we to condemn a desperation we have helped to cause!

However, as John XXIII pointed out, the "law of fear" is not the only law under which men can live, nor is it really the normal mark of the human condition. To live under the law of fear and to deal with one another by "the methods of beasts" will hardly help world events "to follow a course in keeping with man's destiny and dignity." In order for us to realize this, we must remember that "one of the profound requirements of [our] nature is this: . . . it is not fear that should reign but love—a love that tends to express itself in mutual collaboration."

"Love" is unfortunately a much misused word. It trips easily off the Christian tongue—so easily that one gets the impression it means others ought to love us for standing on their necks.

A theology of love cannot afford to be sentimental. It cannot afford to preach edifying generalities about charity, while identifying "peace" with mere established power and legalized violence against the oppressed. A theology of love cannot be allowed merely to serve the interests of the rich and powerful, justifying their wars, their violence and their bombs, while exhorting the poor and underprivileged to practice patience, meekness, long-suffering and to solve their problems, if at all, nonviolently.

The theology of love must seek to deal realistically with the evil and injustice in the world, and not merely to compromise with them. Such a theology will have to take note of the ambiguous realities of politics, without embracing the specious myth of a "realism" that merely justifies force in the service of established power. Theology does not exist merely to appease the already too untroubled conscience of the powerful and the established. A theology of love may also conceivably turn out to be a theology of revolution. In any case, it is a theology of *resistance,* a refusal of the evil that reduces a brother to homicidal desperation.

On the other hand, Christian faith and purity of intention—the simplicity of the dove—are no guarantee of political acumen, and theological insight is no substitute for the wisdom of the serpent which is seldom acquired in Sunday school. Should the theologian or the priest be too anxious to acquire that particiular kind of wisdom? Should he be too ambitious for the achievements of a successful political operator? Should he be more careful to separate authentic Christian witness from effectiveness in political maneuvering? Or is the real place of the priest the place which Fr. Camilo Torres took, with the Colombian guerrillas?

This book cannot hope to answer such questions. But it can at least provide a few materials for a theology, not of pacifism and nonviolence in the sense of *nonresistance,* but for a theology of resistance which is at the same time *Christian* resistance and which therefore emphasizes reason and humane communication rather than force, but which also admits the possibility of force in a limit situation when everything else fails.

Such a theology could not claim to be Christian if it did not retain at least some faith in the meaning of the Cross and of the redemptive death of Jesus who, instead of using force against his accusers, took all the evil upon himself and overcame that evil by his suffering. This is a basic Christian pattern, but a realistic theology will, I believe, give a new practical emphasis to it. Instead of preaching the Cross *for others* and advising them to suffer patiently the violence which we sweetly impose on them, with the aid of armies and police, we might conceivably recognize the right of the less fortunate to use force, and study more seriously the practice of nonviolence and humane methods on our own part when, as it happens, we possess the most stupendous arsenal of power the world has ever known.

General MacArthur was no doubt sincerely edified when the conquered Japanese wrote into their constitution a clause saying they would never again arm and go to war. He warmly congratulated them for their wisdom. But he never gave the slightest hint of thinking the United States ought to follow their example. On the contrary, he maintained to the end that for *us* there could be no other axiom than that "there is no substitute for victory." Others have come after him with even more forceful convictions. They would probably be glad to see all Asian nations disarm on the spot; but failing that, we can always bomb them back to the stone age. And there is no reason to believe that the United States may not eventually try to do so.

The title of this book is *Faith and Violence*. This might imply several interesting possibilities. The book might, for instance, study the violence of believers—and this, as history shows, has sometimes been considerable. The disciples of the King of Peace have sometimes managed to prove themselves extremely bloodthirsty, particularly among themselves. They have rather consistently held, in practice, that the way to prove the sincerity of faith was not so much nonviolence as the generous use of lethal weapons. It is a curious fact that in this present century there have been two world wars of unparalleled savagery in which Christians, on both sides, were exhorted to go out and kill each other if not in the name of Christ and faith, at least in the name of "Christian duty." One of the strange facts about this was that, in the Second World War, German Christians were exhorted by their pastors to die for a government that was not only non-Christian but anti-Christian and which had evident intentions of getting rid of the Church. An official theology which urged Christians, as a matter of Christian duty, to fight for such a government surely calls for examination. And we shall see that few questioned it. Few question it still. One man did, and we shall devote a few pages to his unusual case. Possibly he was what the Catholic Church might conceivably call a "saint." If so, it was because he dared to refuse military service under the Fuehrer whom his bishop told him he was obliged to obey.

In the case of Franz Jägerstätter we have a faith that stood up against an unjust but established power and refused to practice in the service of that power. On the other side, we have Simone Weil who was a French pacifist before World War II and who later joined the French resistance against the Nazis. Simone was not a Christian in the official sense of the word, but no matter; her motives and reservations were Christian, and the limits which she set to force when she decided to resist were also Christian.

Father Delp, Franz Jägerstätter and Simone Weil all resisted the same evil, the same violent, destructive and antihuman political force of Nazism, and they all resisted it for the same motives. Their resistance took somewhat different forms. But one can see in them three possible examples of Christian resistance. In each case the resistance was more or less nonviolent. It might conceivably have involved a use of force (as in the case of those Christians who plotted against Hitler's life—as Father Delp was accused of doing). The point to be emphasized, however, is not only that these Christians were nonviolent but that they *resisted*. They refused to submit to a force which they recognized as antihuman and utterly destructive. They refused to accept this evil and to palliate it under the guise of "legitimate authority." In doing so they proved themselves better theologians than the professionals and the pontiffs who supported that power and made others obey it, thus cooperating in the evil.

The first section of this book studies various aspects of nonviolent resistance to the evil of war as waged by the "large bands of robbers." Its approach assumes that nonviolent resistance can be an effective means of conflict resolution, perhaps more effective than the use of force. At no point in these pages will the reader find the author trying to prove that evil should not be resisted. The reason for emphasizing nonviolent resistance is this: he who resists force with force in order to seize power may become contaminated by the evil which he is resisting and, when he gains power, may be just as ruthless and unjust a tyrant as the one he has dethroned. A nonviolent victory, while far more difficult to achieve, stands a better chance of curing the illness instead of contracting it.

There is an essential difference here, for nonviolence seeks to "win" not by destroying or even by humiliating the adversary, but by *convincing him* that there is a higher and more certain common good than can be attained by bombs and blood. Nonviolence, ideally speaking, does not try to overcome the adversary by winning over him, but to turn him from an adversary into a collaborator by winning him over. Unfortunately, nonviolent resistance as practiced by those who do not understand it and have been trained in it is often only a weak and veiled form of psychological aggression.

The second part of the book, devoted to Vietnam, takes into account the fact that the use of force in Vietnam is curing and settling nothing. With incredible expense and complication, and with appalling consequences to the people we claim to be helping, we are inexorably destroying the country we want to "save." The Third Part considers the racial conflict in the United States, where nonviolence was first adopted as the best method and later discredited as ineffective, in favor of an appeal to force. The last section considers the rather ambiguous "death of God" which has curiously coincided with these other events and may perhaps cast some light on them.

At any rate, faith itself is in crisis along with the society which was once officially Christian, officially supported by God and his representatives, and which is now seeking to consolidate itself by an ever more insistent appeal to violence and brute power.

In brief: without attempting a systematic treatment of that theology of love which, in crisis situations, may become a theology of resistance, we will examine principles and cases all of which help us to see the unacceptable ambiguities of a theology of "might makes right" masquerading as a Christian theology of love.

Part Two: The Vietnam War: An Overwhelming Atrocity

> No country may unjustly oppress others or unduly meddle in their affairs.
>
> (*Pacem in Terris,* n.120)

> As men in their private enterprises cannot pursue their own interests to the detriment of others, so too states cannot lawfully seek that development of their own resources which brings harm to other states and unjustly oppresses them.
>
> (*Pacem in Terris,* n.92)

In 1967 several young members of the International Volunteer Service in Vietnam resigned and returned to America, in protest against the way the war was, in their opinion, needlessly and hopelessly ravaging the country.

The International Volunteer Service is a nonprofit organization meant to help American youth to contribute to international goodwill by person-to-person contracts and service programs in other countries. Ambassador Lodge had called it "one of the success stories of American assistance," and obviously the men serving in Vietnam were in very close touch with the people, knew the language, and were perhaps better able to judge the state of affairs than most other Americans. As they said, they "dealt with people, not statistics," and they were in a position to know that the story of the Vietnam war is a very different one when it is learned from women and children whose flesh has been burned by napalm than it is when those same women and children appear in statistics as "enemy" casualities.

At this point, in case the reader is not fully aware of what napalm is, we might quote from a report of four American physicians on "Medical Problems of South Vietnam":

> Napalm is a highly sticky inflammable jelly which clings to anything it touches and burns with such heat that all oxygen in the area is exhausted within moments. Death is either by roasting or suffocation. Napalm wounds are often fatal (estimates are 90%). Those who survive face a living death. The victims are frequently children.

Another American physician wrote (Dr. R. E. Perry, *Redbook*, January, 1967):

> I have been an orthopedic surgeon for a good number of years with rather a wide range of medical experience. But nothing could have prepared me for my encounters with Vietnamese women and children burned by napalm. It was shocking and sickening even for a physician to see and smell the blackened and burned flesh.

By their resignation and by the statement they issued in an open letter to President Johnson, these men attempted to get through to the American public with a true idea of what the war really means to the Vietnamese—our allies, the ones we are supposedly "saving" from Communism. The attitude and feelings of the Vietnamese *people* (as distinct from the government) are too little known in the United States. They have been systematically ignored. Pictures of GIs bestowing candy bars upon half-naked "native" children are supposed to give us all the information we need in this regard. These are happy people who love our boys because we are saving them from the Reds and teaching them "democracy." It is of course important, psychologically and politically, for the public to believe this because otherwise the war itself would be questioned, and as a matter of fact it *is* questioned. Never was there a war in American history that was so much questioned! The official claim that such questioning is "betrayal" is a transparently gross and authoritarian attack on democratic liberty.

According to these Americans in the International Volunteer Service, men who cannot be considered leftists, still less as traitors, the American policy of victory at any price is simply destroying Vietnam. It is quite possible that the United States may eventually "win," but the price may be so high that there will be few left around to enjoy the fruits of victory and democracy in a country which we will, of course, obligingly reconstruct according to ideas of our own.

The people of South Vietnam have already had some experience of this kind of resettlement and reconstruction. Having seen their own homes burned or bulldozed out of existence, their fields and crops blasted with defoliants and herbicides, their livelihood and culture destroyed, they have been forcibly transplanted into places where they cannot live as they would like or as they know how, and forced into a society where, to adapt and be "at home" one has to be a hustler, a prostitute, or some kind of operator who knows how to get where the dollars are.

The people we are "liberating" in Vietnam are caught between two different kinds of terrorism, and the future presents them with nothing but a more and more bleak and hopeless prospect of unnatural and alienated existence. From their point of view, it doesn't matter much who wins. Either way it is going to be awful: but at least if the war can stop before everything is destroyed, and if they can somehow manage their own destiny, they will settle for that.

This, however, does not fit in with our ideas. We intend to go on bombing, burning, killing, bulldozing and moving people around while the numbers of plague victims begin to mount sharply and while the "civilization" we have brought becomes more and more rotten. The people of South Vietnam believe that we are supporting a government of wealthy parasites they do not and cannot trust. They believe that the 1967 election was rigged, and they know that the two newspapers which protested about it were immediately silenced and closed down by the "democratic" government which we are supporting at such cost.

To put it plainly, according to the men who resigned from the International Volunteer Service the people of South Vietnam are hardly grateful for "democracy" on such terms, and while they are quite willing to accept our dollars when they have a chance, they do not respect us or trust us. In point of fact, they have begun to hate us.

Far from weakening Communism in Asia by our war policy, we are only strengthening it. The Vietnamese are no lovers of China, but by the ruthlessness of our war for "total victory" we are driving them into the arms of the Red Chinese. "The war as it is now being waged," say the Volunteers, "is self-defeating." They support their contentions by quoting people they have known in Vietnam.

A youth leader: "When the Americans learn to respect the true aspirations in Vietnam, true nationalism will come to power. Only true nationalists can bring peace to the South, talk to the North and bring unification."

While a Catholic bishop in the United States was soothing President Johnson with the assurance the war in Vietnam is "a sad and heavy obligation imposed by the mandate of love," a Buddhist nun said in Vietnam: "You Americans come to help the Vietnamese people, but have brought only death and destruction. Most of us Vietnamese hate from the bottom of our hearts the Americans who have brought the suffering of this war. . . ." After which she burned herself to death. That, too, was a drastic act of violence. Whether or not we may agree with it, we must admit that it lends a certain air of seriousness to her denunciation! Unfortunately, such seriousness does not seem to get through to those Americans who most need to hear and understand it.

Meanwhile Billy Graham declared that the war in Vietnam was a "spiritual war between good and evil." A plausible statement, certainly, but not in the way in which he meant it. At the same time a Saigon Catholic Youth leader gave another view of the picture: "We are caught in a struggle between two power blocs. . . . Many people told me you cannot trust Americans, but I never accepted it. Now I am beginning to believe it. You come to help my people, but they will hate you for it."

The tragic thing about Vietnam is that, after all, the "realism" of our program there is so unrealistic, so rooted in myth, so completely out of touch with the needs of the people whom we know only as statistics and to whom we never manage to listen, except where they fit in with our psychopathic delusions. Our external violence in Vietnam is rooted in an inner violence which simply ignores the human reality of those we claim to be helping. The result of this at home has been an ever-mounting desperation on the part of those who see the uselessness and inhumanity of the war, together with an increasing stubbornness and truculence on the part of those who insist they want to win, regardless of what victory may mean.

What will the situation be when this book appears in print? Will the 1968 presidential election force the issue one way or another? Will the candidates *have to* make sense out of this in spite of everything? We are getting to the point where American "victory" in Vietnam is becoming a word without any possible human meaning. What matters is the ability and willingness to arrive at some kind of workable solution that will save the identity of the nation that still wants to survive in spite of us, in spite of Communism, in spite of the international balance of power. This cannot be arrived at unless the United States is willing to deescalate, stop bombing the North, stop destroying crops, and recognize the NLF as among those with whom we have to deal if we want to make peace. Obviously a perfect solution is impossible but some solution can be realized and lives can be saved.

It is still possible to learn something from Vietnam: and above all we should recognize that the United States has received from no one the mission to police every country in the world or to decide for them how they are to live. No single nation has the right to try to run the world according to its own ideas. One thing is certain, the Vietnam war is a tragic error and, in the words of the resigned volunteers, "an overwhelming atrocity."

How do we explain such atrocities? Obviously, they are well-meant and the Americans who support the war are, for the most part, convinced that it is an inescapable moral necessity. Why? For one thing, as the more sophisticated reader is well aware, the picture of the war given by the mass media and the official version of what is happening are both extremely one-sided and oversimplified, to say the least. Some claim that the public has been deliberately misinformed. In any case, Americans do not seem to realize what effect the war is really having. The hatred of America which it is causing everywhere (analogous to the hatred of Russia after the violent suppression of the Hungarian revolt in 1956) is not just the result of Red propaganda. On the contrary, the Communists could never do such a fine job of blackening us as we are doing all by ourselves.

There is another, deeper source of delusion in the popular mythology of our time. One example of this popular mythology is examined in the first chapter of this section. It is the myth that all biological species in their struggle for survival must follow a law of aggression in which the stronger earns the right to exist by violently exterminating all his competitors. This pseudoscientific myth is simply another version of the cliché that "might makes right" and of course it was explicitly used and developed by the ideologists of Nazism. This canonization of violence by pseudoscience has come to be so much taken for granted, that when Konrad Lorenz in his carefully thought out study *On Aggression* sought to qualify it in very important ways, his book has simply been lumped with others, like Mr. Ardrey's, as one more rationalization of the aggression theory. Thus in *The New York Times Book Review* (Christmas issue, 1967) the paperback edition of *On Aggression* is summarized with approval in this one line: "Like all other animals man is instinctively aggressive." True, of course, up to a point. But this contains the same implicit false conclusion ("therefore he *has to* beat up and destroy members of his own kind") and explicitly ignores the real point of Lorenz's book. The point is that man is the *only species*, besides the rat, who wantonly and cruelly turns on his own kind in *unprovoked* and murderous hostility. Man is the only one who deliberately seeks to *destroy* his own kind (as opposed to merely resisting encroachment).

To quote a prominent Dutch psychoanalyst who, among other things, has studied the mentality of Nazi war criminals:

> What we usually call hatred or hostility is different from normal self-assertive aggression. The former are hypercharged fantasy products, mixed with reactions to frustrations. They form an aura of intense anticipation of revenge and greater discharge in the future. . . . This finds its most paradoxical action in the hatred of those who want to break out into history. They destroy because they want to be remembered. NO OTHER ANIMAL AVAILS HIMSELF OF PLANS FOR MOBILIZATION AND FUTURE ATTACK. However, man gets caught in his own trap, and what he once dreamed up in a fatal hour often takes possession of him so that he is finally compelled to act it out.[1]

Now this develops the point made by Lorenz in *On Aggression.* Lorenz *distinguishes* the destructive hostility of men and of rats from the natural self-assertive aggression common to all species, and indicates that far from pointing to the "survival of the fittest" this drive toward intraspecific aggression may perhaps lead to the self-destruction of the human race. That is the thesis developed in detail by Dr. Meerloo. Mr. Ardrey's book, like so much other popular mythology on the subject, serves to contribute to those "hypercharged fantasies" by which modern man at once excuses and foments his inner hostilities until he is compelled to discharge them, as we are now doing, with immense cost for innocent and harmless people on the other side of the globe.[2]

It is because of these obsessions and fantasies that we continue to draft our young men into the army when in fact a professional army of enlisted men would suffice, along with our fabulous nuclear arsenal, to meet any conceivable need for national defense. The Vietnam war has called the legality and justice of the draft law into question, and rightly. Our young men feel that they are simply being imposed upon and that their lives are being stupidly sacrificed, not to defend the country but to act out the manias of politicians and manufacturers who think they have a mission to police the world and run the affairs of smaller countries in the interests of American business. The draft law ought to be abolished. That would somewhat lessen the temptation

1. I am grateful to my friend Dr. Joost A. M. Meerloo for permission to quote from his unpublished manuscript of the English version of *Homo Militants.*

2. I have examined elsewhere the psychological connection between the Indian wars of extermination in the last century, and the Vietnam war. See: "Ishi: A Meditation," in the *Catholic Worker,* March, 1967.

to get involved in any more "overwhelming atrocities" like the one in Vietnam.

Part Three: From Nonviolence to Black Power

Violence is as American as cherry pie.
(H. Rap Brown)

The Nonviolent Civil Rights movement has practically ceased to exist. The nonviolent struggle for integration was won on the law books—and was lost in fact. Integration is more myth than real possibility. The result has been that nonviolence both as tactic and as mystique has been largely rejected as irrelevant by the American Negro. At the same time, the struggle for racial recognition has taken on an entirely new and more aggressive character.

First of all, Frantz Fanon has replaced Martin Luther King as the prophet of Black America, and Malcolm X has become its martyr. Fanon was a black psychoanalyst from the French colony of Martinique. He joined in the Algerian conflict and preached a mystique of violence as necessary for the Third World to recover its identity and organize for revolutionary self-liberation. The Black Power movement in America has accepted this doctrine as simpler, and more effective, and more meaningful than Christian nonviolence.

It must be admitted that for the majority of black Americans, Christian nonviolence remained highly ambiguous. The Negro felt himself imprisoned in the fantasy image of him devised by the white man: an image of subservient, subhuman, passive tutelage and minority. Part of this image was the assumption that the Negro was there to be beaten over the head. Whether he chose to accept his beating with Christian dignity and herioc, self-sacrificial motives was a matter of supreme indifference to people like Bull Connor.

It is true that the Montgomery bus strike and the Birmingham demonstrations did communicate to the whole nation an image of Negro dignity, maturity and integrity—an example of restraint and nobility which should not have been lost on a culture with our professed ideals. It was unfortunately soon forgotten when black people in the North began to ask for open housing. Northern liberals might admire black dignity at a distance, but they still did not want all that nobility right next door: it might affect property values. Nobility is one thing and property values quite another.

Second, the Vietnam war has had a great deal to do with the new trend to Black Power. The Negroes have been more keenly aware than anyone else of the war's ambiguities. They have tended to identify themselves with the Vietnamese—indeed with the Vietcong—and have not paid much heed to the official rhetoric of Washington. They have. on the contrary, seen the Vietnam war as another manifestation of

Whitey's versatility in beating down colored people. They have naturally concluded that white America is not really interested in nonviolence at all.

Rap Brown's statement that "violence is as American as cherry pie" is steeped in the pungent ironies which characterize the new language or racial conflict. (One is tempted to explore possible psychoanalytic insights in the droll image used. Orality, mother love, hate of brother . . .) Yes, violence is thoroughly American and Rap Brown is saying that it is in fact the real American language. Perhaps so, perhaps not. But in any event, it is the language the Black American has now elected to speak. Oddly enough, he instantly got himself a much better hearing when he did so.

America sat up and began paying a great deal of attention. "Black Power" became an explosive and inexhaustible theme in the white media. It turned out to be a much better money-maker than nonviolence (indeed nonviolence was found to interest the American public only insofar as it could be seen as an obscure, perverse form of violence—a dishonest and so to speak "inverted" violence—hence the persistent snide allusions attempting to link nonviolence with passivity and homosexuality). Black Power was clearly a message that somehow white America *wanted* to hear. Not of course that white America was not scared, it was deliciously afraid. And glad. Because now things were so much simpler. One had perfectly good reasons to call out the cops and the National Guard.

Well, the blacks wanted it that way too. It was also simpler for them. And they turned it into a self-justifying weapon. There is a lot of truth in this arraignment of white America by Rap Brown:

> You sit out there and you pretend violence scares you, but you watch TV every night and you can't turn it on for five minutes without seeing somebody shot to death or karated to death. Violence is part of your culture. There's no doubt about it. You gave us violence and this is the only value that black people can use to their advantage to end oppression. . . . Johnson says every day if Vietnam don't come round, Vietnam will burn down. I say that if America don't come round America should be burned down. *It's the same thing.*

My reason for quoting these lines is not necessarily to approve a program of arson, but to make the point that it is, quite literally *the same thing* and to congratulate Rap Brown on the firm and acute justice of his ironic insight.

An America that destroys Vietnamese noncombatants with napalm has no right to object when blacks at home burn down their slums. Indeed, if there is a difference, it is that the second case is more justifiable than the first: it is a protest against real injustice.

It is perfectly logical that the America of LBJ should be at once the

America of the Vietnam war and the Detroit riots. It's the same America, the same violence, the same slice of mother's cherry pie. (Or maybe it's mammy's pie, I don't know).

The people who have been most shocked by the Black Power movement are the white liberals. And of course they are right, because the whole impact of the movement is directed against *them.* It is a rejection of their tender and ambiguous consciences, their taste for compromise, their desire to eat momma's cherry pie and still have it, their semiconscious proclivity to use the Negro for their own sentimental, self-justifying ends. The black man has definitely seen through and summarily rejected the white liberal. The overtones of racism in the Black Power program are, in their way, an acknowledgment that the Negro feels the white segregationist to be more honest, in his way, than the liberal. Of course this infuriates the liberal, because it is supposed to do just that. And for that reason it is not to be taken too seriously.

The Black Power movement is not just racism in reverse. This racist suggestion is of course a built-in ambiguity which is at once a strength and a weakness of the movement. For two reasons it has to *appear* racist: to help the black man consolidate his sense of identity, and to rebuff the sentimental and meddling integrationism of the white liberal. There is also a third reason: to get the liberals off the black man's back, and to make it quite clear that the Negro wants to run his own liberation movement from now on, without being told what to do by someone who cannot really understand his situation. If the white liberal wants to help, let him do so indirectly. Let him help poor whites, and let him try to show poor whites that they have much the same problems as the blacks, and that they therefore should not mess with the blacks or oppose them.

It is of course to the interests of white society and in particular of the white mass media to confuse and mishandle the whole Black Power issue. The more it can be treated as an eruption of berserk violence and African bloodlust the better the story will be and the more the white public will be charmed into gooseflesh by it. The frank exploitation of this sensationalist aspect of the race crisis is illustrated by the way *Esquire* got William Worthy to write on Black Power and then, against his will, gave his contribution a highly slanted and misleading publicity campaign (emphasizing "racist" implications). For which Worthy then sued the magazine.

This wilful distortion and exploitation make it completely impossible for the average reader to be properly informed about Black Power. He is predisposed to violent and panic reactions, and it can be said that the whole of America is now primed for an explosion of anarchic destructiveness and aimless slaughter. The fault does not lie with Black Power, or not entirely. The Black Power movement has simply elected to act as catalyst, in order that what is deeply hidden in American society may come out into the open. And evidently it will.

The essays that follow cannot pretend to be anything like adequate to the present situation. The first one is by now completely dated: it represents a provisional view of things in 1964. The one on the summer of 1967 is also provisional, but a few sentences here may serve to retrace the same outlines with firmer and more definite strokes, thanks to better information and to more mature reflection.

The Black Power movement is not really a racist movement, but it is definitely revolutionary. As Rap Brown says, again: "We are not an anti-white movement, we are anti-anybody who is anti-black." It is a frankly violent movement. It is an antiliberal movement, because it takes as axiomatic the belief that liberals are in favor of the established power institutions and of all liberal ideologies which covertly or otherwise aim at preserving these. Black Power claims it wants to destroy white institutions but in this it is perhaps ambiguous. Doubtless there are many in the Black Power movement who are frankly revolutionary, and passionately desire to destroy the American capitalist system. Others, on the other hand, are already moving toward more sophisticated (or more corrupt?) establishment positions, and are accused of careerism, of professorial rhetoric, and of complicity with the government-supported intellectuals. In fact they are accused of *becoming* establishment intellectuals. It is not my place here to say whether or not this is true, but it is obviously a familiar development. It is altogether possible that the American establishment will be smart enough to neutralize Black Power by simply sucking the leaders into the government or academic machine, as was done before with the older and less radical Negro organizations. The question then is: how long before Rap Brown becomes another Uncle Tom?

The Black Power movement is explicitly identified with and involved in the world revolutionary ferment in the Third World. "We are members of the Third World." "The liberation of oppressed people across the world depends on the liberation of black people in this country."

Is Black Power a Marxist movement? No. At least not yet. In fact, the danger of the leaders being sucked into a Marxist establishment is just as great as that of their being absorbed by the American establishment. In either case Black Power will become a white movement again —dominated by white ideologies, plugged in to a white tradition. In which case it will be neutralized in a different way.

Black Power thus claims to be relevant not only to American black people but to people of all colors, everywhere, who are held down in tutelage and subservience by the big white powers—whether American, European or Russian. It claims to be relevant also to the dissatisfied and disengaged within U.S. society (the hippies). *It is part of a world movement of refusal and rejection of the value system we call Western culture.* It is therefore at least implicitly critical of Christianity as a white man's religion and accepts Christianity only as somewhat radically revised: "Christ was (literally and historically) a black man!" (Actually, there is a certain typological point to this, but I cannot discuss it here).

What is to be said about Black Power? What does it mean to a serious—therefore radical—Christian? I for one do not believe a radical Christian has a moral obligation to manufacture Molotov cocktails in the cellar and smuggle them into the ghetto. Nor do I believe he has a moral obligation to convert the Black Power movement back to nonviolence (which is unlikely anyhow).

I do believe that the Christian is obligated, by his commitment to Christ, to seek out effective and authentic ways of peace in the midst of violence. But merely to demand support and obedience to an established disorder which is essentially violent through and through will not qualify as "peacemaking."

There are no easy and simple solutions to this problem, but in the long run the evil root that has to be dealt with is the root of violence, hatred, poison, cruelty and greed which is part of the system itself. The job of the white Christian is then partly a job of diagnosis and criticism, a prophetic task of finding and identifying the injustice which is the cause of *all* the violence, both white and black, which is also the root of war, and of the greed which keeps war going in order that some might make money out of it.

The delicacy and difficulty of the task are due, of course, to the fact that, in spite of all good intentions, Christians themselves have at times come to identify this evil of greed and power with "Christian order." They have confused it with peace, with right, with justice and with freedom, not distinguishing what really contributes to the good of man and what simply panders to his appetite for wealth and power.

We do not have to go and burn down the slums: but perhaps we might profitably consider whether some of our own venerable religious institutions are not, without our realizing it, supporting themselves in part by the exploitation of slum real estate, or capitalizing in some other way on a disastrous and explosive situation.

In any case, we have to make a clear decision. Black Power or no Black Power, I for one remain *for* the Negro. I trust him, I recognize the overwhelming justice of his complaint, I confess I have no right whatever to get in his way, and that as a Christian I owe him support, not in his ranks but in my own, among the whites who refuse to trust him or hear him, who want to destroy him.

Part Four: Violence and the Death of God: Or God as Unknown Soldier

Since the essays in this section spell out some of the things I have against the "Death of God" theology, it is only fair that I begin by saying what I think can be said *for* it.

First of all, the radical "Death of God" theologians are not only to be taken very seriously as Christians, but they are characteristic products of a real theological revival. The present time, for all its confusions and ambiguities, is certainly one of theological ferment: it is one of the most active periods in the history of theological thought. This fruitfulness and creativity have been due largely to men like Karl Barth, Paul Tillich, Karl Rahner, Jacques Maritain, Rudolf Bultmann and the other well-known names of the first half of the century. There are many others appearing on all sides after the Council. The Honest to God set in England is perhaps overly naïve, and it is their popular theology that I have tended to question most. In America, there is no coherent, still less unanimous, Death of God movement. There is quite a lot of variety in the thinking of Altizer (often hard to follow), Hamilton (apostle of the Playboy type) and Vahanian, a serious iconoclast with whom I tend most consistently to agree. In what follows, I am considering the "Death of God" chiefly from the viewpoint of Vahanian.

The basic premise of the Death of God theology is not, of course, the old and outworn scientific atheism of the nineteenth century. For this radical theology, the whole question of God's objective existence is completely irrelevant. The approach is altogether different: man's capacity to experience and to apprehend religious thought and concepts of God. Traditional theology has tended to assume that man experienced in himself a need for ultimate certitude which could only be satisfied by God's manifestation of himself in revealed truth. The Death of God starts by taking it as axiomatic that no modern man in good faith can really have an authentic religious experience that is not an experience of God's *absence*. Traditional theology posits God's hidden presence and works to make that presence manifest. In the light of God's presence and of his love, everything else becomes clear. God is the key to everything. The Death of God theology begins with a claim that this whole approach has utterly failed: to argue that man feels in himself a need for God, to go on to speak of the presence of God, and to explain everything else in this light is, it believes, simply to substitute ideas about God for gratuitously assumed "presence" of God and thus to make him all the more inexorably absent. In other words, it is not only that traditional theology proves nothing, but it antagonizes and alienates modern man and makes it all the more difficult for him to find any meaning whatever in the concept of God.

Now this is no new or revolutionary discovery. The approach to God "as unknown" has always had a recognized place in Catholic theology, and Protestantism also asserted from the beginning that a too sophisticated intellectual and rational structure in theology might neutralize the living and personal encounter with the inscrutable God of revelation in faith. Traditional theology itself has always recognized the insufficiency of propositions *about* God and *about* redemption which tend to objectify God and set him off at arm's length so that he can be "used" and "manipulated." Such a god becomes completely unreal—a mere convenience, serving man's purposes, a social commodity, a cosmic tranquillizer to be packaged and marketed along with any other product. The Death of God is a necessary iconoclastic protest against every form of popular religion which has blasphemed God by trying to sell him on the same terms as next year's Chevrolet.

Furthermore, the accusation runs (and I run right with it), this conceptualizing of God has tended more and more to identify the God of the Bible and of the Church with the Angel of the West—the Power or principality which is the "Guiding Spirit" of European-American civilization. The hidden God "whom no man shall see and live" and whose only manifestation is "in Christ" has been claimed as visible and present in the spirit, the ethos, the inner drive and the whole cultural outlook of the Western world. Thus the ways and attitudes of the post-Roman, medieval, then Renaissance, then enlightenment, then technological West have come to be seen as the vesture and even as the Face of God. Europe and America became the only true locus of his epiphany. Western man became in fact the manifestation of God in and as Christ. Hence the whole problem of the salvation of the world could be reduced to the task of turning everybody else into a more or less plausible replica of Western man. More grossly, to make Africa Christian, one needed only to make it Belgian, German, English, French. More grossly still, to save the soul of the African one needed only to baptize him and enslave him, thus killing two birds with one stone: gaining black souls for heaven and making a fortune out of Alabama cotton.

In other words, the saving knowledge of God in Christ was simply a matter of incorporation, however rudimentary, in some limb of Western "Christian" culture. Obviously the Church was not conscious of doing this, and the tension between Church and culture, Church and state, Church and world, was always maintained at least in theory. But how real was that tension? In actual fact, while "the world" was habitually and consistently denigrated, at least in words, the tension between it and the Church was more and more relaxed. In proportion as the world proved itself able to get along without the Church, the Church became less and less demanding, Christianity issued less and less of a challenge, until finally the Church would allow you practically anything as long as you continued to obey and to conform. A few difficult and symbolic issues like birth control, clerical celibacy, one permanent marriage, remained longer than any other, but are now being corroded away too. More and more the demands of the Church resolved themselves into demands for formal and exterior gestures of pious allegiance to God alone with rather more firm commitments to the claims of Caesar.

The clearest example of this has been in war. The French revolution put the Church in a new position *vis-à-vis* the state. The state now became hostile and demanding. The position of the Church was increasingly defensive—a matter of difficult concordats which guaranteed at least the integrity of the Church *as institution.* In order to protect these guarantees, the faithful had to be ready to meet the demands of the state in other areas. The State was now in need of larger armies. Conscription was becoming more and more universal. Even clerics, even religious, exempt by their very vocation to follow the counsels of perfection, were required to waive that exemption, when necessary to protect the interests of the Church institution in an anticlerical nation (such as France). In other words, one of the ways in which the Church protected her institutional structures in potentially hostile countries was to support the nation in its wars.

One of the few real demands for heroic sacrifice still made by the Church was that the faithful put aside their scruples and fears and obey the nation without question when it summoned them to go to war, even against other supposedly "Christian" nations. Theirs not to reason why. The government knew best. They did not have to inquire too minutely into the causes of the war or into the ways by which it was being waged. Suffice it that the bishops, by their approval, implied that the war and everything about it was "just." And the bishops, in their turn, as good patriots, left all these technicalities to the Ministry of War.

Thus it happened that the Christian gave heroic witness to his God and his faith by a meek, unquestioning obedience even unto death in submission to a Church authority that ordered him to submit to a civil authority that was not necessarily Christian—perhaps even anti-Christian.

Thus in fact God was drafted into all the armies and invited to get out there and kill himself.

As far as Europe was concerned, these rites were already thoroughly solemnized in World War I, but the Second World War guaranteed their full and complete efficacy. The nihilism and black despair of French literary and atheistic existentialism after World War II gave conclusive evidence that God had been a casualty of the war. He had died in it as one—or all—of its soldiers, both known and unknown. For the United States—which underwent a brief spasm of popular religion after World War II—the immolation has proceeded in Korea and most especially in Vietnam.

The effect of this more or less complete identification of God with "Western civilization" and with "Western society" regarded as still implicitly Christian has been of course that the crisis of Western civilization has also been necessarily a crisis of Christianity and of Christian faith. In this crisis, the Christian position has been one of more and more intolerable ambiguity, since in fact the last remaining elements of Christianity in Western culture have all but bled away.

The reaction of Christians has been somewhat frantic—where there has been any real reaction at all. One tended to lash out wildly against "materialism" and "secularism" and other scapegoat ideas, and to adopt a rather rigid posture of belief in order to maintain some coherent sense of Christian identity. But now that theologians and churchmen themselves are celebrating the praises of matter and of the secular city, this identity has been further undermined.

The true believers in this state of insecurity and frustration have only manifested more clearly and more pitifully the contradiction of their inner state. They have come out vociferously for the most bizarre, the most fanatical, the most aberrant causes in politics and culture. You can now find the most ardent Christians lined up in the most ridiculous, regressive, irrational parades. If they were concerned only with flying saucers and conversations with the departed it would not be so bad: but they are also deeply involved in racism, in quasi-Fascist nationalism, in every shade of fanatical hate cult, and in every semilunatic pressure group that is all the more self-congratulatory in that it is supported by the affluent as well as by the clergy. Such Christianity is of course a mere monstrosity and tends to make us believe that our Christian institutions are, in Vahanian's words, only "the lips with which we praise God while our hearts are far from him." He says:

> The survival of the Christian tradition is handicapped rather than helped by the existence of structures that are Christian in name only. It was doubtless easier to make the conversion from pre-Christian to Christian than it is from post-Christian to Christian. . . .
>
> Ultimately, organized religion, with its variegated paraphernalia, by trying to show how pertinent faith is, blunts it and mummifies it; [this leads to] the cultural annexation of God or a deliquescence of faith into religiosity. . . .
>
> (*Wait Without Idols*)

In such a situation, who needs atheists? The unbelief of believers is amply sufficient to make God repugnant and incredible.

Here we have to take account of the positive Christian affirmation made by the Death of God theologians. It is this: the deformation of God, due to the manipulative exploitation of him in the official concepts, is self-destroying. "God is man's failure." The intentness with which official Christianity seeks to make God relevant to man makes him so irrelevant that there remains but one alternative: to declare him dead. Then the true God, the God who is "absent," comes to life again.

When the god invented by man "dies" (he never really lived) then the true God is once again mysteriously present precisely because "God is absent." For Vahanian, Biblical religion shows us once for all that man's basic obligation to God is iconoclasm. That sounds wild, but it is only a reformulation of the first two commandments.

The chief problem of the Death of God theology as I see it is not that its language is calculatingly and consistently insulting to the

Church, nor that it deliberately makes use of near blasphemy in its contention that the official concept of God has now become blasphemous. All this can be understood when it is seen in the atmosphere of creativity and prophetism which surely is a sign of theology in our time. The real problem is that the Death of God theology too easily falls short of the prophetism to which it lays claim. It is often mere sophomoric antireligion and anticlericalism, and seems to end by subjecting man more completely and more arbitrarily to the massive domination of post-Christian secularism. My feeling is that the Death of God theology simply issues in acquiescence to political totalism, the police state—whether capitalist or Communist makes little difference. Either way, by conventional Christianity or by the Death of God, we seem to end up rendering everything to Caesar.

Nevertheless, the challenge issued by the Death of God theology is not to be evaded. In order to disentangle Christian faith from the crisis and collapse of Western culture, and open it to entirely new world perspectives, we have to be able to renounce the mighty spirit that has let himself be set up in the place of God: the Angel of the West.

Blessed Are the Meek: The Christian Roots of Nonviolence

It would be a serious mistake to regard Christian nonviolence simply as a novel tactic which is at once efficacious and even edifying, and which enables the sensitive man to participate in the struggles of the world without being dirtied with blood. Nonviolence is not simply a way of proving one's point and getting what one wants without being involved in behavior that one considers ugly and evil. Nor is it, for that matter, a means which anyone legitimately can make use of according to his fancy for any purpose whatever. To practice nonviolence for a purely selfish or arbitrary end would in fact discredit and distort the truth of nonviolent resistance.

Nonviolence is perhaps the most exacting of all forms of struggle, not only because it demands first of all that one be ready to suffer evil and even face the threat of death without violent retaliation, but because it excludes mere transient self-interest from its considerations. In a very real sense, he who practices nonviolent resistance must commit himself not to the defense of his own interests or even those of a particular group: he must commit himself to the defense of objective truth and right and above all of *man*. His aim is then not simply to "prevail" or to prove that he is right and the adversary wrong, or to make the adversary give in and yield what is demanded of him.

Nor should the nonviolent resister be content to prove *to himself* that *he* is virtuous and right, and that *his* hands and heart are pure even though the adversary's may be evil and defiled. Still less should he seek for himself the psychological gratification of upsetting the adversary's conscience and perhaps driving him to an act of bad faith and refusal of the truth. We know that our unconscious motives may, at times, make our nonviolence a form of moral aggression and even a subtle provocation designed (without our awareness) to bring out the evil we hope to find in the adversary, and thus to justify ourselves in our own eyes and in the eyes of "decent people." Wherever there is a high moral ideal there is an attendant risk of pharisaism, and nonviolence is no exception. The basis of pharisaism is division: on one hand this morally or socially privileged self and the elite to which it belongs. On the other hand, the "others," the wicked, the unenlightened, whoever they may be, Communists, capitalists, colonialists, traitors, international Jewry, racists, etc.

Christian nonviolence is not built on a presupposed division, but on the basic unity of man. It is not out for the conversion of the wicked to the ideas of the good, but for the healing and reconciliation of man with himself, man the person and man the human family.

The nonviolent resister is not fighting simply for "his" truth or for "his" pure conscience, or for the right that is on "his side." On the contrary, both his strength and his weakness come from the fact that he is fighting for *the* truth, common to him and to the adversary, *the* right which is objective and universal. He is fighting for *everybody.*

For this very reason, as Gandhi saw, the fully consistent practice of nonviolence demands a solid metaphysical and religious basis both in being and in God. This comes *before* subjective good intentions and sincerity. For the Hindu this metaphysical basis was provided by the Vedantist doctrine of the Atman, the true transcendent Self which alone is absolutely real, and before which the empirical self of the individual must be effaced in the faithful practice of *dharma.* For the Christian, the basis of nonviolence is the Gospel message of salvation for *all men* and of the Kingdom of God to which *all* are summoned. The disciple of Christ, he who has heard the good news, the announcement of the Lord's coming and of His victory, and is aware of the definitive establishment of the Kingdom, proves his faith by the gift of his whole self to the Lord in order that *all* may enter the Kingdom. This Christian discipleship entails a certain way of acting, a *politeia,* a *conservatio,* which is proper to the Kingdom.

The great historical event, the coming of the Kingdom, is made clear and is "realized" in proportion as Christians themselves live the life of the Kingdom in the circumstances of their own place and time. The saving grace of God in the Lord Jesus is proclaimed to man existentially in the love, the openness, the simplicity, the humility and the self-sacrifice of Christians. By their example of a truly Christian understanding of the world, expressed in a living and active application of the Christian faith to the human problems of their own time, Christians manifest the love of Christ for men (John 13:35, 17:21), and by that fact make him visibly present in the world. The religious basis of Christian nonviolence is then faith in Christ the Redeemer and obedience to his demand to love and manifest himself in us by a certain manner of acting in the world and in relation to other men. This obedience enables us to live as true citizens of the Kingdom, in which the divine mercy, the grace, favor and redeeming love of God are active in our lives. Then the Holy Spirit will indeed "rest upon us" and act in us, not for our own good alone but for God and his Kingdom. And if the Spirit dwells in us and works in us, our lives will be a continuous and progressive conversion and transformation in which we also, in some measure, help to transform others and allow ourselves to be transformed by and with others, in Christ.

The chief place in which this new mode of life is set forth in detail is the Sermon on the Mount. At the very beginning of this great inaugural discourse, the Lord numbers the beatitudes, which are the theological foundation of Christian nonviolence: Blessed are the poor in spirit . . . blessed are the meek (Matthew 5:3–4).

This does not mean "blessed are they who are endowed with a tranquil natural temperament, who are not easily moved to anger, who are always quiet and obedient, who do not naturally resist." Still less does it mean "blessed are they who passively submit to unjust oppression." On the contrary, we know that the "poor in spirit" are those of whom the prophets spoke, those who in the last days will be the "humble of the earth," that is to say the oppressed who have no human weapons to rely on and who nevertheless are true to the commandments of Yahweh, and who hear the voice that tells them: "Seek justice, seek humility, perhaps you will find shelter on the day of the Lord's wrath" (Sophonias 2:3). In other words they seek justice in the power of truth and of God, not by the power of man. Note that Christian meekness, which is essential to true nonviolence, has this eschatological quality about it. It refrains from self-assertion and from violent aggression because it sees all things in the light of the great judgment. Hence it does not struggle and fight merely for this or that ephemeral gain. It struggles for the truth and the right which alone will stand in that day when all is to be tried by fire (I Corinthians 3:10–15).

Furthermore, Christian nonviolence and meekness imply a particular understanding of the power of human poverty and powerlessness when they are united with the invisible strength of Christ. The Beatitudes indeed convey a profound existential understanding of the dynamic of the Kingdom of God—a dynamic made clear in the parables of the mustard seed and of the yeast. This is a dynamism of patient and secret growth, in belief that out of the smallest, weakest, and most insignificant seed the greatest tree will come. This is not merely a matter of blind and arbitrary faith. The early history of the Church, the record of the apostles and martyrs remains to testify to this inherent and mysterious dynamism of the ecclesial "event" in the world of history and time. Christian nonviolence is rooted in this consciousness and this faith.

This aspect of Christian nonviolence is extremely important and it gives us the key to a proper understanding of the meekness which accepts being "without strength" (*gewaltlos*) not out of masochism, quietism, defeatism or false passivity, but trusting in the strength of the Lord of truth. Indeed, we repeat, Christian nonviolence is nothing if not first of all a formal profession of faith in the Gospel message that the *Kingdom has been established* and that the Lord of truth is indeed risen and reigning over his Kingdom.

Faith of course tells us that we live in a time of eschatological struggle, facing a fierce combat which marshalls all the forces of evil and darkness against the still-invisible truth, yet this combat is already decided by the victory of Christ over death and over sin. The Christian can renounce the protection of violence and risk being humble, therefore *vulnerable,* not because he trusts in the supposed efficacy of a gentle and persuasive tactic that will disarm hatred and tame cruelty, but because he believes that the hidden power of the Gospel is demanding to be manifested in and through his own poor person. Hence in perfect obedience to the Gospel, he effaces himself and his own interests and even risks his life in order to testify not simply to "the truth" in a sweeping, idealistic and purely platonic sense, but to the truth that is incarnate in a concrete human situation, involving living persons whose rights are denied or whose lives are threatened.

Here it must be remarked that a holy zeal for the cause of humanity in the abstract may sometimes be mere lovelessness and indifference for concrete and living human beings. When we appeal to the highest and most noble ideals, we are more easily tempted to hate and contemn those who, so we believe, are standing in the way of their realization.

Christian nonviolence does not encourage or excuse hatred of a special class, nation or social group. It is not merely *anti*-this or that. In other words, the evangelical realism which is demanded of the Christian should make it impossible for him to generalize about "the wicked" against whom he takes up moral arms in a struggle for righteousness. He will not let himself be persuaded that the adversary is totally wicked and can therefore never be reasonable or well-intentioned, and hence need never be listened to. This attitude, which defeats the very purpose of nonviolence—openness, communication, dialogue—often accounts for the fact that some acts of civil disobedience merely antagonize the adversary without making him willing to communicate in any way whatever, except with bullets or missiles. Thomas à Becket, in Eliot's play *Murder in the Cathedral,* debated with himself, fearing that he might be seeking martyrdom merely in order to demonstrate his own righteousness and the King's injustice: "This is the greatest treason, to do the right thing for the wrong reason."

Now all these principles are fine and they accord with our Christian faith. But once we view the principles in the light of current *facts,* a practical difficulty confronts us. If the "gospel is preached to the poor," if the Christian message is essentially a message of hope and redemption for the poor, the oppressed, the underprivileged and those who have no power humanly speaking, how are we to reconcile ourselves to the fact that Christians belong for the most part to the rich and powerful nations of the earth? Seventeen percent of the world's population control eighty percent of the world's wealth, and most of these seventeen percent are supposedly Christian. Admittedly those Christians who are interested in nonviolence are not ordinarily the wealthy ones. Nevertheless, like it or not, they share in the power and privilege of the most wealthy and mighty society the world has ever known. Even with the best subjective intentions in the world, how can they avoid a certain ambiguity in preachng nonviolence? It this not a mystification?

We must remember Marx's accusation that "the social principles of Christianity encourage dullness, lack of self-respect, submissiveness, self-abasement, in short all the characteristics of the proletariat." We must frankly face the possibility that the nonviolence of the European or American preaching Christian meekness may conceivably be adulterated by bourgeois feelings and by an unconscious desire to preserve the status quo against violent upheaval.

On the other hand, Marx's view of Christianity is obviously tendentious and distorted. A real understanding of Christian nonviolence (backed up by the evidence of history in the Apostolic Age) shows not only that it is a *power,* but that it remains perhaps the only really effective way of transforming man and human society. After nearly fifty years of communist revolution, we find little evidence that the world is improved by violence. Let us however seriously consider at least the *conditions* for relative honesty in the practice of Christian nonviolence.

1. Nonviolence must be aimed above all at the transformation of the present state of the world, and it must therefore be free from all occult, unconscious connivance with an unjust use of power. This poses enormous problems—for if nonviolence is too political it becomes drawn into the power struggle and identified with one side or another in that struggle, while if it is totally apolitical it runs the risk of being ineffective or at best merely symbolic.

2. The nonviolent resistance of the Christian who belongs to one of the powerful nations and who is himself in some sense a privileged member of world society will have to be clearly not *for himself* but *for others,* that is for the poor and underprivileged. (Obviously in the case of Negroes in the United States, though they may be citizens of a privileged nation, their case is different. They are clearly entitled to wage a nonviolent struggle for their rights, but even for them this struggle should be primarily for *truth itself*—this being the source of their power.)

3. In the case of nonviolent struggle for peace—the threat of nuclear war abolishes all privileges. Under the bomb there is not much distinc-

tion between rich and poor. In fact the richest nations are usually the most threatened. Nonviolence must simply avoid the ambiguity of an unclear and *confusing protest* that hardens the warmakers in their self-righteous blindness. This means in fact that *in this case above all nonviolence must avoid a facile and fanatical self-righteousness,* and refrain from being satisfied with dramatic self-justifying gestures.

4. Perhaps the most insidious temptation to be avoided is one which is characteristic of the power structure itself: this fetishism of immediate visible results. Modern society understands "possibilities" and "results" in terms of a superficial and quantitative idea of efficacy. One of the missions of Christian nonviolence is to restore a different standard of practical judgment in social conflicts. This means that the Christian humility of nonviolent action must establish itself in the minds and memories of modern man not only as *conceivable* and *possible,* but as *a desirable alternative* to what he now considers the only realistic possibility: namely political technique backed by force. Here the human dignity of nonviolence must manifest itself clearly in terms of a freedom and a nobility which are able to resist political manipulation and brute force and show them up as arbitrary, barbarous and irrational. This will not be easy. The temptation to get publicity and quick results by spectacular tricks or by forms of protest that are merely odd and provocative but whose human meaning is not clear may defeat this purpose.

The realism of nonviolence must be made evident by humility and self-restraint which clearly show frankness and open-mindedness and invite the adversary to serious and reasonable discussion.

Instead of trying to use the adversary as leverage for one's own effort to realize an ideal, nonviolence seeks only to enter into a dialogue with him in order to attain, together with him, the common good of *man.* Nonviolence must be realistic and concrete. Like ordinary political action, it is no more than the "art of the possible." But precisely the advantage of nonviolence is that it has a *more Christian and more humane notion of what is possible.* Where the powerful believe that only power is efficacious, the nonviolent resister is persuaded of the superior efficacy of love, openness, peaceful negotiation and above all of truth. For power can guarantee the interests of *some men* but it can never foster the good of *man.* Power always protects the good of some at the expense of all the others. Only love can attain and preserve the good of all. Any claim to build the security of *all* on force is a manifest imposture.

It is here that genuine humility is of the greatest importance. Such humility, united with true Christian courage (because it is based on trust in God and not in one's own ingenuity and tenacity), is itself a way of communicating the message that one is interested only in truth and in the genuine rights of others. Conversely, our authentic interest in the common good above all will help us to be humble, and to distrust our own hidden drive to self-assertion.

5. Christian nonviolence, therefore, is convinced that the manner in which the conflict for truth is waged will itself manifest or obscure the truth. To fight for truth by dishonest, violent, inhuman, or unreasonable means would simply betray the truth one is trying to vindicate. The absolute refusal of evil or suspect means is a necessary element in the witness of nonviolence.

As Pope Paul said before the United Nations Assembly in 1965, "Men cannot be brohers if they are not humble. No matter how justified it may appear, pride provokes tensions and struggles for prestige, domination, colonialism and egoism. In a word *pride shatters brotherhood.*" He went on to say that the attempts to establish peace on the basis of violence were in fact a manifestation of human pride. "If you wish to be brothers, let the weapons fall from your hands. You cannot love with offensive weapons in your hands."

6. A test of our sincerity in the practice of nonviolence is this: are we willing to *learn something from the adversary*? If a *new truth* is made known to us by him or through him, will we accept it? Are we willing to admit that he is not totally inhumane, wrong, unreasonable, cruel, etc.? This is important. If he sees that we are completely incapable of listening to him with an open mind, our nonviolence will have nothing to say to him except that we distrust him and seek to outwit him. Our readiness to see some good in him and to agree with some of his ideas (though tactically this might look like a weakness on our part), actually gives us power: the power of sincerity and of truth. On the other hand, if we are obviously unwilling to accept any truth that we have not first discovered and declared ourselves, we show by that very fact that we are interested not in the truth so much as in "being right." Since the adversary is presumably interested in being right also, and in proving himself right by what he considers the superior argument of force, we end up where we started. Nonviolence has great power, provided that it really witnesses to truth and not just to self-righteousness.

The dread of being open to the ideas of others generally comes from our hidden insecurity about our own convictions. We fear that we may be "converted"—or perverted—by a pernicious doctrine. On the other hand, if we are mature and objective in our open-mindedness, we may find that viewing things from a basically different perspective —that of our adversary—we discover our own truth in a new light and are able to understand our own ideal more realistically.

Our willingness to take *an alternative approach* to a problem will perhaps relax the obsessive fixation of the adversary on his view, which he believes is the only reasonable possibility and which he is determined to impose on everyone else by coercion.

It is the refusal of alternatives—a compulsive state of mind which one might call the "ultimatum complex"—which makes wars in order to force the unconditional acceptance of one oversimplified interpretation of reality. This mission of Christian humility in social life is not merely to edify, but to *keep minds open to many alternatives.* The rigidity of a certain type of Christian thought has seriously impaired this capacity, which nonviolence must recover.

Needless to say, Christian humility must not be confused with a mere desire to win approval and to find reassurance by conciliating others superficially.

7. Christian hope and Christian humility are inseparable. The quality of nonviolence is decided largely by the purity of the Christian hope behind it. In its insistence on certain human values, the Second Vatican Council, following *Pacem in Terris,* displayed a basically optimistic trust *in man himself.* Not that there is not wickedness in the world, but today trust in God cannot be completely divorced from a certain trust in man. The Christian knows that there are radically sound possibilities in every man, and he believes that love and grace always have the power to bring out those possibilities at the most unexpected moments. Therefore if he has hopes that God will grant peace to the world it is because he also trusts that man, God's creature, is not basically evil: that there is in man a potentiality for peace and order which can be realized provided the right conditions are there. The Christian will do his part in creating these conditions by preferring love and trust to hate and suspiciousness. Obviously, once again, this "hope in man" must not be naïve. But experience itself has shown, in the last few years, how much an attitude of simplicity and openness can do to break down barriers of suspicion that had divided men for centuries.

It is therefore very important to understand that Christian humility implies not only a certain wise reserve in regard to one's own judgments—a good sense which sees that we are not always necessarily infallible in our ideas—but it also cherishes positive and trustful expectations of others. A supposed "humility" which is simply depressed about itself and about the world is usually a false humility. This negative, self-pitying "humility" may cling desperately to dark and apocalyptic expectations, and refuse to let go of them. It is secretly convinced that only tragedy and evil can possibly come from our present world situation. This secret conviction cannot be kept hidden. It will manifest itself in our attitudes, in our social action and in our protest. It will show that in fact we despair of reasonable dialogue with anyone. It will show that we expect only the worst. Our action seeks only to block or frustrate the adversary in some way. A protest that from the start declares itself to be in despair is hardly likely to have valuable results. At best it provides an outlet for the personal frustrations of the one protesting. It enables him to articulate his despair in public. This is not the function of Christian nonviolence. This pseudo-prophetic desperation has nothing to do with the beatitudes, even the third. No blessedness has been promised to those who are merely sorry for themselves.

In résumé, the meekness and humility which Christ extolled in the Sermon on the Mount and which are the basis of true Christian nonviolence are inseparable from an eschatological Christian hope which is completely open to the presence of God in the world and therefore to the presence of our brother who is always seen, no matter who he may be, in the perspectives of the Kingdom. Despair is not permitted to the meek, the humble, the afflicted, the ones famished for justice, the merciful, the clean of heart and the peacemakers. All the beatitudes "hope against hope," "bear everything, believe everything, hope for everything, endure everything" (I Corinthians 13:7). The beatitudes are simply aspects of love. They refuse to despair of the world and abandon it to a supposedly evil fate which it has brought upon itself. Instead, like Christ himself, the Christian takes upon his own shoulders the yoke of the Savior, meek and humble of heart. This yoke is the burden of the world's sin with all its confusions and all its problems. These sins, confusions and problems are our very own. We do not disown them.

Christian nonviolence derives its hope from the promise of Christ: "Fear not, little flock, for the Father has prepared for you a Kingdom" (Luke 12:32).

The hope of the Christian must be, like the hope of a child, pure and full of trust. The child is totally available in the present because he has relatively little to remember, his experience of evil is as yet brief, and his anticipation of the future does not extend very far. The Christian, in his humility and faith, must be as totally available to his brother, to his world, in the present, as the child is. But he cannot see the world with childlike innocence and simplicity unless his memory is cleared of past evils by forgiveness, and his anticipation of the future is hopefully free of craft and calculation. For this reason, the humility of Christian nonviolence is at once patient and uncalculating. The chief difference between nonviolence and violence is that the latter depends entirely on its own calculations. The former depends entirely on God and on His word.

At the same time the violent or coercive approach to the solution of human problems considers man in general, in the abstract, and according to various notions about the laws that govern his nature. In other words, it is concerned with man as subject to necessity, and it seeks out the points at which his nature is consistently vulnerable in order to coerce him physically or psychologically. Nonviolence on the other hand is based on that respect for the human person without which there is no deep and genuine Christianity. It is concerned with an appeal to the liberty and intelligence of the person insofar as he is able to transcend nature and natural necessity. Instead of forcing a decision upon him from the outside, it invites him to arrive freely at a decision of his own, in dialogue and cooperation, and in the presence of that truth which Christian nonviolence brings into full view by its sacrificial witness. The key to nonviolence is the willingness of the nonviolent resister to suffer a certain amount of accidental evil in order to bring about a change of mind in the oppressor and awaken him to personal openness and to dialogue. A nonviolent protest that merely seeks to gain publicity and to show up the oppressor for what he is, without opening his eyes to new values, can be said to be in large part a failure. At the same time, a nonviolence which does not rise to the level of the personal, and remains confined to the consideration of nature and natural necessity, may perhaps make a deal but it cannot really make sense.

It is understandable that the Second Vatican Council, which placed such strong emphasis on the dignity of the human person and the freedom of the individual conscience, should also have strongly approved "those who renounce the use of violence in the vindication of their rights and who resort to methods of defense which are otherwise available to weaker parties too" (*Constitution on the Church in the Modern World*, n. 78). In such a confrontation between conflicting parties, on the level of personality, intelligence and freedom, instead of with massive weapons or with trickery and deceit, a fully human solution becomes possible. Conflict will never be abolished but a new way of solving it can become habitual. Man can then act according to the dignity of that adulthood which he is now said to have reached—and which yet remains, perhaps to be conclusively proved. One of the ways in which it can, without doubt, be proved is precisely this: man's ability to settle conflicts by reason and arbitration instead of by slaughter and destruction.

The distinction suggested here, between two types of thought—one oriented to nature and necessity, the other to person and freedom—calls for further study at another time. It seems to be helpful. The "nature-oriented" mind treats other human beings as objects to be manipulated in order to control the course of events and make the future for the whole human species conform to certain rather rigidly determined expectations. "Person-oriented" thinking does not lay down these draconian demands, does not seek so much to *control* as to *respond*, and to *awaken response*. It is not set on determining anyone or anything, and does not insistently demand that persons and events correspond to our own abstract ideal. All it seeks is the openness of free exchange in which reason and love have freedom of action. In such a situation the future will take care of itself. This is the truly Christian outlook. Needless to say that many otherwise serious and sincere Christians are unfortunately dominated by this "nature-thinking" which is basically legalistic and technical. They never rise to the level of authentic interpersonal relationships outside their own intimate circle. For them, even today, the idea of building peace on a foundation of war and coercion is not incongruous—it seems perfectly reasonable!

Christian Action in World Crisis

A death struggle can also be a struggle for life, a new birth. One is sometimes tempted to think the present crisis is the final sickness unto death: there is plenty of evidence that it might be so. Or perhaps it is the birth agony of a new world. Let us hope that it is. No one can dare to predict what is about to be born of our confusion, our frenzy, our apocalyptic madness. Certainly the old order is changing, but we do not know what is to come. All we know is that we see the many-crowned and many-headed monsters rising on all sides out of the deep, from the ocean of our own hidden and collective self. We do not understand them, and we cannot. We panic at the very sight of their iridescent scales, their deadly jaws that flame with nuclear fire. But they pursue us relentlessly, even into absurd little caves fitted out with battery radios and hand-operated blowers. We find no security even in the spiritual cave of forgetfulness, the anaesthesia of the human mind that finally shuts out an unbearable truth, and goes about the business of life in torpor and stoical indifference.

And yet the monsters do not have to come to life. They are not yet fully objective like the world around us. They do not have the substance which is given to things by the creative power of God: they are the spiritual emanations of our own sick and sinful being. They exist in and by us. They are from us. They cannot exist without us. They are our illusions. They are nightmares which our incredible technological skill can all too easily actualize. But they are also dreams from which we can awaken before it is too late. They are dreams which we can still, perhaps, choose not to dream.

The awful problem of our time is not so much the dreams, the monsters, which may take shape and consume us, but the moral paralysis in our own souls which leaves us immobile, inert, passive, tongue-tied, ready and even willing to succumb. The great tragedy is in the cold, silent waters of moral death which climb imperceptibly within us, blinding conscience, drowning compassion, suffocating faith and extinguishing the Spirit. The progressive extinction of conscience, of judgment and of compassion is the inexorable work of the cold war. When the work is completed, then . . .

One thing is getting to be more and more certain. The balance of terror, which dictates all the policies of the two great armed power blocs, cannot stay "balanced" much longer. It will crash. It may crash very soon. Napoleon said you cannot sit on bayonets. You have to use them, if you have them around. This is a thousand times more true of the monstrous weapons which offer an overwhelming advantage to the one who strikes first and who strikes hardest, who smashes everything the enemy has before the enemy can wake up to his danger.

The slightest false move, the most innocent miscalculation, an ill-chosen word, a misprint, a trivial failure in the mechanism of a computer, and one hundred million people evaporate, burn to death, go up in radioactive dust, or crawl about the face of the earth howling for death to release them from agony.

We are not good at resisting sin, even under the best conditions. But under the most violent provocation, under the most diabolical pressures, when we have abdicated all morality, when we have frankly gone back to the law of the jungle, how much chance is there, humanly speaking, that we can live without disaster?

Two things are clear. First, the enemy is not just one side or the other. The enemy is not just Russia, or China, or Communism, or Castro, or Khrushchev, or capitalism, or imperialism. The enemy is on both sides. The enemy is in all of us. The enemy is war itself, and the root of war is hatred, fear, selfishness, lust. Pius XII said in 1944, "If ever a generation has known in the depths of his being the cry of 'War on war' it is our own!" As long as we arm only against Russia, we are fighting for the real enemy and against ourselves. We are fighting to release the monster in our own soul, which will devour the world. We are fighting for the demon who strives to re-assert his power over mankind. We have got to arm not against Russia but against war. Not only against war, but against hatred. Against lies. Against injustice. Against greed. Against every manifestation of these things, wherever they may be found.

Yet at the same time we cannot attempt to ignore the spiritual border line that separates the nations of the West, with their Christian background, from the officially atheistic Communist bloc. We must avoid two extremes: seeing all good on our side and all evil on their side, or, on the contrary, dismissing both sides as totally evil. The fact remains that although the Communists have explicitly rejected the Christian ethical tradition, there may still remain in Communist-dominated countries strong surviving elements of that tradition. And although we of the West appeal to the Christian tradition in favor of our own cause, and do this quite legitimately, yet nevertheless there are materialistic and atheistic elements at work among us just as powerful and just as destructive of our tradition as the materialism and atheism of the official Communist ideology.

On both sides there are powerful and fanatical pressure groups dominated by their political obsessions, who drive towards nuclear war. On both sides the vast majority desire nothing but peace. The extremists on both sides are very much alike though they regard one another as opposites. The moderates on both sides also have very much in common. One sometimes wonders if the real dividing line is not to be drawn between the fanatics (whether Russian or American) and the moderate, ordinary people of both sides.

In any case the policy-makers and propagandists are more and more clearly and cynically espousing the cause of what they call "realism": that is to say an all-out preemptive nuclear attack involving mass destruction of civilians. This policy is clearly unacceptable by Christian moral standards. In effect, the extreme bellicosity which leads each of the great power blocs to depend more and more on the threat of a preemptive attack, with no limit to the megatonic impact of the nuclear weapons and no discrimination between civil and military objectives, *is equally immoral on both sides, equally inhuman and incompatible with Christian ethics.*

In this restricted sense it may indeed be possible to find the same demonic evil at work, perhaps in different degrees, on both sides. Once one adopts the policy of nuclear "realism" which is purely and simply a policy of annihilation, then one abandons the moral advantage of fighting for freedom, justice and democracy. None of these values are likely to survive an all-out nuclear war. Even if one nation manages to win such a war, the conditions will be such that social, moral and spiritual values with which we are familiar, and which we should certainly be prepared to defend with our lives, will no longer be recognizable in the moral debacle. Such at least is the belief of Pope Pius XII and of John XXIII.

The conclusion is, then, that we must defend freedom and sanity against the bellicose fanaticism of all war-makers, whether "ours" or "theirs," and that we must strive to do so not with force but with the spiritual weapons of Christian prayer and action. But this action must be at once nonviolent and decisive. Good intentions and fond hopes are not enough.

The present world crisis is not merely a political and economic conflict. It goes deeper than ideologies. It is a crisis of man's spirit. It is a great religious and moral upheaval of the human race, and we do not really know half the causes of this upheaval. We cannot pretend to have a full understanding of what is going on in ourselves and in our society. That is why our desperate hunger for clear and definite solutions sometimes leads us into temptation. We oversimplify. We seek the cause of evil and find it here or there in a particular nation, class, race, ideology, system. And we discharge upon this scapegoat all the virulent force of our hatred, compounded with fear and anguish, striving to rid ourselves of our fear by destroying the object we have arbitrarily singled out as the embodiment of all evil. Far from curing us, this is only another paroxysm which aggravates our sickness.

The moral evil in the world is due to man's alienation from the deepest truth, from the springs of spiritual life within himself, to his alienation from God. Those who realize this try desperately to persuade and enlighten their brothers. But we are in a radically different position from the first Christians, who revolutionized an essentially religious world of paganism with the message of a new religion that had never been heard of. We are on the contrary living in an irreligious world in which the Christian message has been repeated over and over until it has come to seem empty of all intelligible content to those whose ears close to the word of God even before it is uttered. Christianity is no longer identified with newness and change, but only with the static preservation of outworn structures.

This should teach us that though the words of the Gospel still objectively retain all the force and freshness of their original life, it is not enough now for us to make them known and clarify them. It is not enough to announce the familiar message that no longer seems to be news. Not enough to teach, to explain, convince. Now above all it is the time to embody Christian truth in action even more than in words. No matter how lucid, how persuasive, how logical, how profound our theological and spiritual statements may be, they are often wasted on anyone who does not already think as we do. That is why the serene and almost classic sanity of moralists exposing the traditional teaching of Catholic theologians on the "just war" is almost total loss in the general clamor and confusion of half truths, propaganda slogans, and pernicious clichés. Who will listen and agree, except another professional theologian? What influence can such statements have in preserving sanity, clear and logical though they may be?

What is needed now is the Christian who manifests the truth of the Gospel in social action, with or without explanation. The more clearly his life manifests the teaching of Christ, the more salutary will it be. Clear and decisive Christian action explains itself and teaches in a way that words never can.

What is wanted now is therefore not simply the Christian who takes an inner complacency in the words and example of Christ, but who seeks to follow Christ perfectly, not only in his own personal life, not only in prayer and penance, but also in his political commitments and in all his social responsibilities. There is little point, today, in a morality which seeks by refined casuistical reasoning to justify conduct which comes as close as possible to sin without actually sinning. Still less is it justifiable for Christian moralists to seek to justify and permit as much as possible of force and terror, in international politics and in war, instead of struggling in every way to restrain force and bring into being a positive international authority which can effectively prevent war and promote peace.

We are at a point of momentous choice. Either our frenzy of desperation will lead to destruction, or our patient loyalty to truth, to God and to our fellow man will enable us to perform the patient, heroic task of building a world that will thrive in unity and peace. At this point, Christian action will be decisive. That is why it is supremely important for us to keep our heads and refuse to be carried away by the wild projects of fanatics who seek an oversimplified and immediate solution by means of inhuman violence.

Christians have got to speak by their actions. Their political action must not be confined to the privacy of the polling booth. It must be clear and manifest to everybody. It must speak loudly and plainly the Christian truth, and it must be prepared to defend that truth with sacrifice, accepting misunderstanding, injustice, calumny, and even imprisonment or death. It is crucially important for Christians today to adopt a clear position and back it up with everything they have got. This means an unremitting fight for justice in every sphere—in labor, in race relations, in the "third world" and above all in international affairs.

This means (to adopt a current military cliché) closing the gap between our interior intentions and our exterior acts. Our social actions must conform to our deepest religious principles. Beliefs and politics can no longer be kept isolated from one another. It is no longer possible for us to be content with abstract and hidden acts of "purity of intention" which do nothing to make our outward actions different from those of atheists or agnostics.

Nor can we be content to make our highest ideal the preservation of a minimum of ethical rectitude prescribed by natural law. Too often the nobility and grandeur of natural law have been debased and deformed by the manipulations of theorists until natural law has become indistinguishable from the law of the jungle, which is no law at all. Hence those who complacently prescribe the duty of national defense on the basis of "natural law" often forget entirely the norms of justice and humanity without which no war can be permitted. Without those norms, natural law becomes mere jungle law, that is to say crime.

The Popes have repeatedly pleaded with Christian people to show themselves in all things disciples of Christ the Prince of Peace, and to embody in their lives their faith in His teaching. "All His teaching is an invitation to peace," says Pope John XXIII in the 1961 Christmas message. Deploring the ever increasing selfishness, hardness of heart, cynicism and callousness of mankind, as war becomes once again more and more imminent, Pope John says that Christian goodness and charity must permeate all the activity, whether personal or social, of every Christian. The Pontiff quotes Saint Leo the Great in a passage which contrasts natural ethics with the nonviolent ethic of the Gospel:

"To commit injustice and to make reparation—this is the prudence of the world. On the contrary, *not to render evil for evil is the virtuous expression of Christian forgiveness.*" These words, embodying the wisdom of the Church and the heart of her moral teaching, are heard without attention and complacently discussed even by Catholics.

Too often, in practice, we tend to assume that the teaching of Christian forgiveness and meekness applies only to the individual, not to nations or collectivities. The state can go to war and exert every form of violent force, while the individual expresses his Christian meekness by shouldering his gun without resistance and obeying the command to go out and kill. This is not Pope John's idea at all. He utters a solemn warning to rulers of nations: "With the authority we have received from Jesus Christ we say: *Shun all thought of force; think of the tragedy of initiating a chain reaction of acts, decisions and resentments which could erupt into rash and irreparable deeds.* You have received great powers not to destroy but to build, not to divide but to unite, not to cause tears to be shed but to provide employment and security."

Christian action is based on the Christian conscience, and conscience has to be informed by moral truth. What are the moral options open to the Catholic in regard to nuclear war? This has seldom been made clear, and it is tragic to observe that many Catholics are in a state of ignorance and confusion on some very important points. The vague statement that "a Catholic cannot be a pacifist" (a statement that requires a great deal of clear interpretation) is taken to signify that a Catholic is bound in conscience to accept passively every form of war and military force that his government may decide to use against an enemy. According to this view, a good Christian is one who shrinks from no work of violent destruction commanded by the state in war. How far that would be from the primitive idea that the good Christian normally refused military service and suffered violence in himself rather than inflicting it on others. Such a misconception could lead to the awful conclusion that a Catholic commanded by a new Hitler to operate the furnaces of another Dachau would be only "doing his duty" if he obeyed. The noble Christian concept of duty and sacrifice must not be debased to the point where the Christian becomes the passive and servile instrument of inhuman governments.

Succinctly: A Catholic is permitted to hold the following views of nuclear war:

a. Many sound theologians have taught that the traditional conditions of a just war cannot be fully realized today and that, as Pope Pius XII himself said, "the theory of war as an apt and proportionate means of solving international conflicts is now out of date." In practice, what has been called "relative pacifism" can very certainly be held and is held by many Catholics. Without rejecting the traditional teaching that a "just war" can theoretically be possible under certain well-defined conditions, this view holds that nuclear war is by its very nature beyond the limits of the traditional doctrine. This is supported by very clear statements of Cardinal Ottaviani and Pope Pius XII. Hence, though it is not the definitive "teaching of the Church" it is certainly not only a tenable doctrine but seems to be the soundest and most traditional opinion.

b. Though absolute pacifism in a completely unqualified form has been reproved, nevertheless today the pacifist standpoint pure and simple tends in practice to rejoin the above view, since a Catholic can be a pacifist in a particular case when there are very serious reasons for believing that even a limited war may be unjust, or may "escalate" to proportions which violate justice. It is to be noted that *when a war is evidently unjust* a Catholic not only *may* refuse to serve but he is *morally obliged to refuse to participate* in it.

c. Catholic tradition has always admitted the legality of a defensive war where there is a just cause, right intention and use of the right means. It is argued that a limited nuclear war for defensive purposes can fulfill the requirements of a just war, and that therefore it is right and just to possess stockpiles of nuclear weapons and to threaten retaliation for a nuclear attack. This may be and is held by many Catholics, and it is probably the majority opinion among Catholics in the United States. But it can be said that this position, while specious and reasonable in theory, becomes very dangerous when we consider the actual facts. All theologians agree that the unrestricted use of nuclear weapons for the simple purpose of annihilation of civilian centers is completely immoral. It is nothing but murder and is never permitted, any more than a nuclear preemptive strike on civilian centers would be permitted by Christian ethics.

Could a preemptive attack on the military installations of the enemy be admitted as a "just" defensive measure? To do so would seem very rash in view of the disastrous consequences of the retaliatory war that would inevitably be unleashed, and would inevitably entail the total mass destruction of great centers of population. The statement quoted above from Pope John XXIII, while not formally declaring such an action intrinsically evil, is a solemn warning not to initiate, by any form of aggression, a chain of acts of war and violence. While it may be all very well for theologians to theorize about a limited nuclear war, it is quite evident in actual practice that the international policies of both the United States and Russia are frankly built on the threat of an all-out war of annihilation.

In such a situation our Christian duty is clear. Though no Catholic is clearly obliged to adhere to a policy of immediate nuclear disarmament, whether multilateral or unilateral, he is certainly obliged to do everything he can, in his own situation, to work for peace. It is difficult to see how one can work for peace without ultimately seeking disarmament. If he holds one of the above opinions which are tenable, he becomes obliged to a course of action which will promote peace in accordance with the view he takes. If he is one who believes, as the Popes themselves seem quite clearly to believe, that a nuclear war will most probably be a completely unjust war because its destructive effects cannot be controlled, and that it is in any case unreasonable and totally undesirable, then he will be obliged to base his political activity on the belief that war must be prevented here and now, and that we must try as best we can to work for its eventual abolition. This does not mean necessarily an all-out campaign to "ban the bomb" immediately. But it certainly does mean an insistence on peaceful means of settling international disputes. If a Catholic feels himself obliged in conscience to oppose all nuclear armaments and to demand even immediate unilateral disarmament as the best way to peace, though his director of conscience may not agree with his politics he cannot forbid him to hold this view.

There are many reasons to believe that the social action of someone like Dorothy Day, who is willing to refuse cooperation even in civil defense drills and ready to go to jail for her belief in peace, is far more significantly Christian than the rather subtle and comfy positions of certain casuists. When I consider that Dorothy Day was confined to a jail cell in nothing but a light wrap (her clothes having been taken from her) and that she could only get to Mass and Communion in the prison by dressing in clothes borrowed from prostitutes and thieves in the neighboring cells, then I lose all inclination to take seriously the self-complacent nonsense of those who consider her kind of pacifism sentimental.

Note on Civil Disobedience and Nonviolent Revolution

(Submitted at the request of the National Commission on the Causes and Prevention of Violence)

---

1. I am asked to submit some remarks on "the theory and practice of civil disobedience," the implication being that this is one of the areas of "violence" which the commission is worried about. Though this is not really my field, I have done some reading in it and have formulated some ideas which have been published chiefly in books like *Seeds of Destruction, Faith and Violence* and *Gandhi on Non-Violence*. In these books and related articles I have studied what might be called the "classical" approach to nonviolent conflict resolution, exemplified by Mahatma Gandhi and Martin Luther King (as well as by Tolstoy, Thoreau and other precursors). This "classical" approach has the following important characteristics:

a. It is the expression of a religious humanism and seeks to apply the ideals of traditionally religious civilizations to the resolution of conflict and the solution of social problems for which conventional political means seem to have proved inadequate.

b. It claims that instead of having recourse to revolutionary violence and to the overthrow of established systems by force, a more efficacious method is to appeal to the deepest moral idealism of a civilized tradition. It is a way of reform rather than of revolution.

c. It appeals above all to the highest ethical motivations and far from advocating the violent destruction of civilized and traditional structures as such, it bases itself on a fundamental respect for social order. This means that a scrupulous distinction is made between the unjust law, pinpointed as a source of inevitable disorder, and the essential legality of structures. Thus the theory of civil disobedience in this classic context permits only disobedience of a law that has been shown to be unjust, and at the same time it affirms respect for law and order as such by accepting punishment for the act of disobedience. This aspect of civil disobedience is often overlooked.

d. In other words, the "classical" theory of nonviolence claims to respect the values and structures of civilization even more than does the establishment, which (they claim) has become involved in the routine of retaining power and making money. Classic nonviolence questions an establishment which negates civilized values while claiming to defend them and engages in corrupt dealings which in fact are the real source of conflict and disorder. Thus, rightly or wrongly, classic nonviolence seeks to defend all that is regarded as best and highest in civilization. It is essentially a religious humanism and a mystique of reform. In this lie both its strength and its weakness.

e. This classic theory of nonviolent social change is attacked vehemently both by Marxists and by professional revolutionaries committed to the use of force in the struggle for political power, and by conservative establishments. Both these oppositions seek to discredit the classic theory of nonviolence. Because of its attachment to traditional and religious values, classic nonviolence is attacked by Marxists as essentially "bourgeois" and conservative. Because of its advocation of reform and its protest against disorders, it is attacked by the establishment as "anarchy," and sinister links with Marxists are hinted at (seldom proved because they seldom exist).

2. At this present moment, 1968, we have already passed a point of crucial decision. It can be said that the classical approach to nonviolence is no longer the dominant and guiding force in radical efforts to achieve reform and conflict resolution. The events of the past few years have inexorably built up a new polarization of violent forces and those who have hitherto been disposed to nonviolence are being forced more and more toward the violent positions of extremists. This is not so much the result of their own choice as the effect of inexorable pressures: on one hand, in the area of civil rights, the trend toward militancy and the repudiation of anything savoring of nonviolent approach is more and more represented as weak and cowardly. Nevertheless, the Peace Movement is still predominantly nonviolent and although acts of civil disobedience are becoming markedly more aggressive, the Peace Movement has not committed itself to violence—and with good reason, for it would thus tend to contradict itself. Unfortunately, the increasing use of force and the numerous complaints of brutality and police repression in the effort to stifle the voice of protest against the Vietnam war are having a disastrous effect on the Peace Movement. Though by and large the Peace Movement is still made up of nonviolent, love-affirming types who place a high premium on gentleness, conciliation, mutual understanding, dialogue, etc., they are being driven to a kind of despair of traditional civilized humanistic attitudes. Some still believe in the power of love and peaceful conciliation to effect a change in the violent and hostile adversary. Others are simply becoming convinced that the police, the military and the establishment are blindly

opposed to any reasonable expression of protest, that they refuse to listen to civilized argument, that they represent essential corruption and injustice. For instance, the young people in the Peace Movement are not especially impressed by appeals to respect law and order when they believe that the Vietnam war itself is a flagrant example of illegality and contempt for international order. When they are accused of trying to "take the law into their own hands," they answer, rightly or wrongly, that this is precisely what President Johnson and the Pentagon are doing in Asia. I am not of course espousing these arguments here: I am just citing them as examples of what the young people believe to be bad faith on the part of their elders and of authority.

It is these people who are now beginning to talk revolution. I say *talk* revolution because it is almost entirely talk (as far as I can tell). But if they feel themselves continually singled out for what they conceive to be brutal, unjust, uncomprehending treatment, they will be driven more and more to identify themselves somewhat romantically with typological figures like Che Guevara. The whole psychology of this situation calls for careful study and, I might add, sympathetic study.

3. I might say quite frankly that in my opinion one of the reasons for the current swing toward violence is that the classic nonviolent position has been consistently misrepresented, misunderstood and subjected to more and more brutal repression. The people who were at first attracted to this approach have thus been disillusioned not only with the established structures but also (more tragically) with the whole civilized tradition of religious humanism. Thus they are turning more and more not only to revolution but to a new pragmatic mystique of revolutionary humanism. To put it bluntly, the kind of brutal and incomprehending repression to which they find themselves subjected, in the name of "civilized tradition," "law and order," etc., makes them more and more convinced that there is no authentic humanism that is not militantly revolutionary. In other words, they are moving more and more toward the Marxist position. They are being driven to the Marxist position by a sort of self-fulfilling prophecy. If they are beaten over the head long enough and hard enough, they will end up as full-fledged Marxists, and then the police can say, "We told you so," and everyone can start shooting with a "clear conscience." Needless to say, I regard this as tragic futility, and in my opinion it brings us closer and closer to a particular kind of totalitarian state. It may not reproduce the crude patterns of European Gestapo culture, but it will nevertheless mean the end of real democracy and freedom for the United States of America.

4. To sum up: I ask myself this rather disquieting question: Will the commission concentrate on the suppression of nonviolent protest and disregard the real murderers, the extremists and fanatics who are already explicitly committed to violence, bloodshed, murder and destruction? The assassins are not—at least not yet—to be looked for

chiefly among the rioting students and peaceniks who burn their draft cards. And the real focus of American violence is not in esoteric groups but in the very culture itself, its mass media, its extreme individualism and competitiveness, its inflated myths of virility and toughness, and its overwhelming preoccupation with the power of nuclear, chemical, bacteriological and psychological overkill. If we live in what is essentially a culture of overkill, how can we be surprised at finding violence in it? Can we get to the root of the trouble? In my opinion, the best way to do it would have been the classic way of religious humanism and nonviolence exemplified by Gandhi. That way seems now to have been closed. I do not find the future reassuring.

Note for Ave Maria

There seems to be a general impression that nonviolence in America has been tried and found wanting. The tragic death of Martin Luther King is supposed to have marked the end of an era in which nonviolence could have any possible significance, and the Poor People's March has been described as a sort of post mortem on nonviolence. From now on, we hear, it's violence only. Why? Because nonviolence not only does not get results, but it is not even effective as communication.

I might as well say clearly that I do not believe this at all. And in spite of the fact that the Montgomery bus boycott, for instance, was a great example of the effective use of nonviolence both as tactic and as communication, in spite of the freedom rides, Birmingham, Selma, etc., I don't think America has yet begun to look at nonviolence or to really understand it. It is not my business to tell the SNCC people how to manage their political affairs. If they feel that they can no longer make good use of nonviolence, let them look to it. There are certainly reasons for thinking that a seemingly passive resistance may not be what the Black people of America can profitably use. Nor do I think, incidentally, that "Black Power" means nothing but mindless and anarchic violence. It is more sophisticated than that.

But we are considering the Peace Movement.

The napalming of draft records by the Baltimore nine is a special and significant case because it seems to indicate a borderline situation: as if the Peace Movement too were standing at the very edge of violence. As if this were a sort of "last chance" at straight nonviolence and a first step toward violent resistance. Well, we live in a world of escalation in which no one seems to know how to deescalate, and it does pose a problem. The Peace Movement may be escalating beyond peaceful protest. In which case it may also be escalating into self-contradiction. But let me make it clear that I do not think the Baltimore nine have done this.

What were the Berrigans and the others trying to do?

It seems to me this was an attempt at prophetic nonviolent provocation. It bordered on violence and was violent to the extent that it meant pushing some good ladies around and destroying some government property. The nine realized that this was a criminal act and knew that they could go to jail for it. They accepted this in the classic nonviolent fashion. The standard doctrine of nonviolence says that you can disobey a law you consider unjust but you have to accept the punishment. In this way you are distinguished from the mere revolutionary. You protest the purity of your witness. You undergo redemptive suffering for religious—or anyway ethical—motives. You are "doing penance" for the sin and injustice against which you have protested. And in the case of the Berrigans, I would say there is present a sort of "jail mystique," as a way of saying dumbly to the rest of the country that in our society nobody is really free anyway. That we are all prisoners of a machinery that takes us inevitably where we don't want to go. Presumably *everyone* in the country wants peace in one way or other. But most Americans have prior commitments—or attachments—to other things which make peace impossible. Most people would rather have war and profits than peace and problems. Or so it seems. In such a situation, we speak peace with our lips but the answer in the heart is war, and war only. And there is a certain indecency involved when Christians, even prelates, canonize this unpleasant fact by saying that the war in Vietnam is an act of Christian love. Small wonder that certain more sensitive and more questioning people are driven to extremities.

The evident desperation of the Baltimore nine has, however, frightened more than it has edified. The country is in a very edgy psychological state. Americans feel terribly threatened, on grounds which are party rational, partly irrational, but in any case very real. The rites of assassination recur at more and more frequent intervals, and there is less and less of a catharsis each time. The shocking thing about the murder of another Kennedy is that we seem to have such a terrible propensity to destroy the things and people we admire, the very ones we identify with. (I say "we" insofar as we all have a real stake in the society which makes such things not only possible but easy.) There is, then, a real fear, a deep ambivalence, about our very existence and the order on which we think it depends. In such a case, the use of nonviolence has to be extremely careful and clear. People are not in a mood for clear thinking: their fears and premonitions have long ago run away with their minds before anyone can get to them with a cool nonviolent statement. And it has long ago become automatic to interpret nonviolence as violence merely because it is resistance.

The classic (Gandhian) doctrine of nonviolence, even in a much less tense and explosive situation, always emphasized respect for the just laws in order to highlight clearly and unambiguously the injustice of the unjust law. In this way, nonviolence did not pose a sort of free-floating psychological threat, but was clearly pinpointed, directed to what even the adversary had to admit was wrong. Ideally, that is what nonviolence is supposed to do. But if nonviolence merely says in a very loud voice "*I don't like this damn law,*" it does not do much to make the adversary admit that the law is wrong. On the contrary, what he sees is an apparently arbitrary attack on law and order, dictated by emotion or caprice—or fanaticism of some sort. His reply is obviously going to be: "Well, if you don't like law and order you can go to jail where you belong." And he will send you to jail with a firm and righteous conviction that the law is just. He will not even for a moment have occasion to question its justice. He will be too busy responding to what he feels to be aggressive and indignant in your near-violent protest.

It seems to me that the protest and resistance against the Selective Service Law is all oriented to the affirmation of the rightness, the determination and the conviction of the protesters, and not to the injustice of the law itself. In other words, people who are protesting against the draft seem to be communicating, before everything else, their own intense conviction that the law is wrong, rather than pointing out where and how the law is wrong. It boils down to saying "We don't like this law and feel strongly that it is bad." To which the opposition is content to reply: "The real reason why you don't like the draft is that you are a coward."

What is to be done? First, on a short-term and emergency basis, the whole Vietnam problem has to be solved even if it demands a certain political compromise. It is idiotic to hold out for negotiations in which the position of the other side is completely ignored. Senator McCarthy seems to me to be the only presidential candidate who has the remotest idea of how to end the war, and he is the only one for whom I personally, in conscience, can vote. The war being ended, I think it is necessary that we realize the draft law is unjust, useless and an occasion of further interference in the affairs of small countries we cannot understand. It should be abolished. It has no relation to the real defense needs of the country. On a long term basis, I think the Peace Movement needs to really study, practice and use nonviolence in its classic form, with all that this implies of religious and ethical grounds. The current facile rejection of nonviolence is too pragmatic. You point to one or two cases where it does not seem to have got results and you say it has completely failed.

But nonviolence is useless if it is merely pragmatic. The whole point of nonviolence is that it rises above pragmatism and does not consider whether or not it pays off politically. *Ahimsa* is defense of and witness to *truth,* not efficacy. I admit that may sound odd. Someone once said, did he not, "What is truth?" And the One to whom he said it also mentioned, somewhere: "The truth shall make you free." It seems to me that this is what really matters.

War and the Crisis of Language

The Romans, to speak generally, rely
on force in all their enterprises and
think it incumbent upon them to carry
out their projects in spite of all,
and that nothing is impossible when
they have once decided upon it.
POLYBIUS

I

Long before George Steiner pointed out that the German language was one of the casualties of Naziism and World War II, Brice Parain in France had studied the "word sickness" of 1940, the mortal illness of journalese and political prose that accompanied the collapse of France. In proportion as the country itself accepted the denatured prose of Vichy—in which peace meant aggression and liberty meant oppression—it lost its identity and its capacity for valid action. It succumbed to "a full armed language without practical application." This, Parain reflected, had already happened before, in World War I, when words meant one thing in the trenches and another behind the lines.[1]

The reflections that follow are random and spontaneous insights—less of a philosopher than of a poet. For poets are perhaps the ones who, at the present moment, are most sensitive to the sickness of language—a sickness that, infecting all literature with nausea, prompts us not so much to declare war on conventional language as simply to pick up and examine intently a few chosen pieces of linguistic garbage. But of course, one does not have to be endowed with a peculiar poetic sensibility, still less with political genius, to recognize that official statements made in Washington, about the Vietnam war, for instance, are symptoms of a national—indeed worldwide—illness. Nor is it very

1. See Sartre's essay on Parain in *Situations I* (Paris, 1947), p. 192.

hard to see that race riots and assassinations are also symptoms of the same illness, while they are also (and this is more important) a kind of universal language. Perhaps one might better call them an anti-language, a concrete expression of something that is uttered in fire and bullets rather than in words. And this in itself expresses an acute awareness of the gap between words and actions that is characteristic of modern war, because it is also characteristic of political life in general.

The malaise is universal. There is no need to quote a Swedish poet to prove it. But these lines from Gunnar Ekelöf may serve as an apéritif for what is to follow. He begins his poem "Sonata For Denatured Prose" in these words:

> *crush the alphabet between your teeth yawn*
> *vowels, the fire is burning in hell vomit and*
> *spit now or never I and dizziness you or never*
> *dizziness now or never.*
>
> *we will begin over.*
>
> *crush the alphabet macadam and your teeth*
> *yawn vowels, the sweat runs in hell I am dying*
> *in the convolutions of my brain vomit now or*
> *never dizziness I and you. . . .*[2]

There is no need to complete the poem. It is an angry protest against contemporary, denatured language. Ironically, it declares that ordinary modes of communication have broken down into banality and deception. It suggests that violence has gradually come to take the place of other, more polite, communications. Where there is such a flood of words that all words are unsure, it becomes necessary to make one's meaning clear with blows; or at least one explores this as a valid possibility.

The incoherence of language that cannot be trusted and the coherence of weapons that are infallible, or thought to be: this is the dialectic of politics and war, the prose of the twentieth century. We shall see at the end of the chapter that awareness of this fact has made a crucial difference in the racial conflict in the United States, and everywhere else.

II

Meanwhile, it is interesting to observe that religion too has reacted to the same spastic upheaval of language. I do not here refer to the phenomenon of a radical "God is Dead" theology—which in effect is

2. Gunnar Ekelöf: *Late Arrival on Earth,* Selected Poems, trans. Robert Bly & Christine Paulston (London: 1967), p. 13.

our effort to reshape the language of religion in a last-minute attempt to save it from a plague of abstractness and formalism. This phenomenon is of course important. And so much has been said about it already—perhaps a great deal more than the subject deserves. I merely want to point out, in passing, that the fifties and sixties of our century have witnessed a curious revival of *glossolalia*—"speaking in tongues." Without attempting to evaluate this as charisma, I will at least say that it is significant in a context of religious and linguistic spasm. It is in its own way an expression of a curious kind of radicalism, a reaction to a religious language that is (perhaps obscurely) felt to be inadequate. But it is also, it seems to me, a reaction to something else. Glossolalia has flowered most abundantly in the United States, in fundamentalist and Pentecostal sects of white Protestants, and perhaps most often in the South about the time of the Freedom Rides and nonviolent civil rights demonstrations. (I do not have much information on what has taken place most recently.) This was also the time when the cold war was finally building up to the Cuba Crisis and the U.S. intervention in Vietnam was about to begin. Surely there is something interesting about this. At a time when the churches were at last becoming uneasily aware of a grave responsibility to *say something* about civil rights and nuclear war, the ones who could be least expected to be articulate on such subjects (and who often had solid dogmatic prejudices that foreclosed all discussion) began to cry out in unknown tongues.

At precisely the same moment, the Roman Catholic Church was abandoning its ancient liturgical language, the medieval Latin that was unknown to most of its members, and speaking out in a vernacular that many critics found disconcertingly banal and effete. If I refer to these things, it is not in scorn or in criticism. They are simply further expressions of a universal uneasiness about *language*—a sense of anxiety lest speech become entirely deceptive and unreal.

Can this apply to glossolalia? Of course. Fundamentalist religion assumes that the "unknown language" spoken "in the Spirit" is (though unintelligible) *more real* than the ordinary tired everyday language that everybody knows too well. Whether or not one believes that simple Texas housewives can burst out in the dialects of New Guinea head-hunters, under direct inspiration from God, there is here a significant implication that ordinary language is not good enough, and that there is something else which is at once more *real* and less comprehensible. Has ordinary language somehow failed?

I do not wish to hazard all sort of incompetent guesses about something I have not studied and do not intend to study. But one thing is quite evident about this phenomenon. He who speaks in an unknown tongue can safely speak without fear of contradiction. His utterance is *definitive* in the sense that it forecloses all dialogue. As St. Paul complained, if you utter a blessing in a strange language the congregation cannot answer "Amen" because it does not know it has been blessed.

Such utterance is so final that nothing whatever can be done about it.[3] I wish to stress this unconscious aspiration to *definitive* utterance, to which there can be no rejoinder.

III

Now let us turn elsewhere, to the language of advertisement, which at times approaches the mystic and charismatic heights of glossolalia. Here too, utterance is final. No doubt there are insinuations of dialogue, but really there is no dialogue with an advertisement, just as there was no dialogue between the sirens and the crews they lured to disaster on their rocks. There is nothing to do but be hypnotized and drown, unless you have somehow acquired a fortunate case of deafness. But who can guarantee that he is deaf enough? Meanwhile, it is the vocation of the poet—or anti-poet—*not* to be deaf to such things but to apply his ear intently to their corrupt charms. An example: a perfume advertisement from *The New Yorker* (September 17, 1966).

I present the poem as it appears on a full page, with a picture of a lady swooning with delight at her own smell—the smell of *Arpège.* (Note that the word properly signifies a sound—*arpeggio.* Aware that we are now smelling music, let us be on our guard!)

For the love of Arpège . . .
There's a new hair spray!
The world's most adored fragrance
now in a hair spray. But not hair spray
as you know it.

A delicate-as-air-spray
Your hair takes on a shimmer and sheen
that's wonderfully young.
You seem to spray new life and bounce
right into it. And a coif of Arpège has
one more thing no other hair spray has.
It has Arpège.

One look at this masterpiece and the anti-poet recognizes himself beaten hands down. This is beyond parody. It must stand inviolate in its own victorious rejection of meaning. We must avoid the temptation to dwell on details: interior rhyme, suggestions of an esoteric cult (the use of our product, besides making you young again, is also a kind of gnostic initiation), of magic (our product gives you a hat of smell—a "coif"—it clothes you in an aura of music-radiance-perfume). What I want to point out is the logical *structure* of this sonata: is is a fool-proof tautology, locked tight upon itself, impenetrable, unbreakable,

3. See I Corinthians 14.

irrefutable. It is endowed with a finality so inviolable that it is beyond debate and beyond reason. Faced with the declaration that "Arpège has Arpège," reason is reduced to silence (I almost said despair). Here again we have an example of speech that is at once totally trivial and totally definitive. It has nothing to do with anything real (although of course the sale of the product is a matter of considerable importance to the manufacturer!), but what it says, it says with utter finality.

The unknown poet might protest that he (or she) was not concerned with truth alone but also with beauty—indeed with love. And obviously this too enters into the structure and substance (so to speak) of the text. Just as the argument takes the form of a completely self-enclosed tautological cliché, so the content, the "experience," is one of self-enclosed narcissism woven of misty confusion. It begins with the claim that a new hair spray exists solely for love of itself and yet also exists for love of *you,* baby, because you are somehow subtly identified with Arpège. This perfume is so magic that it not only makes you smell good, it "coifs" you with a new and unassailable identity: it is you who are unassailable because it is you who have somehow become a tautology. And indeed we are reminded that just as Arpège is—or has—Arpège, so, in the popular psychology of women's magazines, "you are eminently lovable because you are just *you.*" When we reflect that the ultimate conceptions of theology and metaphysics have surfaced in such a context—hair spray—we no longer wonder that theologians are tearing their hair and crying that God is dead. After all, when every smell, every taste, every hissing breakfast food is endowed with the transcendental properties of being . . . But let us turn from art, religion, and love to something more serious and more central to the concerns of our time: war.

IV

A classic example of the contamination of reason and speech by the inherent ambiguity of war is that of the U.S. major who, on February 7, 1968, shelled the South Vietnamese town of Bentre "regardless of civilian casualties . . . to rout the Vietcong." As he calmly explained, "It became necessary to destroy the town in order to save it." Here we see, again, an insatiable appetite for the tautological, the definitive, the *final.* It is the same kind of language and logic that Hitler used for his notorious "final solution." The symbol of this perfect finality is the circle. An argument turns upon itself, and the beginning and end get lost: it just goes round and round its own circumference. A message comes in that someone thinks there might be some Vietcong in a certain village. Planes are sent, the village is destroyed, many of the people are killed. The destruction of the village and the killing of the people earn for them a final and official identity. The burned huts become "enemy structures"; the dead men, women, and children become

"Vietcong," thus adding to a "kill ratio" that can be interpreted as "favorable." They were thought to be Vietcong and were therefore destroyed. By being destroyed they became Vietcong for keeps; they entered "history" definitively as our enemies, because we wanted to be on the "safe side," and "save American lives"—as well as Vietnam.

The logic of "Red or dead" has long since urged us to identify destruction with rescue—to be "dead" is to be saved from being "Red." In the language of melodrama, our grandparents became accustomed to the idea of a "fate worse than death." A schematic morality concluded that if such and such is a fate worse than death, then to prefer it to death would surely be a heinous sin. The logic of war-makers has extended this not only to the preservation of one's own moral integrity but to the fate of others, even of people on the other side of the earth, whom we do not always bother to consult personally on the subject. We weigh the arguments that they are not able to understand (perhaps they have not even heard that arguments exist!). And we decide, in their place, that it is better for them to be dead—killed by us—than Red, living under our enemies.

The Asian whose future we are about to decide is either a bad guy or a good guy. If he is a bad guy, he obviously has to be killed. If he is a good guy, he is on our side and he ought to be ready to die for freedom. We will provide an opportunity for him to do so: we will kill him to prevent him falling under the tyranny of a demonic enemy. Thus we not only defend his interests together with our own, but we protect his virtue along with our own. Think what might happen if he fell under Communist rule *and liked it!*

The advantages of this kind of logic are no exclusive possession of the United States. This is purely and simply the logic shared by all war-makers. It is the logic of *power*. Possibly American generals are naïve enough to push this logic, without realizing, to absurd conclusions. But all who love power tend to think in some such way. Remember Hitler weeping over the ruins of Warsaw after it had been demolished by the Luftwaffe: "How wicked these people must have been," he sobbed, "to make me do this to them!"

Words like "pacification" and "liberation" have acquired sinister connotations as war has succeeded war. Vietnam has done much to refine and perfect these notions. A "free zone" is now one in which anything that moves is assumed to be "enemy" and can be shot. In order to create a "free zone" that can live up effectively to its name, one must level everything, buildings, vegetation, everything, so that one can clearly see anything that moves, and shoot it. This has very interesting semantic consequences.

> An American Captain accounts for the levelling of a new "Free Zone" in the following terms: "We want to prevent them from moving freely in this area. . . . From now on anything that moves around here is going to be automatically considered

> V.C. and bombed or fired on. The whole Triangle is going to become a Free Zone. These villagers here are all considered hostile civilians."
>
> How did the Captain solve the semantic problem of distinguishing the hostile civilian from the refugee? "In a V.C. area like this there are three categories. First there are the straight V.C. . . . Then there are the V.C. sympathizers. Then there's the . . . There's a third category. . . . I can't think of the third just now but . . . there's no middle road in this war." [4]

"Pacification" or "winning the hearts" of the undecided is thus very much simplified. "Soon" says a news report,[5] "the Government will have no need to win the hearts and minds of Bensuc. There will be no Bensuc." But there are further simplifications. A "high-ranking U.S. Field commander is quoted as saying: 'If the people are to the guerrillas as oceans are to the fish . . . we are going to dry up that ocean.' " [6] Merely by existing, a civilian, in this context, becomes a "hostile civilian." But at the same time and by the same token he is our friend and our ally. What simpler way out of the dilemma than to destroy him to "save American lives"?

V

So much for the practical language of the battlefield. Let us now attend to the much more pompous and sinister jargon of the war mandarins in government offices and military think-tanks. Here we have a whole community of intellectuals, scholars who spend their time playing out "scenarios" and considering "acceptable levels" in megadeaths. Their language and their thought are as esoteric, as self-enclosed, as tautologous as the advertisement we have just discussed. But instead of being "coifed" in a sweet smell, they are scientifically antiseptic, businesslike, uncontaminated with sentimental concern for life—other than their own. It is the same basic narcissism, but in a masculine, that is, managerial, mode. One proves one's realism along with one's virility by toughness in playing statistically with global death. It is this playing with death, however, that brings into the players' language itself the corruption of death: not physical but mental and moral extinction. And the corruption spreads from their talk, their thinking, to the words and minds of everybody. What happens then is that the political and moral values they claim to be defending are destroyed by the *contempt* that is more and more evident in the language in which they talk about such things. Technological strategy becomes an end in

4. See Jonathan Schell in *The New Yorker* (July 15, 1967), p. 59.
5. *The New York Times,* January 11, 1967.
6. Quoted in the *New Statesman* (March 11, 1966).

itself and leads the fascinated players into a maze where finally the very purpose strategy was supposed to serve is itself destroyed. The ambiguity of official war talk has one purpose above all: to mask this ultimate unreason and permit the game to go on.

Of special importance is the *style* of these nuclear mandarins. The technological puckishness of Herman Kahn is perhaps the classic of this genre. He excels in the sly understatement of the inhuman, the apocalyptic, enormity. His style is esoteric, allusive, yet confidential. The reader has the sense of being a privileged eavesdropper in the councils of the mighty. He knows enough to realize that things are going to happen about which he can do nothing, though perhaps he can save his skin in a properly equipped shelter where he may consider at leisure the rationality of survival in an unlivable world. Meanwhile, the cool tone of the author and the reassuring solemnity of his jargon seem to suggest that those in power, those who turn loose these instruments of destruction, have no intention of perishing themselves, that consequently survival must have a point. The point is not revealed, except that nuclear war is somehow implied to be good business. Nor are H-bombs necessarily a sign of cruel intentions. They enable one to enter into communication with the high priests in the enemy camp. They permit the decision-makers on both sides to engage in a ritual "test of nerve." In any case, the language of escalation is the language of naked power, a language that is all the more persuasive because it is proud of being ethically illiterate and because it accepts, as realistic, the basic irrationality of its own tactics. The language of escalation, in its superb mixture of banality and apocalypse, science and unreason, is the expression of a massive death wish. We can only hope that this death wish is only that of a decaying Western civilization, and that it is not common to the entire race. Yet the language itself is given universal currency by the mass media. It can quickly contaminate the thinking of everybody.

VI

Sartre speaks of the peculiar, expert negligence of the language used by European mandarins (bankers, politicians, prelates), the "indolent and consummate art" they have of communicating with one another in double-talk that leaves them always able to escape while their subordinates are firmly caught.[7] On others, ambiguous directives are imposed with full authority. For others, these are final and inescapable. The purpose of the language game is then to maintain a certain balance of ambiguity and of authority so that the subject is caught and the official is not. Thus the subject can always be proved wrong and the official is always right. The offical is enabled to lie in such a way that

7. *Op. cit.*, p. 202.

if the lie is discovered, a subordinate takes the blame. So much for European democracy. The same has been true in America in a somewhat different context—that of wheeler-dealing and political corruption rather than the framework of authoritarian and official privilege. But power in America, we find, can become mean, belligerent, temperamental. American power, while paying due respect to the demands of plain egalitarian folksiness, has its moments of arbitrary bad humor. But lest this bad humor become too evident, and lest repression begin to seem too forceful, language is at hand as an instrument of manipulation. Once again, the use of language to extol freedom, democracy, and equal rights, while at the same time denying them, causes words to turn sour and to rot in the minds of those who use them. In such a context, the effort of someone such as Lenny Bruce to restore to language some of its authentic impact was a service despairingly offered to a public that could not fully appreciate it. One might argue that the language of this disconcerting and perhaps prophetic comedian was often less obscene than the "decent" but horrifying platitudes of those who persecuted him.

VII

Michel Foucault has described the evolution of the dialogue between medicine and madness in the Age of Reason.[8] Therapeutic experiments with manic-depressives in the eighteenth century assumed a certain inner consistency in the delirium of the mad and, working within the suppressed framework of this consistency, sought to suggest to the madman an alternative to his madness—or, rather, to push the "logic" of his madness to a paroxysm and crisis in which it would be confronted with itself and "forced to argue against the demands of its own truth." Thus, for instance, in cases of religious mania and despair, patients who believed themselves damned were shown a theatrical tableau in which the avenging angel appeared, punished, and then gave assurance that guilt was now taken away. Patients who were dying of starvation because, believing themselves dead, they would not eat were shown representations of dead persons eating and were thus brought face to face with an unexpected syllogism: you claim you are dead and cannot eat, but dead men can eat. . . . The beauty of Foucault's book is that we become fascinated by the way in which the "reason" of the Age of Englightenment unconsciously shared so much of the madness with which it was in dialogue.

Reading of this dialogue between reason and madness, one is reminded of the language of power and war. In the deliberate, realistic madness of the new language we find an implicit admission that words, ordinary discourse, won't do—not exactly that language itself has

8. Michel Foucault, *Madness and Civilization* (New York: 1967), p. 188.

broken down, is no longer valid as such. But the enemy is at once so perverse and so irrational—such a psychopathic liar in fact—that he has to be cleverly treated as a beast or as a maniac. We all know that it is customary for one who resorts to violence to do so on the ground that the adversary "does not understand anything else." The "language of escalation" is a more sophisticated application of this principle, but on a massive scale implemented by the threat of a nuclear strike. It seems, indeed, that since the adversary understands nothing but force, and since force means everything up to and including the use of H-bombs, we will eventually get beyond the mere threat of a nuclear strike: one of us will actually strike. This will demonstrate that if you face an enemy with the conviction that he understands nothing but force, you will yourself necessarily behave as if you understood nothing but force. And in fact it is highly probable that if you say he understands nothing but force, it is because you yourself are already in the same plight.

In any case, it is quite obvious that the military on whatever side must be quite convinced of the superior efficacy of force, or they would not be military. If they worry about this at all, they can always reason that force is necessary because we are faced by various bunches of madmen who understand nothing else. The dialogue then proceeds in a way that reminds us of Foucault:

1. Rational discourse with the enemy is useless. He does not understand rational discourse and makes negotiation an opportunity for lying and pathological trickery. He *has to* cheat.

2. Therefore he has to be dealt with solely in the framework of his madness and wickedness, his propensity to lie and cheat. One does not bargain with such a one, because bargaining implies the acceptance, on both sides, of conditions. He must be pushed to the point where his surrender is unconditional in terms of his own madness. To grant him reasonable conditions would be to treat a madman as a rational being, which would be the worst possible kind of mistake and indeed (if you believe in sin) a sin.

3. His madness has roots in guilt, because he is, after all, wicked. He understands *punishment*. But the punishment must be shown to him in terms of his own madness. He must see that his own destructive violence will lead inexorably to one consequence: his own annihilation. But to translate this into words would lead to confusion. The message must be got to him in the unmistakable language of force itself. Of course, verbal formulas have to be resorted to, in order to define what force is all about, to set conditions, etc. But the verbal formulas must be kept deliberately ambiguous, unclear. The clear and unmistakable message is not that of the *terms offered* but of the escalation itself. In other words there is an *appearance* of dialogue on the verbal and political level. But the real dialogue is with weapons and may be a complete contradiction of what appears to be said in the prose of politics.

The effect of this, of course, is a vicious circle: it begins with a tacit admission that negotiation is meaningless, and it does in fact render the language of negotiation meaningless. War-makers in the twentieth century have gone far toward creating a political language so obscure, so apt for treachery, so ambiguous, that it can no longer serve as an instrument for peace: it is good only for war. But why? Because the language of the war-maker is *self-enclosed in finality*. It does not invite reasonable dialogue, it uses language to silence dialogue, to block communication, so that instead of words the two sides may trade divisions, positions, villages, air bases, cities—and of course the lives of the people in them. The daily toll of the killed (or the "kill ratio") is perfunctorily scrutinized and decoded. And the totals are expertly managed by "ministers of truth" so that the newspaper reader may get the right message.

Our side is always ahead. He who is winning must be the one who is right. But we are right, therefore we must be winning. Once again we have the beautiful, narcissistic tautology of war—or of advertising. Once again, "Arpège has Arpège." There is no communicating with anyone else, because anyone who does not agree, who is outside the charmed circle, is wrong, is evil, is already in hell.

VIII

It is a dictum of Marxism that a word is true if it can be verified by being carried out in action. But this idea is not a monopoly of the Communists. It is now universal. It is everybody's property. Modern politics is a matter of defining how you think things ought to be and then making them come out that way by cunning or by force. If you aren't strong enough or smart enough to verify your ideas by putting them into effect, then you have no business saying how things should be in the first place: follow somebody else who has the necessary power! The strange thing is that this idea is not so modern after all. In fact it is quite ancient. Another word for it is magic, or witchcraft.

Of course, the shaman and the medicine man in primitive society did not possess the advantages of a technological skill that would enable them to say that white was black and then prove the point by turning white into black. Yet even unlimited power does not always succeed in making one's own words come true—as the Vietnam war has conclusively shown.

One of the most curious things about the war in Vietnam is that it is being *fought to vindicate the assumptions upon which it is being fought*. Now it turns out that these American assumptions are quite wrong: the White House and the Pentagon have consistently interpreted the war as a military invasion of South Vietnam by the North. In other words it is the Korean War over again, a "conventional limited war" in which the problems are above all military and can be handled in terms of bombing, sending in more troops, wiping out areas in which the enemy tends to concentrate, cutting supply lines, etc. By the escalation of the war and the bombing of North Vietnam (after the "Tonkin Bay Incident," which has now been shown to have been exaggerated if not actually faked) the United States did actually turn the war into the kind of war it was supposed to be in America—apart from the fact that the aggression was the other way around. But this did nothing to alter the fact that the war in the South remained essentially a revolutionary guerrilla struggle that could not be adequately handled by conventional military operations.

Alastair Buchan, analyzing this curious fact in *Encounter*,[9] wonders how it was possible for such a policy to be accepted when the U.S. government relies on "a wide range of research institutes and universities to give greater depth and accuracy to its own operational and political analysis." He hazards a guess that the unassailable self-confidence of science somehow contributed to the error: "Probably technology (helicopters, new small arms, infra-red sensors and all the rest) was the element that corrupted judgement, making it seem possible that the Americans could do what the natives (i.e. the South Vietnamese army) or the old colonial powers (e.g. the French) could not." In other words, there is a certain hubris built into technological thinking that encloses it within itself and its own suppositions and makes it fatally ignore decisive realities that do not fit those suppositions.

However, in such a situation, power can still vindicate itself by *declaring* that its estimate was the correct one and that it is still winning. Since statistics can be made to prove anything, it adduces statistics to show that its words are in fact coming true. Unfortunately, the Tet offensive of the Vietcong in 1968 made it finally clear that no amount of juggling with words or figures could make this "politics of inadvertence" (the words of Arthur Schlesinger's) come out level with reality. Lyndon Johnson is certainly well versed in all the appropriate skills, and yet in this instance he turned out to be a singularly failed witch.

What needs to be noted is that the massive effort of the United States to gain acceptance for its own version of the Vietnam war by doing all in its power to turn that version into accomplished fact has had profoundly significant effects. And these effects are not what was intended. Confidence in the Washington government, in the American political system, in the credibility of American officials, even in the basic human integrity and sincerity of the American Establishment is now seriously undermined at home and abroad. The *political language* of the United States, which was suspect before, has now been fatally denatured. It has probably lost all its value as intellectual currency. The crisis of the dollar is intimately connected with the crisis of human communication that has resulted from the sinister double-talk of the American Establishment about itself, about the war, about the

9. January–February, 1968.

race situation, about the urgent domestic problems that are being ignored or set aside while the government puts more and more money and manpower into the war. The tragedy is not so much that America has come out of its pristine isolationism but that it has decided to rule the world without paying serious attention to anybody else's view of what the world is all about. Language has been distorted and denatured in defense of this solipsistic, this basically isolationist and sometimes even paranoid, attitude.

IX

What next? The illness of political language—which is almost universal and is a symptom of a Plague of Power that is common to China and America, Russia and Western Europe—is characterized everywhere by the same sort of double-talk, tautology, ambiguous cliché, self-righteous and doctrinaire pomposity, and pseudoscientific jargon that mask a total callousness and moral insensitivity, indeed a basic contempt for man. The self-enclosed finality that bars all open dialogue and pretends to impose absolute conditions of one's own choosing upon everybody else ultimately becomes the language of totalist dictatorship, if it is not so already. Revolt against this is taking the form of another, more elemental and anarchistic, kind of violence, together with a different semantic code. Space does not permit us to study this other language, but it must be acknowledged as immensely popular and influential all over the world. It is the language of Che Guevara, of Régis Debray, of Frantz Fanon: the violent language and the apocalyptic myth of the guerrilla warrior, the isolated individual and the small group, enabled by revolutionary charisma to defy all the technological might of the biggest powers in the world. In spite of the failure of Che in Bolivia—a failure that only resulted in his canonization as a martyr of the post-colonial revolution—the Vietnam war has had the result of awakening revolutionary hopes all over the world, from Harlem to Angola. Che Guevara called for Vietnams everywhere, and the Black Power movement, introducing the language of Fanon into American political life, is set on making the inner cities of the United States "other Vietnams." At the moment, when the full tragedy has not yet manifested itself, this might to some seem an inspiring revolt against the inhuman pride of technological white power. But the hopes of Fanon—which may have some basis in the jungles of Africa—are couched in the same terms of magic and witchcraft that assert something and then proceed to make it so in fact, thereby vindicating their own prophecy. If this went wrong for U.S. power in Vietnam, it may also go wrong in the American ghettos, where, unfortunately, the Negro does not have miles of swamp and jungle to maneuver in but is enclosed in a small and highly vulnerable area in which he can easily be destroyed or arrested and taken off to concentration camps.

However that may be, the revolutionary tactic that tends to harass and immobolize the Goliath of technological military power and bring it down largely by its own elephantine weight has at the same time created a new language that mocks the ponderous and self-important utterances of the Establishment. This new language, racy, insolent, direct, profane, iconoclastic, and earthy, may have its own magic incantation and myth. It may be involved in its own elaborate set of illusions. But at least it represents a healthier and more concrete style of thought. It does not reduce everything to abstractions, and though it is fully as intransigent as the language of the Establishment, it still seems to be more in contact with relevant experience: the hard realities of poverty, brutality, vice, and resistance.

Yet, flexible though it might be in some respects, it remains another language of power, therefore of self-enclosed finality, which rejects dialogue and negotiation on the axiomatic supposition that the adversary is a devil with whom no dialogue is possible.

Ishi: A Meditation

Genocide is a new word. Perhaps the word is new because technology has now got into the game of destroying whole races at once. The destruction of races is not new—just easier. Nor is it a specialty of totalitarian regimes. We have forgotten that a century ago white America was engaged in the destruction of entire tribes and ethnic groups of Indians. The trauma of California gold. And the vigilantes who, in spite of every plea from Washington for restraint and understanding, repeatedly took matters into their own hands and went out slaughtering Indians. Indiscriminate destruction of the "good" along with the "bad"—just so long as they were Indians. Parties of riffraff from the mining camps and saloons suddenly constituted themselves defenders of civilization. They armed and went out to spill blood and gather scalps. They not only combed the woods and canyons—they even went into the barns and ranch houses, to find and destroy the Indian servants and hired people, in spite of the protests of the ranchers who employed them.

The Yana Indians (including the Yahi or Mill Creeks) lived around the foothills of Mount Lassen, east of the Sacramento River. Their country came within a few miles of Vina, where the Trappist monastery in California stands today. These hill tribes were less easy to subdue than their valley neighbors. More courageous and more aloof, they tried to keep clear of the white man altogether. They were not necessarily more ferocious than other Indians, but because they kept to themselves and had a legendary reputation as "fighters," they were more feared. They were understood to be completely "savage." As they were driven further and further back into the hills, and as their traditional hunting grounds gradually narrowed and emptied of game, they had to raid the ranches in order to keep alive. White reprisals were to be expected, and they were ruthless. The Indians defended themselves by guerrilla warfare. The whites decided that there could be no peaceful coexistence with such neighbors. The Yahi, or Mill Creek Indians, as they were called, were marked for complete destruction.

Hence they were regarded as subhuman. Against them there were no restrictions and no rules. No treaties need be made, for no Indian could be trusted. Where was the point in "negotiation"?

Ishi, the last survivor of the Mill Creek Indians, whose story was published by the University of California at Berkeley three years ago,[1] was born during the war of extermination against his people. The fact that the last Mill Creeks were able to go into hiding and to survive for another fifty years in their woods and canyons is extraordinary enough. But the courage, the resourcefulness, and the sheer nobility of these few stone-age men struggling to preserve their life, their autonomy and their identity as a people rises to the level of tragic myth. Yet there is nothing mythical about it. The story is told with impeccable objectivity—though also with compassion—by the scholars who finally saved Ishi and learned from him his language, his culture, and his tribal history.

To read this story thoughtfully, to open one's heart to it, is to receive a most significant message: one that not only moves, but disturbs. You begin to feel the inner stirrings of that pity and dread which Aristotle said were the purifying effect of tragedy. "The history of Ishi and his people," says the author, Theodora Kroeber, "is inexorably part of our own history. We have absorbed their lands into our holdings. Just so must we be the responsible custodians of their tragedy, absorbing it into our tradition and morality." Unfortunately, we learned little or nothing about ourselves from the Indian wars!

"They have separated murder into two parts and fastened the worse on me"—words which William Carlos Williams put on the lips of a Viking exile, Eric the Red. Men are always separating murder into two parts: one which is unholy and unclean: for "the enemy." Another which is a sacred duty: "for our side." He who first makes the separation, in order that he may kill, proves his bad faith. So too in the Indian wars. Why do we always assume the Indian was the aggressor? We were in *his* country, we were taking it over for ourselves, and we likewise refused even to share any with him. We were the people of God, always in the right, following a manifest destiny. The Indian could only be a devil. But once we allow ourselves to see all sides of the question, the familiar perspectives of American history undergo a change. The "savages" suddenly become human and the "whites," the "civilized," can seem barbarians. True, the Indians were often cruel and inhuman (some more than others). True, also the humanity, the intelligence, the compassion and understanding which Ishi met with in his friends the scholars, when he came to join our civilization, restore the balance in our favor. But we are left with a deep sense of guilt and shame. The record is there. The Mill Creek Indians, who were once seen as bloodthirsty devils, were peaceful, innocent and

1. Theodora Kroeber, *Ishi in Two Worlds:* A biography of the last wild Indian in North America (Berkeley & Los Angeles, U. of California Press, 1961).

deeply wronged human beings. In their use of violence they were, so it seems, generally very fair. It is we who were the wanton murderers, and they who were the innocent victims. The loving kindness lavished on Ishi in the end did nothing to change that fact. His race had been barbarously, pointlessly destroyed.

The impact of the story is all the greater because the events are so deeply charged with a natural symbolism: the structure of these happenings is such that it leaves a haunting imprint on the mind. Out of that imprint come disturbing and potent reflections.

Take, for example, the scene in 1870 when the Mill Creeks were down to their last twenty or thirty survivors. A group had been captured. A delegation from the tiny remnant of the tribe appeared at a ranch to negotiate. In a symbolic gesture, they handed over five bows (five being a sacred number) and stood unarmed waiting for an answer. The gesture was not properly understood, though it was evident that the Indians were trying to recover their captives and promising to abandon all hostilities. In effect, the message was: "Leave us alone, in peace, in our hills, and we will not bother you any more. We are few, you are many, why destroy us? We are no longer any menace to you." No formal answer was given. While the Indians were waiting for some kind of intelligible response, one of the whites slung a rope over the branch of a tree. The Indians quietly withdrew into the woods.

From then on, for the next twelve years, the Yahi disappeared into the hills without a trace. There were perhaps twenty of them left, one of whom was Ishi, together with his mother and sister. In order to preserve their identity as a tribe, they had decided that there was no alternative but to keep completely away from white men, and have nothing whatever to do with them. Since coexistence was impossible, they would try to be as if they did not exist for the white man at all. To be there as if they were not there.

In fact, not a Yahi was seen. No campfire smoke rose over the trees. Not a trace of fire was found. No village was discovered. No track of an Indian was observed. The Yahi remnant (and that phrase takes on haunting biblical resonances) systematically learned to live as invisible and as unknown.

To anyone who has ever felt in himself the stirrings of a monastic or solitary vocation, the notion is stirring. It has implications that are simply beyond speech. There is nothing one can say in the presence of such a happening and of its connotations for what our spiritual books so glibly call "the hidden life." The "hidden life" is surely not irrelevant to our modern world: nor is it a life of spiritual comfort and tranquillity which a chosen minority can happily enjoy, at the price of a funny costume and a few prayers. The "hidden life" is the extremely difficult life that is forced upon a remnant that has to stay completely out of sight in order to escape destruction.

This so-called long concealment of the Mill Creek Indians is not romanticized by any means. The account is sober, objective, though it cannot help being an admiring tribute to extraordinary courage and ingenuity of these lost stone-age people. Let the book speak for itself.

> The long concealment failed in its objective to save a people's life but it would seem to have been brilliantly successful in its psychology and techniques of living. . . . Ishi's group was a master of the difficult art of communal and peaceful coexistence in the presence of alarm and in a tragic and deteriorating prospect. . . . It is a curious circumstance that some of the questions which arise about the concealment, are those for which in a different context psychologists and neurologists are trying to find answers for the submarine and outer space services today. Some of these are: what makes for morale under confining and limiting life-conditions? What are the presumable limits of claustrophobic endurance? . . . It seems that the Yahi might have qualified for outer space had they lasted into this century.

There is something challenging and awe-inspiring about this thoughtful passage by a scientifically trained mind. And that phrase about "qualifying for outer space" has an eerie ring about it. Does someone pick up the half-heard suggestion that the man who wants to live a normal life span during the next two hundred years of our history must be the kind of person who is "qualified for outer space"? Let us return to Ishi! The following sentences are significant:

> In contrast to the Forty-niners . . . whose morality and morale had crumbled, Ishi and his band remained incorrupt, humane, compassionate, and with their faith intact even unto starvation, pain and death. The questions then are: what makes for stability? For psychic strength? For endurance, courage, faith?

The answers given by the author to these questions are mere suggestions. The Yahi were on their own home ground. This idea is not developed. The reader should reflect a little on the relation of the Indian to the land on which he lived. In this sense, most modern men never know what it means to have a "home ground." Then there is a casual reference to the "American Indian mystique" which could also be developed. William Faulkner's hunting stories, particularly "The Bear," give us some idea of what this "mystique" might involve. The word "mystique" has unfortunate connotations: it suggests an emotional icing on an ideological cake. Actually the Indian lived by a deeply religious wisdom which can be called in a broad sense mystical, and that is certainly much more than "a mystique." The book does not go into religious questions very deeply, but it shows us Ishi as a man sustained by a deep and unassailable spiritual strength which he never discussed.

Later, when he was living "in civilization" and was something of a celebrity as well as an object of charitable concern, Ishi was questioned about religion by a well-meaning lady. Ishi's English was liable to be unpredictable, and the language of his reply was not without its own ironic depths of absurdity:

> "Do you believe in God?" the lady inquired.
> "Sure, Mike!" he retorted briskly.

There is something dreadfully eloquent about this innocent short-circuit in communication.

One other very important remark is made by the author. The Yahi found strength in the incontrovertible fact that they were in the right. "*Of very great importance to their psychic health was the circumstance that their suffering and curtailments arose from wrongs done to them by others.* They were not guilt-ridden."

Contrast this with the spectacle of our own country with its incomparable technological power, its unequalled material strength, and its psychic turmoil, its moral confusion and its profound heritage of guilt which neither the righteous declarations of Cardinals nor the moral indifference of "realists" can do anything to change! Every bomb we drop on a defenseless Asian village, every Asian child we disfigure or destroy with fire only adds to the moral strength of those we wish to destroy for our own profit. It does not make the Vietcong cause just; but by an accumulation of injustice done against innocent people we drive them into the arms of our enemies and make our own ideals look like the most pitiful sham.

Gradually the last members of the Yahi tribe died out. The situation of the survivors became more and more desperate. They could not continue to keep up their perfect invisibility: they had to steal food. Finally the hidden camp where Ishi lived with his sister and sick mother was discovered by surveyors who callously walked off with the few objects they found as souvenirs. The mother and sister died and finally on August 29, 1911, Ishi surrendered to the white race, expecting to be destroyed.

Actually, the news of this "last wild Indian" reached the anthropology department at Berkeley and a professor quickly took charge of things. He came and got the "wild man" out of jail. Ishi spent the rest of his life in San Francisco, patiently teaching his hitherto completely unknown (and quite sophisticated) language to experts like Sapir. Curiously enough, Ishi lived in an anthropological museum where he earned his living as a kind of caretaker and also functioned, on occasion, as a live exhibit. He was well treated, and in fact the affection and charm of his relations with his white friends are not the least moving part of his story. He adapted to life in the city without too much trouble and returned once, with his friends, to live several months in his old territory, under his natural conditions, showing them how the Yahi had carried out the fantastic operation of their invisible survival. But he finally succumbed to one of the diseases of civilization. He died of TB in 1916, after four and a half years among white men.

For the reflective reader who is—as everyone must be today—deeply concerned about man and his fate, this is a moving and significant book, one of those unusually suggestive works that *must* be read, and perhaps more than once. It is a book to think deeply about and take notes on not only because of its extraordinary factual interest but because of its special quality as a kind of parable.

One cannot help thinking today of the Vietnam war in terms of the Indian wars of a hundred years ago. Here again, one meets the same myths and misunderstandings, the same obsession with "completely wiping out" an enemy regarded as diabolical. The language of the vigilantes had overtones of puritanism in it. The backwoods had to be "completely cleaned out," or "purified" of Indians—as if they were vermin. I have read accounts of American GIs taking the same attitude toward the Vietcong. The jungles are thought to be "infested" with Communists, and hence one goes after them as one would go after ants in the kitchen back home. And in this process of "cleaning up" (the language of "cleansing" appeases and pacifies the conscience) one becomes without realizing it a murderer of women and children. But this is an unfortunate accident, what the moralists call "double effect." Something that is just too bad, but which must be accepted in view of something more important that has to be done. And so there is more and more killing of civilians and less and less of the "something more important" which is what we are trying to achieve. In the end, it is the civilians that are killed in the ordinary course of events, and combatants only get killed by accident. No one worries any more about double effect. War is waged against the innocent to "break enemy morale."

What is most significant is that Vietnam seems to have become an extension of our old Western frontier, complete with enemies of another, "inferior" race. This is a real "new frontier" that enables us to continue the cowboys-and-Indians game which seems to be part and parcel of our national identity. What a pity that so many innocent people have to pay with their lives for our obsessive fantasies!

One last thing. Ishi never told anyone his real name. The California Indians apparently never uttered their own names, and were very careful about how they spoke the name of others. Ishi would never refer to the dead by name either. "He never revealed his own private Yahi name," says the author. "It was as though it had been consumed in the funeral pyre of the last of his loved ones."

In the end, no one ever found out a single name of the vanished community. Not even Ishi's. For Ishi means simply MAN.

III

INCIDENTAL WRITINGS

In Acceptance of the Pax Medal, 1963

First I want to thank you most sincerely for the honor you have bestowed on me in awarding me this prize, and to apologize for not being present in person. In fact, my inability to be there might almost seem to disqualify me from receiving such an honor. But if I were to make much out of my being "out of the world" and "in a monastery" I would certainly waste your time and mine, and would also be unfaithful to the demands of the present situation.

A monastery is not a snail's shell, nor is religious faith a kind of spiritual fallout shelter into which one can plunge to escape the criminal realities of an apocalyptic age.

Never has the total solidarity of all men, either in good or in evil, been so obvious and so unavoidable. I believe we live in a time in which one cannot help making decisions for or against man, for or against life, for or against justice, for or against truth.

And according to my way of thinking, all these decisions rolled into one (for they are inseparable) amount to a decision for or against God.

I have attempted to say this in the past as opportunity has permitted, and opportunity has not permitted as much as I would have liked. But one thing I must admit: to say these things seems to me to be only the plain duty of any reasonable being. Such an attitude implies no heroism, no extraordinary insight, no special moral qualities, and no unusual intelligence.

It seems to me perfectly obvious and beyond dispute that *"the arms race ought to cease, that nuclear weapons should be banned, that an effective program of gradual disarmament should be agreed upon by all nations,"* and this as soon as possible because the danger of global war remains always proximate and imminent, *"and nothing is lost by peace, yet everything may be lost by war."*

These propositions, which are as obvious, and clear as daylight, are all taken word for word from Pope John's encyclical *Pacem in Terris*. For my part I have said nothing that Pope John did not say. If I said it before *Pacem in Terris* that still does not make me terribly original, because the same things were said long ago by Popes before Pope John, and by Theologians, and by the Fathers of the Church, and by the Gospels themselves.

This puts me in the rather awkward position of receiving a prize for doing what is only the plain and obvious duty of a reasonable human being who also happens to be a Christian. It is like getting a medal for going to work in the morning, or stopping at traffic lights, or paying one's bills.

And yet you know that I am really not ignorant of the actual situation. I know very well that in giving me this prize you are trying to say that in reality today most reasonable men, most professed Christians, and most of the clergy in this country have *not* as yet clearly and unequivocally committed themselves on this point.

Pacem in Terris is a magnificent document. It has been acclaimed by everyone. But, as is not unusual, these acclamations are accompanied, in practice, by a continued reluctance to act according to the norms laid down by Pope John in the name of reason.

If I am correct in thinking that you have some such thought in mind in awarding me this prize, then it becomes a matter of conscience for me to accept. By accepting I am publicly affirming that *Pacem in Terris* as I understand it was written in order to prevent nuclear war, and indeed to rule out all further consideration of war as a reasonable and just means of settling international disputes. As a consequence *Pacem in Terris* is a reminder to the conscience of every reasonable human being on the face of the earth that each one of us has a strict obligation to work for world peace, for the peaceful arbitration of all disputes, and for the peaceful settlement of the social, international, interracial, religious, economic and political problems in which we may be directly or indirectly involved.

I repeat, I don't think I deserve a medal for affirming such obvious and commonsense truths. But if by receiving the medal I can publicly declare these to be my convictions, then I most gladly and gratefully accept.

Retreat, November, 1964: Spiritual Roots of Protest

We are hoping to reflect together during these days on our common grounds for *religious dissent and commitment* in the face of the injustice and disorder of a world in which total war seems at times inevitable, in which few seek any but violent solutions to economic and social problems more critical and more vast than man has ever known before.

What we are seeking is not the formulation of a program, but a deepening of roots.

Roots in the "ground" of all being, in God, through His word.

Standing in the presence of His word knowing that we are judged by it.

Bringing our inner motives into line with this judgement.

Protest: Against whom or what?
For what? *By what right?*
How?
Why?

It would help if in our meetings we could show our various ways of answering these questions, thus helping one another to attain new perspectives. We can help one another to a new *openness.* We will not necessarily cling to sectarian programs and interpretations. We will think, speak and act as brothers, conscious that one same Spirit works in us, according to the gifts of each, for the manifestation of the justice and truth of God in the world, through Christ. But what do we mean by this? Does it mean only meditation on familiar themes or the awakening of a new (eschatological?) conscience?

Emphasis has been placed on the question "*By what right* do we assume that we are called to protest, to judge, and to witness?" If we once (in the past) had a clear right, have we now forfeited it? And are we simply assuming such a "right" or "mandate" by virtue of our insertion in a collective program of one sort or another? An institution? A "movement"?

It is suggested that at each of our meetings, someone might act as leader of the discussion after himself starting off with a talk on any aspect of the question that seems relevant to him. For example:

Wednesday Afternoon: T. Merton, "The Monastic Protest. The voice in the wilderness."
Thursday Morning: A. J. Muste
Thursday Afternoon: John H. Yoder
Friday Morning: Fr. Daniel Berrigan, S.J.

Further points:
Among the special problems that might be kept in mind, we might consider the *nature of technological society,* whether such a society is by its very nature oriented to self-destruction, or whether it can on the contrary be regarded as a source of hope for a new "sacral" order, a millenial "city" in which God will be manifested and praised in the freedom and enlightenment of man. . . .

In any case, technology is not at present in a state that is morally or religiously promising. Does this call for reaction and protest; if so, what kind? What can we really do about it?

The question of accurate information and the formation of a lucid and moral public opinion: or even the possibility of forming a really straight personal conscience? (Problem of mass media and our own means of *communication.*)
The relevance of our preaching and of our worship in the present social context?
The relevance of traditional forms of social and political action?

The relevance and validity of the interior life? The question of "asceticism," "contemplation" or the "prophetic witness," intercessory prayer?

The meaning of *metanoia,* total personal renewal, as a prerequisite for valid nonviolent action? The role of sacrifice and suffering in (redemptive) nonviolent protest.
The question of reparatory sacrifice for the sins of racism, war, etc.

Message aux Amis de Gandhi

le 31 janvier, 1965

Voici un frère lointain qui vous addresse un message de solidarité et d'amitié. Mais, étant donné que je ne suis pas du nombre de ceux qui écrivent habituellement des messages pereils, je vous prie de m'excuser si ces paroles ne conforment pas exactement au style que je connais mal.

Je me contente de partager avec vous une pensée qui me préoccupe, et qui n'est pas du tout originelle. Elle est du regretté ami de Gandhi, l'Abbé Monchanin. Il a dit de Gandhi qu'il était "de ceux qui comme Socrate, Platon ou Saint Augustin, ont retrouvé les sources, de ceux qui ont ramené l'homme à son âme, qui ont désensablé les puits que les philistins avaient comblés."

Il me semble en effet que c'est là l'aspect le plus important de notre tâche commune, de notre mission dans le monde de la technologie moderne.

Nous voyons autour de nous les effets, soits bons, soit mauvais, qui procèdent de causes que le monde ne voit pas. Nous sommes de ceux qui boivent, comme tous nos contemporains, l'eau trouble d'un fleuve qui nous est étranger: "A quoi bon partir en Assyrie pour boire l'eau du fleuve?" (Jérémie 2:18). A quoi bon nous bâtir des citernes qui ne tiennent pas d'eau? C'est ce que Gandhi nous a rappelé, comme aussi des amis de Gandhi comme Louis Massignon.

Le mouvement non-violent doit être tout d'abord un mouvement de vérité, donc de "désensablement des puits comblés par l'ambition, la violence, l'appétit de la puissance, la haine, le revanchisme [*sic*]. Cherchons toujours a nous entr'aider dans cette tâche, a nous ramener les uns les autres aux sources de la liberté authentique pour que nous puissions avant tout "être amis" et ainsi donner au monde moderne le témoignage d'une simplicité qui ne craint pas la violence des forts puisqu'elle est elle-même plus forte.

Je prie pour vous tous. Priez aussi pour moi, dans l'amour d'une même vérité.

Nhat Hanh Is My Brother

This is not a political statement. It has no "interested" motive, it seeks to provoke no immediate reaction "for" or "against" this or that side in the Vietnam war. It is on the contrary a human and personal statement and an anguished plea for the Vietnamese Buddhist monk Thich Nhat Hanh who is my brother. He is more my brother than many who are nearer to me by race and nationality, because he and I see things exactly the same way. He and I deplore the war that is ravaging his country. We deplore it for exactly the same reasons: human reasons, reasons of sanity, justice and love. We deplore the needless destruction, the fantastic and callous ravaging of human life, the rape of the culture and spirit of an exhausted people. It is surely evident that this carnage serves no purpose that can be discerned and indeed contradicts the alleged intentions of the mighty nation that has constituted itself the "defender" of the people it is destroying.

Certainly this statement cannot help being a plea for peace. But it is also a plea for my brother Nhat Hanh. He represents the least "political" of all the movements in Vietnam. He is not directly associated with the Buddhists who are trying to use political manipulation in order to save their country. He is by no means a Communist. The Vietcong is deeply hostile to him. He refuses to be identified with the established government which hates and distrusts him. He represents the young, the defenseless, the new ranks of youth who find themselves with every hand turned against them except those of the peasants and the poor, with whom they are working. Nhat Hanh speaks truly for the people of Vietnam, if there can be said to be a "people" still left in Vietnam.

Nhat Hanh has left his country and has come to us in order to present a picture which is not given us in our newspapers and magazines. He has been well received—and that speaks well for those who have received him. His visit to the United States has shown that we are a people who still desire the truth when we can find it, and still decide in favor of *man* against the political machine when we get a fair chance to do so. But when Nhat Hanh goes home, what will happen to him? He is not in favor with the government which has suppressed his writings. The Vietcong will view with disfavor his American contacts. To have pleaded for an end to the fighting will make him a traitor in the eyes of those who stand to gain personally as long as the war goes on, as long as their countrymen are being killed, as long as they can do business with our military. Nhat Hanh may be returning to imprisonment, torture, even death. We cannot let him go back to Saigon to be destroyed while we sit here, cherishing the warm humanitarian glow of good intentions and worthy sentiments about the ongoing war. We who have met and heard Nhat Hanh, or who have read about him, must also raise our voices to demand that his life and freedom be respected when he returns to his country. Furthermore, we demand this not in terms of any conceivable political advantage, but purely in the name of those values of freedom and humanity in favor of which our armed forces declare they are fighting the Vietnam war.

Nhat Hanh is a free man who has acted as a free man in favor of his brothers and moved by the spiritual dynamic of a tradition of religious compassion. He has come among us as many others have, from time to time, bearing witness to the spirit of Zen. More than any other he has shown us that Zen is not an esoteric and world-denying cult of inner illumination, but that it has its rare and unique sense of responsibility in the modern world. Wherever he goes he will walk in the strength of his spirit and in the solitude of the Zen monk who sees beyond life and death. It is for our own honor as much as for his safety that we must raise our voices to demand that his life and personal integrity be fully respected when he returns to his smashed and gutted country, there to continue his work with the students and peasants, hoping for the day when reconstruction can begin.

I have said Nhat Hanh is my brother, and it is true. We are both monks, and we have lived the monastic life about the same number of years. We are both poets, both existentialists. I have far more in common with Nhat Hanh than I have with many Americans, and I do not hesitate to say it. It is vitally important that such bonds be admitted. They are the bonds of a new solidarity and a new brotherhood which is beginning to be evident on all the five continents and which cuts across all political, religious and cultural lines to unite young men and women in every country in something that is more concrete than an ideal and more alive than a program. This unity of the young is the only hope of the world. In its name I appeal for Nhat Hanh. Do what you can for him. If I mean something to you, then let me put it this way: do for Nhat Hanh whatever you would do for me if I were in his position. In many ways I wish I were.

Notes for a Statement on Aid to Civilian War Victims in Vietnam

1. Most of the war victims in Vietnam are noncombatants. It is estimated that for every enemy combatant killed, five noncombatants are killed. The proportion of wounded is probably larger. These noncombatants are in most cases supposed to be people we are "defending" against Communism. Thousands of women, children and old people have been most cruelly destroyed, maimed or disfigured by the latest and most destructive of "conventional" weapons devised by our technology.

2. The death and wounding of these noncombatants could be avoided without difficulty and without harming our war effort. The continued destruction of villages in North and South Vietnam may be rationalized in various ways, but apparently one of the reasons why this destruction continues is that systematic terrorism is being used to break all further resistance. Such methods were used by the Nazis in World War II and were universally condemned as criminal. The whole world today regards the U.S. destruction of Vietnam villages as part of a deliberate program of terrorism and of planned atrocities.

3. The situation is such that for Americans now to offer aid to the victims of our military in Vietnam might seriously be regarded as pure hypocrisy. However, the objective fact remains: whatever the reason, whatever the policy, thousands of innocent Vietnamese civilians, including a very high proportion of children, have, though absolutely defenseless, been destroyed or ruined and maimed by American bombs. There is debt of justice owing to them: a debt which cannot be evaded without further sin on our part. These people must be helped, no matter what the difficulty and no matter what the cost. But in fact there should be no difficulty in helping the thousands of wounded in areas under U.S. control, and by no stretch of the imagination could this be

called "helping the enemy." Yet obstacles are being placed by our government in the way of this aid to people who are supposed to be our friends, people we are supposed to be "defending."

4. Even the most morally insensitive individual must be able to see that there is something revolting and shameful in the spectacle of the world's greatest superpower smashing with all the force of its most modern weapons into the utterly defenseless villages of a primitive and nonwhite people—and destroying their crops into the bargain. Even the most politically stupid individual ought to be capable of realizing the effect this has on the nonwhite majority in the world today. How can American protestations of justice, humanity and liberty be credible under such conditions? And what is the effect when the Name of Christ Our Savior is invoked to "bless" these atrocities? Though some may sincerely be convinced that this is a "holy war," they must admit that the massive horror visited upon noncombatants would stand a better chance of being construed as holy rather than diabolical, if we would do more to take care of those unfortunate victims that have some hope of recovery and of survival.

5. If we are content to rationalize and excuse what is in fact a systematic use of terror and a policy of nihilism carried out by our military in Asia, we need not be surprised if we wake up one day to find fire and violence in our own front yards here in America. If the fire of hatred and violent anarchy happens to break out in some of our cities (as it can surely be expected to do sooner or later), we will simply be getting a taste—perhaps only a very slight taste—of our own medicine.

6. In the face of these facts, as Christians, and quite apart from any political considerations regarding the Vietnam war, we must admit:

a) That we have a grave moral responsibility before God to help the innocent victims of our military venture in Vietnam.

b) That in any case such help can hardly be considered an act of disloyalty to America. Opposition to it on such grounds is not only a further injustice and inhumanity but is completely irrational.

c) That in this situation of utter shame for our nation, we have an opportunity to salvage at least a vestige of our Christian decency by acts of humanity which, in any case, are demanded by the moral law.

d) We also have an opportunity to show our sorrow for the immense harm that has been done, and to make some kind of reparation to those we have harmed—and to God who abhors injustice done to the poor and the helpless.

e) Therefore as Christians we have an urgent obligation to do all we can both to send aid to the victims of war and to persuade those in control to remove all obstacles to the sending of such aid.

7. To conclude: one might aptly paraphrase some words that were written in a similar case by Albert Camus concerning the war in Algeria:

"Some people are not aware of the real horror of the situation: these have no business trying to make a judgment. Others are aware, but they go on heroically insisting that our brothers must perish rather than our obsessions. Such people I can admire only from a distance." (See Camus, *Actuelles iii, Avant Propos.*)

February 22, 1967

Prayer for Peace

Almighty and merciful God, Father of all men, Creator and Ruler of the Universe, Lord of History, whose designs are inscrutable, whose glory is without blemish, whose compassion for the errors of men is inexhaustible, in your will is our peace!

Mercifully hear this prayer which rises to you from the tumult and desperation of a world in which you are forgotten, in which your name is not invoked, your laws are derided and your presence is ignored. Because we do not know you, we have no peace.

From the heart of an eternal silence, you have watched the rise of empires and have seen the smoke of their downfall.

You have seen Egypt, Assyria, Babylon, Greece and Rome, once powerful, carried away like sand in the wind.

You have witnessed the impious fury of ten thousand fratricidal wars, in which great powers have torn whole continents to shreds in the name of peace and justice.

And now our nation itself stands in imminent danger of a war the like of which has never been seen!
This nation dedicated to freedom, not to power,
Has obtained, through freedom, a power it did not desire.

And seeking by that power to defend its freedom, it is enslaved by the processes and policies of power.
Must we wage a war we do not desire, a war that can do us no good,
And which our very hatred of war forces us to prepare?

A day of ominous decision has now dawned on this free nation.
Armed with a titanic weapon, and convinced of our own right,

We face a powerful adversary, armed with the same weapon, equally convinced that he is right.

In this moment of destiny, this moment we never foresaw, we cannot afford to fail.
Our choice of peace or war may decide our judgment and publish it in an eternal record.

In this fatal moment of choice in which we might begin the patient architecture of peace
We may also take the last step across the rim of chaos.

Save us then from our obsessions! Open our eyes, dissipate our confusions, teach us to understand ourselves and our adversary!
Let us never forget that sins against the law of love are punished by loss of faith,
And those without faith stop at no crime to achieve their ends!

Help us to be masters of the weapons that threaten to master us.
Help us to use our science for peace and plenty, not for war and destruction.
Show us how to use atomic power to bless our children's children, not to blight them.

Save us from the compulsion to follow our adversaries in all that we most hate, confirming them in their hatred and suspicion of us.
Resolve our inner contradictions, which now grow beyond belief and beyond bearing.
They are at once a torment and a blessing: for if you had not left us the light of conscience, we would not have to endure them.

Teach us to be long-suffering in anguish and insecurity.

Teach us to wait and trust.
Grant light, grant strength and patience to all who work for peace,
To this Congress, our President, our military forces, and our adversaries.

Grant us prudence in proportion to our power,
Wisdom in proportion to our science,
Humaneness in proportion to our wealth and might.
And bless our earnest will to help all races and peoples to travel, in friendship with us,
Along the road to justice, liberty and lasting peace:
But grant us above all to see that our ways are not necessarily your ways,
That we cannot fully penetrate the mystery of your designs

And that the very storm of power now raging on this earth
Reveals your hidden will and your inscrutable decision.
Grant us to see your face in the lightning of this cosmic storm,
O God of holiness, mercifuul to men:
Grant us to seek peace where it is truly found!

In your will, O God, is our peace!
Amen

This prayer, written by T. Merton, was read in the House of Representatives by Congressman Frank Kowalski (D. Connecticut) on April 12, 1962 (Wednesday in Holy Week).